Clinical Considerations in Child and Adolescent Mental Health with Diverse Populations

Editors

WARREN YIU KEE NG
ALEXANDRA CANETTI
DENISE LEUNG

CHILD AND ADOLESCENT PSYCHIATRIC CLINICS OF NORTH AMERICA

www.childpsych.theclinics.com

Consulting Editor
JUSTINE LARSON

October 2022 • Volume 31 • Number 4

ELSEVIER

1600 John F. Kennedy Boulevard • Suite 1800 • Philadelphia, Pennsylvania, 19103-2899

http://www.theclinics.com

CHILD AND ADOLESCENT PSYCHIATRIC CLINICS OF NORTH AMERICA Volume 31, Number 4
October 2022 ISSN 1056–4993, ISBN-13: 978-0-323-93859-4

Editor: Megan Ashdown
Developmental Editor: Arlene Campos

Child and Adolescent Psychiatric Clinics of North America (ISSN 1056-4993) is published quarterly by Elsevier Inc., 360 Park Avenue South, New York, NY 10010-1710. Months of issue are January, April, July, and October. Business and Editorial Offices: 1600 John F. Kennedy Boulevard, Suite 1800, Philadelphia, PA 19103-2899. Periodicals postage paid at New York, NY and additional mailing offices. Subscription prices are $358.00 per year (US individuals), $869.00 per year (US institutions), $100.00 per year (US & Canadian students), $399.00 per year (Canadian individuals), $895.00 per year (Canadian institutions), $459.00 per year (international individuals), $895.00 per year (international institutions), and $200.00 per year (international students). International air speed delivery is included in all *Clinics* subscription prices. All prices are subject to change without notice. **POSTMASTER:** Send address changes to *Child and Adolescent Psychiatric Clinics of North America*, Elsevier Health Sciences Division, Subscription Customer Service, 3251 Riverport Lane, Maryland Heights, MO 63043. **Customer Service: 1-800-654-2452 (U.S. and Canada); 314-447-8871 (outside U.S. and Canada). Fax: 314-447-8029. E-mail:** JournalsCustomer Service-usa@elsevier.com **(for print support) or** journalsonlinesupport-usa@elsevier.com **(for online support).**

Reprints. For copies of 100 or more of articles in this publication, please contact the Commercial Reprints Department, Elsevier Inc., 360 Park Avenue South, New York, New York 10010-1710 Tel.: 212-633-3874; Fax: 212-633-3820, E-mail: reprints@elsevier.com.

Child and Adolescent Psychiatric Clinics of North America is covered in *MEDLINE/PubMed (Index Medicus), ISI, SSCI, Research Alert, Social Search, Current Contents,* and *EMBASE/Excerpta Medica.*

Contributors

CONSULTING EDITOR

JUSTINE LARSON, MD, MPH, DFAACAP
Medical Director, Schools and Residential Treatment, Consulting Editor, *Child and Adolescent Psychiatric Clinics of North America*, Sheppard Pratt, Rockville, Maryland, USA

EDITORS

WARREN YIU KEE NG, MD, MPH
Professor of Psychiatry, Columbia University Irving Medical Center, Department of Psychiatry, New York, New York, USA

ALEXANDRA CANETTI, MD
Associate Professor of Psychiatry, Columbia University Irving Medical Center, Department of Psychiatry, New York, New York, USA

DENISE LEUNG, MD
Associate Professor of Psychiatry, Columbia University Irving Medical Center, Department of Psychiatry, New York, New York, USA

AUTHORS

OTEMA A. ADADE, MD, MA
Chief Executive Officer, Lotus: The Center for Behavioral Health and Wellness, Lotus Behavioral Health, Washington, DC, USA

AFIFA ADIBA, MD
Service Chief, Adolescent Mood Disorder Inpatient Unit, Sheppard Pratt Health System, Towson, Maryland, USA; Adjunct Faculty, Yale Child Study Center, Yale School of Medicine, New Haven, Connecticut, USA

KHALID I. AFZAL, MD
Associate Professor, Department of Psychiatry and Behavioral Neuroscience, The University of Chicago, Chicago, Illinois, USA

CHERYL S. AL-MATEEN, MD
Professor, Departments of Psychiatry and Pediatrics, Virginia Commonwealth University School of Medicine, Richmond, Virginia, USA

SEEBA ANAM, MD
Associate Professor, Department of Psychiatry and Behavioral Neuroscience, The University of Chicago, Chicago, Illinois, USA

JOY K.L. ANDRADE, MD
Assistant Professor, Department of Psychiatry, University of Hawaii John A. Burns School of Medicine, Honolulu, Hawaii, USA

SARAH H. ARSHAD, MD
Assistant Professor of Clinical Psychiatry, Department of Child and Adolescent Psychiatry and Behavioral Sciences, Children's Hospital of Philadelphia, Perelman School of Medicine, University of Pennsylvania School of Medicine

ERIN L. BELFORT, MD
Assistant Professor of Psychiatry, Tufts University School of Medicine, Maine Medical Center, Portland, Maine, USA

JAMESHA LEWIS BRYANT, DO, MS
Psychiatry Resident, Post Graduate Year 2, Virginia Commonwealth University, Richmond, Virginia, USA

RICHARD F. CAMINO-GAZTAMBIDE, MD, MA
Medical College of Georgia, Augusta University

MARGARET CARY, MD, MPH
Oregon Health Authority and Yellowhawk Tribal Health Center, Confederated Tribes of the Umatilla, Portland, Oregon, USA

SHINNYI CHOU, MD, PhD
University of Pittsburgh Medical Center, Pittsburgh, Pennsylvania, USA

JACLYN CHUA, DO
Assistant Professor of Clinical Psychiatry, Department of Child and Adolescent Psychiatry and Behavioral Sciences, Children's Hospital of Philadelphia, Perelman School of Medicine, University of Pennsylvania School of Medicine

MAGDOLINE DAAS, MD
Child and Adolescent Psychiatrist, Community Health Network, Assistant Professor, Osteopathic Medical School-Marian University, Indianapolis, Indiana, USA

REBECCA SUSAN DAILY, MD, DLFAPA, DFAACAP
Child and Adolescent Psychiatrist, Behavioral Health, Volunteer Faculty, Oklahoma State University, College of Osteopathic Medicine at the Cherokee Nation, Cherokee Nation, Tahlequah, Oklahoma, USA

VINCENZO DI NICOLA, MPhiL, MD, PhD, FRCPC, DFAPA, FCPA, FCAHS
President, Canadian Association of Social Psychiatry (CASP), President-Elect, World Association of Social Psychiatry (WASP), Professor, Department of Psychiatry and Addictions, University of Montreal, Montreal, Quebec, Canada; Clinical Professor, Department of Psychiatry and Behavioral Sciences, The George Washington University

RASHA ELKADY, MD
Assistant Professor, University of Missouri School of Medicine, Columbia, Missouri, USA

RANA ELMAGHRABY, MD
Child and Adolescent Psychiatrist, Regional Medical Director, Sea Mar Community Health Centers, Vancouver, Washington, USA; Clinical Instructor, University of Washington, Seattle, Washington, USA

ALAA ELNAJJAR, MD
Child and Adolescent Psychiatrist, Bradley Hospital, Clinical Instructor, The Warren Alpert Medical School of Brown University, Providence, Rhode Island, USA

LISA R. FORTUNA, MD, MPH, MDiv
Professor of Clinical Psychiatry, Department of Psychiatry and Behavioral Sciences, University of California, San Francisco, San Francisco, California, USA

TANUJA GANDHI, MD
Assistant Professor, Department of Psychiatry and Human Behavior, The Warren Alpert Medical School at Brown University, Riverside, Rhode Island, USA

GEORGE GIANAKAKOS, MD
Pritzker Department of Psychiatry and Behavioral Health, Ann and Robert H. Lurie Children's Hospital of Chicago, Chicago, Illinois, USA

KIMBERLY GORDON-ACHEBE, MD
Department of Psychiatry, Division of Child and Adolescent Psychiatry, University of Maryland School of Medicine, Baltimore, Maryland, USA

ADITI HAJIRNIS, MD
Assistant Professor, Department of Psychiatry and Human Behavior, The Warren Alpert Medical School at Brown University, Riverside, Rhode Island, USA

CRYSTAL HAN, MD
University of Maryland Medical Center, Baltimore, Maryland, USA

CAMILA HAYNES, MD, PGY-2
Psychiatry Resident, Howard University Hospital

RAKIN HOQ, MD
Clinical Instructor of Psychiatry, NYU School of Medicine, Hassenfeld Children's Hospital at NYU Langone, New York, New York, USA

ARON JANSSEN, MD
Pritzker Department of Psychiatry and Behavioral Health, Ann and Robert H. Lurie Children's Hospital of Chicago, Chicago, Illinois, USA

MANAL KHAN, MD
Child and Adolescent Psychiatry Fellow, Jane and Terry Semel Institute for Neuroscience and Human Behavior, University of California, Los Angeles, Los Angeles, California, USA

NAYLA M. KHOURY, MD, MPH
Assistant Professor, Department of Psychiatry, SUNY Upstate Medical University, Syracuse, New York, USA

QORTNI LANG, MD
NYU Grossman School of Medicine, NYU Langone Health, NYC Health + Hospital–Bellevue Medical Center, New York, New York, USA

RUPINDER K. LEGHA, MD
President, Rupinder K Legha, MD PC, Los Angeles, California, USA

MARISSA LESLIE, MD
Assistant Clinical Professor of Psychiatry, Georgetown University School of Medicine

W. DAVID LOHR, MD
Department of Pediatrics, University of Louisville School of Medicine, Louisville, Kentucky, USA

WYNNE MORGAN, MD
Division of Child and Adolescent Psychiatry, Department of Psychiatry, UMass Chan Medical School, Worcester, Massachusetts, USA

KANYA NESBETH, MD, PGY-2
Psychiatry Resident, Howard University Hospital

JESSICA XIAOXI OUYANG, MD
Georgetown University School of Medicine, MedStar Georgetown University Hospital, Washington, DC, USA

JOHN PRUETT, MD, BCFE, FAPA, DFAACAP
Bellin Health, Green Bay Wisconsin Bellin Psychiatric Center, Green Bay, Wisconsin, USA

TOYA ROBERSON-MOORE, MD
University of Illinois at Chicago College of Medicine, ERC Pathlight Mood and Anxiety Center, Shine Bright Child and Adolescent Behavioral Health, Chicago, Illinois, USA

BARBARA ROBLES-RAMAMURTHY, MD
Assistant Professor, Department of Psychiatry and Behavioral Sciences, University of Texas Health San Antonio, San Antonio, Texas, USA

KENNETH M. ROGERS, MD, MSPH, MMM
South Carolina Department of Mental Health, Columbia, South Carolina, USA

JESSICA F. SANDOVAL, MD
Assistant Professor, Department of Psychiatry and Behavioral Sciences, University of Texas Health San Antonio, San Antonio, Texas, USA

JOHN SARGENT, MD
Professor of Psychiatry and Pediatrics, Tufts University School of Medicine, Tufts Medical Center, Boston, Massachusetts, USA

KRISTIE V. SCHULTZ, PhD
Department of Pediatrics, University of Louisville School of Medicine, Louisville, Kentucky, USA

DEEPIKA SHALIGRAM, MD
Attending Psychiatrist, Department of Psychiatry and Behavioral Sciences, Boston Children's Hospital, Harvard Medical School, Boston, Massachusetts, USA

NEHA SHARMA, DO
Assistant Professor of Psychiatry, Tufts University School of Medicine, Tufts Medical Center, Boston, Massachusetts, USA

MARGARET L. STUBER, MD
University of California, Los Angeles, Los Angeles, California, USA

AMALIA LONDOÑO TOBÓN, MD
National Institutes on Minority Health and Health Disparities, Bethesda, Maryland, USA

RAMESHWARI V. TUMULURU, MD
Associate Professor, University of Pittsburgh School of Medicine, Pittsburgh, Pennsylvania, USA

GEORGE 'BUD' VANA, MD, MA, FAAP, FAPA, FAACAP
Department of Integrated Psychiatry, Volunteer Faculty, University of Washington, Department of Psychiatry and Behavioral Sciences, General Pediatrician, Adult, Child and Adolescent Psychiatrist, Bellingham, Washington, USA

JONATHON W. WANTA, MD
Pritzker Department of Psychiatry and Behavioral Health, Ann and Robert H. Lurie Children's Hospital of Chicago, Chicago, Illinois, USA

STACY-ANN WAYNE, MD
Pediatric Psychiatry Fellow, Virginia Commonwealth University, Richmond, Virginia, USA

WALTER E. WILSON Jr, MD, MHA
HealthPoint Family Care, Inc, Covington, Kentucky, USA

ANNIE SZE YAN LI, MD
NYU Grossman School of Medicine, NYU Langone Health, NYC Health + Hospital–Bellevue Medical Center, NYU Child Study Center, New York, New York, USA

Contents

Clinicians should strive to understand every patient from their own perspective. The authors present tools to help patients narrate their own experiences and elaborate on the context of their symptoms, allowing clinicians to appreciate the cultural influences on a patient and how that affects their symptomatology. This knowledge can then be crafted into a nuanced cultural formulation of the patient, with the goals of not only better understanding the patient's specific, intersectional context but also guiding treatment planning. As a result, the patient is evaluated in a holistic manner, and their specific needs are central in their care.

Child and adolescent psychiatrists (CAPs) work at the intersections of families, cultures, and systems, which affect engagement in care, assessment, and treatment planning. There are several practical strategies that CAPs can apply to practice cultural humility, to join with families, to facilitate difficult conversations and to work through misalignment. Culturally inclusive family-based care can promote greater understanding and lead to stronger outcomes with families as well as help mitigate mental health impact of structural racism and social inequities.

Religion and spirituality (R/S) have been influential in societies' history, daily life, and identity in the past and in today's society. From a sociological perspective, R/S contributes to family development and organization, influences culture, and often contributes to forming opinions, beliefs, and concepts about oneself, family, society, and the world. In addition, R/S help shape individuals, families, and communities' ethical and moral understanding, thus influencing their behavior. This review article aims to provide the clinician with tools to understand, assess, and provide interventions that consider the patients' and their families' R/S. A recent review of the topic focused on general aspects of the R/S but we are unaware of reviews that integrate attachment, moral foundation theory, and forgiveness. This review will integrate these additional features into our understanding of the role of R/S in the delivery of mental health.

education, and juvenile injustice systems, specifically when they intersect with the child mental health system. Relying on bold and radical frameworks, such as abolition, critical race theory, and decolonization, it positions child mental health providers to confront the color of child protection while protecting minoritized children against these systems of harm. These frameworks inspire a daily antiracist practice whereby child mental health providers challenge racist inequities and the historical arcs driving them; protect minoritized children and families against the systems of care designed to harm them; and work toward the longer-term goal of abolishing these systems altogether. In a white supremacist society, child mental health providers have no choice but to engage in such antiracist practices in order to uphold their fundamental oath to first do no harm. The failure to do so amounts to negligence and malpractice.

There is limited literature on Arab American mental health, particularly among youth. This chapter will provide an overview of the Arab American/MENA population, their migration to the United States, traditional Arab culture and values, Arab American youth identity, acculturation and acculturation stress, the impact of discrimination on Arab American youth, mental illness in Arab American youth, and cultural variables to consider in seeking help. This chapter will provide recommendations and cultural considerations when working with Arab American youth.

This article seeks to provide an exploration of the contributors to the mental health of Black and African Americans. We explore the foundations of racism in this country as well as factors leading to systemic racism. It is important to gain an understanding of the multifaceted contributors to disparities in health care and mental health care. Black children and adolescents experience more poverty, discrimination, marginalization, and racism compared with their white counterparts in the United States (APA, 2017). These are factors that greatly impact the mental health of this population. In addition to exploring examples of disparities in diagnosis, treatment, and research on Black youth, we also provide recommendations for clinicians seeking to provide exemplary culturally sensitive care that recognizes the diverse and multifaceted nature of this population.

This article explores the ways East Asian American (EAA) children and adolescents have experienced disparities in the United States throughout the COVID-19 pandemic. The history of racism toward Asian American and Pacific Islanders (AAPI) and the complexities of acculturation are reflected through this contemporary lens. Traditional East Asian (EA) values were disrupted during this period. Implications for children and families are discussed. Persistent underlying xenophobia and racism, such as the model minority myth or perpetual foreigner stereotype, rose to new prominence, furthering emotional distress in EA and EAA youths beyond those already experienced universally by AAPI families during the pandemic.

Clinicians trained to assess and treat child psychopathology are facing an increasing need to expand their clinical expertise outside of traditional frameworks, which have historically focused largely on the child or the child–mother dyad. Clinicians treating children also need to be prepared to assess and address the systems of care that affect a child's mental health, starting with their family. There is a scarcity of Latino mental health providers and limited clinical opportunities or settings that serve this population by incorporating a developmental, cultural, and sociopolitical framework into high quality care of the whole family.

This article provides an overview of the clinical evaluation and clinical treatment on multiple levels of American Indian, Alaskan Native, Native Hawaiian, and Pacific Islander youth, and their families. Included are basic cultural beliefs and practices shared among multiple tribes and nations within this diaspora, where the most important concept is balance and harmony in healing. Readers are provided with current practice approaches to core issues of substance abuse, anxiety, depression, and suicidal ideation including case examples, psychopharmacology, and therapy.

South Asian American (SAA) youth are culturally diverse with respect to migration patterns, language, religion, and social determinants of health. Culturally specific stressors related to family, acculturation, discrimination, and intersectionality converge during developmentally sensitive periods, impacting mental health and identity development. "Model minority" stereotypes and somatic expressions of distress contribute to underdetection and limited perceived need for treatment. SAA families navigate structural barriers, including limited access to culturally tailored services, limited English proficiency, referral bias, and stigma, resulting in underutilization of services. Cultural considerations must be integrated into diagnostic conceptualization and treatment recommendations to effectively engage SAA youth and families in treatment.

CHILD AND ADOLESCENT PSYCHIATRIC CLINICS

SERIES OF RELATED INTEREST

Psychiatric Clinics of North America
https://www.psych.theclinics.com/
Pediatric Clinics of North America
https://www.pediatric.theclinics.com/

AACAP Members: Please go to www.jaacap.org for information on access to the Child and Adolescent Psychiatric Clinics. *Resident* Members of AACAP: Special access information is available at www.childpsych.theclinics.com.

THE CLINICS ARE AVAILABLE ONLINE!
Access your subscription at:
www.theclinics.com

Preface

Clinical Considerations in Working with Youth from Diverse Populations

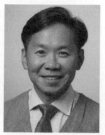 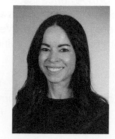 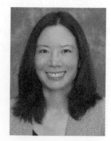

Warren Yiu Kee Ng, MD, MPH   Alexandra Canetti, MD   Denise Leung, MD
Editors

We all should know that diversity makes for a rich tapestry, and we must understand that all the threads of the tapestry are equal in value no matter their color.
—Maya Angelou

The overall racial and ethnic diversity of our nation has continued to increase, and serving our collective communities will require cultural humility, curiosity, and learning. In the 2020 census, nearly 4 out of 10 Americans identified with a race or ethnic group other than white. Additional important dimensions of identity, experience, and culture enrich one another synergistically. Minoritized populations have difficulty accessing mental health care, especially culturally responsive and humble engagement and treatment. This has become more critical as our nation grows more diverse. The nation's pediatric mental health crisis, worsened by the COVID-19 pandemic, has disproportionately impacted communities of color and diverse youth. Given the national state of emergency affecting our youth, clinicians can expect to see more youth from diverse populations and must be able to develop culturally responsive strategies to best engage and treat these children, youth, and families. The goal of this *Child and Adolescent Psychiatric Clinics of North America* issue is to provide the clinician with *both* the cultural dimensions of mental health *and* a problem-based, introspective, and culturally humble approach that places the experiences of the youth and their families at the forefront of treatment. Each of the articles highlights the factors that affect mental health in each diverse population with a focus on strategies for the clinician to be most impactful in treatment. The historic and contemporary effects of immigration, acculturation, racism, structural inequities, discrimination, and other sociocultural factors are

Child Adolesc Psychiatric Clin N Am 31 (2022) xv–xvi
https://doi.org/10.1016/j.chc.2022.07.002
1056-4993/22/© 2022 Published by Elsevier Inc.

woven throughout the articles. The issue starts with an orienting article in creating a cultural formulation that facilitates cultural competence and cultural humility applied throughout the articles (Cultural Formulation Issue, ADDRESSING, and RESPECT-FUL). The clinician can utilize these tools to craft a cultural formulation that further explores the impact of these factors on the youth they are treating and to collaborate on an individualized treatment plan. The following articles in this issue highlight the cultural richness and diversity of our nation's youth and how clinicians can be enriched through their care and treatments to serve them.

We would like to express our sincerest gratitude to the contributors of this *Child and Adolescent Psychiatric Clinics of North America* issue, who have graciously dedicated so much of their time to writing their articles to help us all gain a deeper understanding of the issues critical in treating diverse populations. We dedicate this to the incredible youth who inspire us every day with their courage, vulnerability, and passion by being who they are.

Warren Yiu Kee Ng, MD, MPH
New York Presbyterian Hospital–Columbia University Medical Center
635 West 165th Street El #610
New York, NY 10032, USA

Alexandra Canetti, MD
New York Presbyterian Hospital–Columbia University Medical Center
622 West 168th Street, VC 4 E
New York, NY 10032, USA

Denise Leung, MD
New York Presbyterian Hospital–Columbia University Medical Center
3959 Broadway MSCH North, Room 615A
New York, NY 10032, USA

E-mail addresses:
Yyn2@cumc.columbia.edu (W.Y. Kee Ng)
ac2998@cumc.columbia.edu (A. Canetti)
dl2269@cumc.columbia.edu (D. Leung)

Tools to Craft a Cultural Formulation

Sarah H. Arshad, MD[a],*, Jaclyn Chua, DO[a,1], Stacy-Ann Wayne, MD[b,2], Jamesha Lewis Bryant, DO, MS[c,3], Cheryl S. Al-Mateen, MD[d,e,4]

KEYWORDS

- Outline for cultural formulation • Cultural formulation interview • Culture
- Cultural identity

KEY POINTS

- Cultural formulations are vital to the evaluation and treatment of children and adolescents who present to mental health care, and clinicians should strive to understand youth in their context, including the role of families and other communities and systems in their lives.
- Crafting a cultural formulation is a dynamic process, especially with children and adolescents, and there is a role for gathering collateral from numerous sources, including family, school, and community members.
- The Outline for Cultural Formulation (OCF) is a framework to help clinicians understand their patients' symptoms from their own narration and in their specific, individual, intersectional context to come up with an overall cultural assessment.
- Clinicians can use tools, such as the questions from the Cultural Formulation Interview (CFI) and its Supplementary Modules.
- Clinicians can also use existing frameworks such as *ADDRESSING* and *RESPECTFUL* to better understand patients and families to form a more nuanced cultural assessment and use that to target specific treatment goals.

[a] Department of Child and Adolescent Psychiatry and Behavioral Sciences, Children's Hospital of Philadelphia, Perelman School of Medicine of the University of Pennsylvania School of Medicine, DCAPBS, Floor 12, 3500 Civic Center Boulevard, Philadelphia, PA 19104, USA; [b] Virginia Commonwealth University, Richmond, VA, USA; [c] Post Graduate Year 2, Virginia Commonwealth University, Richmond, VA, USA; [d] Department of Psychiatry, Virginia Commonwealth University School of Medicine, Richmond, VA, USA; [e] Department of Pediatrics, Virginia Commonwealth University School of Medicine, Richmond, VA, USA
[1] Present address: 2326 Alter Street, Philadelphia, PA 19146.
[2] Present address: 1308 Sherwood Avenue, Richmond, VA 23220.
[3] Present address: 1200 East Broad StreetRichmond, VA 23298
[4] Present address: 1308 Sherwood Avenue, Richmond, VA 23220
* Corresponding author. 1815 John F. Kennedy Boulevard Apartment 1116, Philadelphia, PA 19103.
E-mail addresses: Sarah.h.arshad@gmail.com; arshads@chop.edu

Child Adolesc Psychiatric Clin N Am 31 (2022) 583–601
https://doi.org/10.1016/j.chc.2022.05.001
1056-4993/22/© 2022 Elsevier Inc. All rights reserved.
childpsych.theclinics.com

INTRODUCTION: HOW WE GOT HERE

Case 1: Andrew is a 16-year-old white boy with a history of depression and anxiety who presented to the emergency room after a suicide attempt by intentional acetaminophen overdose. He has been admitted to the medical hospital for 3 days but has been minimally engaged with staff. Andrew is not ready to elaborate on his depressive symptoms or suicide attempt and continues to deny the need for mental health treatment, so the admitting team has consulted Psychiatry. Now, the consultants are looking for tools to engage Andrew and his family with a cultural approach.

There are numerous tools that exist to help clinicians conceptualize their patients in a cultural framework, with the overarching goal of crafting a cultural formulation. However, despite the presence of these tools, many clinicians are unaware of or feel uncomfortable using them. Many clinicians may also be unaware that some of their current questions or methods of understanding patient symptoms align with these existing tools. The investigators hope to dispel some myths and discomfort about how to create a cultural formulation by demonstrating how some of these tools can be used practically to formulate a cultural assessment using case examples. These case examples also help shed light on the importance of understanding children and adolescents and families from a cultural lens, as they aid in rapport building, accurate diagnosis, and treatment planning. Specifically, the authors review some of the tools to help clinicians craft a cultural formulation, including the tools in the Diagnostic and Statistical Manual of Mental Disorders (DSM), including the Cultural Formulation Interview (CFI), and two frameworks created by psychologists—*ADDRESSING* and *RESPECTFUL*, in the treatment of children and adolescents.

To broaden cultural proficiency for psychiatrists, the Outline for Cultural Formulation (OCF) was introduced in an appendix of the DSM-IV,[1] showing providers how a patient's culture might influence the manifestation of their symptoms.[2] The elements identified for consideration are in **Table 1**.[1] This addition sanctioned the formal inclusion of cultural factors in the conceptualization of the psychiatric diagnosis for the first time. DSM-III[3] did not mention culture, and DSM-III-R[4] mentioned that the clinician should "apply DSM-III-R with open-mindedness to the presence of distinctive cultural patterns and sensitivity to the possibility of unintended bias because of such differences" (p. xxvi). DSM-IV also introduced the Glossary of Culture-Bound Syndromes in the appendix.[1] DSM-5 moved the OCF out of the Appendix into a section with Emerging Measures and Models.[5] DSM-5-TR has further integrated cultural concepts into a chapter in this section, including important terms, the OCF, Cultural Concepts of Distress, and the CFI, emphasizing that "Individuals and clinicians who seem to share the same cultural background may nevertheless differ in ways that are relevant to care"[6] (p. 863). Cultural concepts and explanations of distress include the different ways of experiencing and communicating personal as well as social concerns and the labels and explanations for the distress. Cultural syndromes are also included.[6] Descriptions of the elements of the OCF are now broadened to more clearly incorporate important concepts, such as intersectionality and social determinants of mental health (see **Table 1**).[6]

The recognition of these cultural concepts is important to "avoid misdiagnosis, to obtain useful clinical information, to improve clinical rapport and engagement, to improve therapeutic efficacy, to guide clinical research, and to clarify cultural epidemiology" (pp. 749–759).[6] To help provide the tools to ask about and create a cultural formulation, the DSM-5 Cross-Cultural Issues Subgroup devised the CFI.[7]

The CFI is a semi-structured interview designed to increase the use of the OCF throughout routine mental health evaluations in any setting.[8] In DSM-5-TR, aspects

Table 1
Outline for cultural formulation elements

OCF Elements DSM-IV (APA 1994)	OCF Elements DSM-5-TR (APA 2022)	Comments
Cultural identity of the individual	Cultural identity of the individual	This emphasizes the need to include *any* "socially and culturally defined characteristics that may influence interpersonal relationships, access to resources, and developmental and current challenges, conflicts, or predicaments" (p. 861), including the aspects prioritized by the individual and the impact of intersectionality.
Cultural explanations of the individual's illness	Cultural concepts of distress	Further normalizes the potential for differences between cultures by changing the phrasing from "cultural reference groups" to "cultural background."
Cultural factors related to the psychosocial environment and functioning	Psychosocial stressors and cultural features of vulnerability and resilience	Specifically identifies the need to identify social determinants of mental health, such as access to resources and opportunities such as housing, transportation, education, employment, and exposure to individual or structural racism and structural violence. Online interactions are included as stressors or supports.
Cultural elements of the relationship between the individual and the clinician.	Cultural features of the relationship between the individual and the clinician, *treatment team and institution* (text in italics is new in DSM-5-TR)	Continues to expand the understanding of the potential for previous experiences of discrimination to impact the clinical encounter, affecting rapport, and development of an effective clinical alliance (p. 862)

(continued on next page)

Table 1 (continued)		
OCF Elements DSM-IV (APA 1994)	OCF Elements DSM-5-TR (APA 2022)	Comments
Overall cultural assessment for diagnosis and care	Overall cultural assessment	Essentially unchanged, this summarizes the implications of the four elements for differential diagnosis, management, and treatment.

Data from American Psychiatric Association. Diagnostic and Statistical Manual of Mental Disorders, Fourth Edition. American Psychiatric Association; 1994 (p.843-844); American Psychiatric Association. Diagnostic and Statistical Manual of Mental Disorders, Fifth Edition, Text Revision. American Psychiatric Association; 2022.p.861.

of background include age, gender, social class, geographic origin, migration, language, religion, sexual orientation, disability, or ethnic or racialized background, and the social network (p. 862).[6] In addition, the culture of the provider and the systemic values and assumptions of the health care organizations are to be considered. It may be used partially or as a whole; the phrasing may be changed.

The CFIs four domains include the following: cultural definition of the problem; cultural perceptions of cause, context, and support; cultural factors affecting self-copying and past help-seeking; and cultural factors affecting current help-seeking. In addition to the core CFI, Supplementary Modules introduced in the DSM-5 include the CFI-Informant version and 12 supplemental modules that incorporate special populations, such as school-age children, immigrants, and refugees.[9] They are available online at: https://www.psychiatry.org/File%20Library/Psychiatrists/Practice/DSM/DSM-5-TR/APA-DSM5TR-CulturalFormulationInterviewSupplementaryModules.pdf .[9] Each module provides a series of questions that clinicians may ask to better understand their patients' symptoms and the context in which the patient is experiencing those symptoms. The clinician is then better equipped to use that knowledge to craft a cultural formulation. Although cultural differences had long been ignored, this more holistic approach to individualized, patient-centered care, as framed in the OCF, now embraces the cultural context in which our patients' behaviors occur.[8] Rousseau has suggested that using interdisciplinary case discussion seminars is a useful way to teach the use of the CFI with children and adolescents, and specifically interdisciplinary discussion can result in more fruitful dialog.[10]

In 2013, the American Academy of Child and Adolescent Psychiatry published a Practice Parameter for Cultural Competence, outlining 13 principles for clinicians to consider cultural aspects of patient care. It recognized the growing diversity of children and adolescents in the United States, highlighted the disparities for "minorities" in the health care system, and recognized that treating diverse youth "requires special expertise and unique approaches" (p. 1101).[11] In addition, culture is not only for ''minorities'' but that it also "affects the clinical encounter for every patient," making culture "an essential component of any comprehensive assessment" (p. 3),[12] hence the efforts of the DSM to incorporate cultural assessments into every interview.

Culture is defined as "shared learned meanings and behaviors that are transmitted from within a social context for purposes of promoting individual and societal adjustment, growth and development."[13] An individual's culture reflects a dynamic process in which he\she interprets reality and, therefore, directly influences the human experience and the manifestation of illness.[13] Factors such as race, ethnicity, sexual orientation, gender identity, religion, spirituality, socioeconomic status, migrant status, and language ability are only some of the cultural identities that should be considered.[14] The interplay of these many social identities at the micro-individual level and macro social-structural level is known as intersectionality.[15] Understanding this interplay is vital for clinicians to be able to craft a cultural formulation.

The questions in the CFI can help professionals incorporate culture into their assessments and thereby provide "culturally responsive care that focuses on the whole person, rather than just their diagnostic symptoms or group level demographic indicators " that "emphasizes the families or patients' needs, as well as strengths, preferences, and values"[16] (p. 3). To make a cultural formulation, the OCF encourages recognizing intersectionality—the many overlapping cultural factors, such as race, ethnicity, gender, sexuality, acculturation, housing, food insecurity, and discrimination experiences, in the overall assessment.[16] This prevents clinicians from assuming that individuals from a particular group are similar and representatives of a standard stereotype of that group, which is an oversimplification of cultural identity. For example, the overall cultural identities of two patients identifying as belonging to the same racial group may be different if they are from different socioeconomic classes, disability status, or if they have different gender identities. Cultural identities, including race and ethnicity, can cause psychological, interpersonal, and intergenerational difficulties but can also be noted as sources of strength and support during diagnostic assessments and treatment; they are important concepts to define in discussing cultural psychiatry, and definitions have been updated in the DSM-5-TR **(Table 2)**.[6]

Appreciating others' cultural perspectives and how this influences emotion and behavior furthers the understanding of both patients and the mental health providers treating them.[2] It is also what most, if not all, providers are already doing—for example, the first question in the CFI, under "cultural definition of the problem," is "what brings you here today?" The second question is to ask "how the patient would describe their problem to friends or family"[5] (p. 752). With the nuanced perspective of the CFI, asking about a patient's chief complaint begins the journey of understanding their cultural definition of their presenting symptoms.

It is imperative to consider the cultural factors and the extent to which this influences a person's beliefs and practices before diagnosis and treatment.[17] Clinically, this can help avoid misdiagnoses and polypharmacy,[8] as this information can add nuance and context to symptom manifestation. Disparities exist with certain minority populations being misdiagnosed with psychiatric diagnoses,[18] and a cultural approach, for example, by using the CFI, to patient care may help providers more accurately assess patients and families and form more robust assessments to aid in treatment planning.

In addition, valuing a patient's distinct psychological experience can promote rapport-building by respectfully incorporating their sociocultural factors into the assessment. For example, generational differences between child and caregiver may be a result of acculturation to a dominant culture, and child psychiatrists may have to separately navigate their patient's understanding of their symptoms from their families' understanding to create a formulation, and use that to align a youth with their family on treatment goals.[19,20] For example, CFI supplementary module nine is for school-age children and adolescents, with an addendum for parents, and module 12 is for caregivers, which providers can use to obtain separate information to create their holistic assessment.[9] Understanding stressors and supports (CFI questions 6 & 7) can help conceptualize the psychosocial context in which the patient is experiencing symptoms, helping the provider incorporate nuance into their formulation. An understanding of self-coping (CFI question 11), past help-seeking (question 12), and barriers (question 13) can help providers partner with patients and families in

Table 2
Important concepts and definitions

Culture	"Culture refers to systems of knowledge, concepts, values, norms, and practices that are learned and transmitted across generations. Culture includes language, religion and spirituality, family structures, life-cycle stages, ceremonial rituals, customs, and ways of understanding health and illness, as well as moral, political, economic and legal systems....Much of culture involves background knowledge, values, and assumptions that remain implicit or presumed and so may be difficult for individuals to describe. These features of culture make it crucial not to over generalize cultural information or stereotype groups in terms of fixed cultural traits. In relation to diagnosis, it is essential to recognize that all forms of illness and distress, including the DSM disorders, are shaped by cultural contexts."
Race	"Race is a social, not a biological construct that divides humanity into groups based on a variety of superficial physical traits...that have been falsely viewed as indicating attributes and capacities assumed to be inherent to the group....The construct of race is important for psychiatry because it can lead to racial ideologies, racism, discrimination, and social oppression and exclusion, which have strong negative effects on mental health. There is evidence that racism can exacerbate many psychiatric disorders, contributing to poor outcomes, and that racial biases can affect diagnostic assessment."
Ethnicity	"Ethnicity is a culturally constructed group identity used to define peoples and communities, rooted in common history, ancestry, geography, language, religion, or other shared characteristics of a group, which distinguish that group from others. Ethnicity may be self-assigned or attributed by outsiders. Increasing mobility, intermarriage, and intermixing of cultural groups have defined newly mixed, multiple, or hybrid ethnic identities. These processes may also lead to the dilution of ethnic identification."

Data from American Psychiatric Association. Diagnostic and Statistical Manual of Mental Disorders, Fifth Edition, Text Revision. American Psychiatric Association; 2022. (p 860).

treatment planning while further incorporating answers about the patient's cultural identity (CFI questions 8–10) and cultural factors affecting current help-seeking" (questions 14–15) to help with adherence.[6]

Moreover, the perceptions of cultural understanding are not always aligned between patient and provider, highlighting the need for providers to actively continue to use tools to understand their patient's cultural perspectives.[20] According to Soto, a clinician's perception of their own "multicultural competence" was not associated with positive therapeutic outcomes, whereas the patient's perception of the provider's competence was.[21] This is further complicated by other factors, including "racial transference" and "self-object transference", which influences the therapeutic relationship via power inequalities reflective of the larger American sociocultural context and the ethnic self-identification of the patient and provider, respectively.[22] Providers can use CFI question 16 "Have you been concerned about this and is there anything that we can do to provide you with the care that you need?"[6] (p. 867), to assess the clinician-patient relationship, and further questions in CFI Supplementary Module 8 to explore this relationship to build rapport and understanding.[9]

It is especially important for child psychiatrists to remember that cultural identity formation begins at an early age and continues to evolve for children and adolescents; as such, it is crucial for clinicians to understand how cultural expectations may impact

parenting styles and reaching developmental milestones or how a child's cultural identity has influenced their personal narratives.[8,14] We will illustrate further that how to (1)
use the CFI by applying its principles to several case examples of children and youth
and (2) use that information to guide a cultural formulation. In general, it is recommended that the interview is modified based on the youth's age and developmental stage
and collateral from significant adults are included.[8]

DISCUSSION: USING CASE EXAMPLES- CHOOSING YOUR TOOLS

There are multiple factors to consider when developing a cultural formulation. Two
useful frameworks that were created by psychologists to help craft a cultural formulation include: *ADDRESSING* by Hays[23] and *RESPECTFUL* by D'Andrea.[24]

The acronym *ADDRESSING* can be used by clinicians to understand cross-cultural
information from two perspectives. The first is that of the provider, including the providers' background, culture, upbringing, their own introspective process, and how that
influences their belief system. The second perspective is from the interpersonal experience with the patient and how the provider understands more about the patient's culture from that direct interaction.[23] Implicit bias, which can lead to a negative evaluation
of a person based on individual characteristics, was early recognized as a factor in
mental health and health care disparities.[18,25,26]

Health care professionals have been shown to exhibit implicit bias that impacts their
assessment of, and interaction with, the patient.[27] A recent image has spoken of identity in a "Wheel of Power/Privilege," encouraging introspection about one's own identity (and perhaps biases). This can help the clinician with the first perspective in
ADDRESSING, and also to think about cultural identity, incorporating an intersectional
array of numerous identity elements (**Fig. 1**).[28]

Table 3 to see how the *ADDRESSING* framework can be used to create a cultural
formulation in Case #2.

The *RESPECTFUL* framework of counseling and development emphasizes the need
for practitioners to manifest an extraordinarily high level of respect for the person with
whom they work. These factors are important because they affect the patient's psychological development and well-being. See **Table 4** for Case #1 to see how this
framework can be used to create a cultural formulation.

It is likely that some questions from the CFI are already a part of your psychiatric
interview. Adding cultural elements to a biopsychosocial formulation of a patient's
psychiatric problem and including collateral from other important figures and systems
in a youth's life can be used to create a cultural formulation. In the case below, during
the initial interview, some parts of cultural identity, including race, religion, family, and
so forth can be identified. In this example case, the cultural formulation interview is
used to provide a framework to ask questions exploring a patient's symptoms and
identity on their terms.

Case 1: Andrew

Let's return to our case: Andrew is a 16-year-old white boy with a history of depression and anxiety who presented to the emergency room after a suicide attempt by
intentional acetaminophen overdose. He has been admitted to the medical hospital
for 3 days but has been minimally engaged with staff. Andrew is not ready to elaborate on his depressive symptoms or suicide attempt and continues to deny the
need for mental health treatment. He refuses to talk with his parents as he is disap-
pointed that he was brought to the hospital. He is currently prescribed 75 mg of
sertraline by his primary care provider but otherwise does not see a therapist.

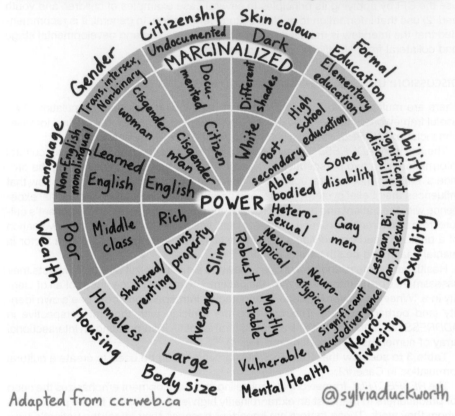

Fig. 1. Wheel of Power/Privilege. Duckworth S. Power/Privilege Wheel. sylviaduckworth. com.

The initial conceptualization was that a 16-year-old white boy with a history of depression and anxiety who presented after a suicide attempt but is reluctant to engage with staff regarding his symptoms or stressors and does not communicate to his parents.

Provider: *I see that you are upset that you are in the hospital; can you tell me what happened that resulted in your admission to the hospital?*

Andrew: *I didn't feel good, and I took pills. My parents think it was a suicide attempt.*

Provider: *People often understand their problems in their own way, which may be similar or different from how doctors describe the problem. How would you describe your problem? [CFI Question 1]*

Andrew: *Well, I feel sad sometimes, well a lot of the time. A few days ago, I was feeling very sad, because I don't feel like my parents understand me. I did take a lot of pills to help me sleep or relax but not to kill myself. I just want to numb my pain.*

Here the provider was able to elicit the patient's core view of his problems or concerns using a question from the CFI. This allows the provider to home in on the aspects of the problem that matter most to the patient and better capture his understanding or his "cultural definition of the problem" of his emotional state.

Table 3	
Use of *ADDRESSING* for Christian (case 2)	
Cultural Influences (ADDRESSING Framework)	**Clinical Information**
Age and generational influences	Christian was an adolescent who appeared easily distracted and active on two electronic devices in addition to his PlayStation
Developmental disabilities	There may have been a concern for distractibility and inattention as Christian was not fully engaged and had noticeable difficulty sitting still, but he had no formal diagnoses
Disabilities acquired later in life	Christian was diagnosed with cystic fibrosis in childhood, including subsequent hepatic Failure
Religion and spiritual orientation	Uncertain
Ethnic and racial identity	Christian is an African American, who appeared to engender subsequent implicit bias by the primary team that he would be "difficult"
Socioeconomic status	Christian was raised by a single African American mother with little financial means and limited support
Sexual orientation	Christian identifies himself as heterosexual
Indigenous heritage	Uncertain
National origin	US citizen
Gender	Male

Data from Hays PA. Connecting Across Cultures: The Helper's Toolkit. In: Connecting Across Cultures: The Helper's Toolkit. Sage Publications; 2013:123. https://doi.org/10.1037/14801-000.

Provider: *What do you think are the causes of your sadness? [CFI Question 4] What things in your life are triggers of sadness?*

Andrew: *Feeling misunderstood by my parents, they just don't understand how I can be stressed.*

Provider: *Sometimes, people have different ways of describing their sadness or depression to their family, friends, or others in their community. How would you describe your problem to them? [CFI Question 2]*

Andrew: *I would tell them I don't feel well, I feel so sick, because I can't be myself.*

Using the CFI allows the provider to delve deeper into the patient's feeling misunderstood by his family and his limited ability to communicate with them about his emotional state or needs. For this adolescent, this not only represents an important element in his biopsychosocial conceptualization but also could be concrete, identifiable target for treatment and safety planning.

Provider: *What do others in your family, your friends, or others in your community think is causing your sadness? [CFI Question 5]*

Andrew: *My parents feel like I can choose to be something I am not. They want me to do things I don't want to do. They think that who I am will make my life worse. Most of my friends are supportive; they think being my true self will help with my depression and pain.*

Provider: *Sometimes, aspects of people's background or identity can make depression or sadness better or worse. By background or identity, I mean, for example, the communities you belong to, the language you speak, or your gender or sexual orientation. Are there aspects of your identity that are causing difficulties for you? [CFI definition of the "role of cultural identity"; Question 10]*

Table 4
Use of *RESPECTFUL* for Andrew (Case 1)

Cultural Influences (RESPECTFUL Framework)	Clinical Information
Religion/spiritual identity	Atheist
Economic class background	Middle class; two-parent household
Sexual identity	Previously gay male; exploring gender identity
Psychological maturity	Appropriate for age
Ethnic/racial identity	Caucasian, Irish, and Scandinavian origins
Chronologic/developmental challenges	None
Trauma and threats to well-being	Experienced bullying for small stature throughout middle school that resulted in physical abuse
Family background	Fourth-generation Irish immigrant family; within the United States; \the Mormon faith
Unique physical characteristics	Thin, petite, ruddy skin with freckles, blue eyes, and dark brown hair; wears glasses
Location of residence and language differences	Resides in Virginia; English-speaking

Data from D'Andrea M, Daniels J. Before You Get Started. In: Ivey AE, D'Andrea M, Ivey MB, Simek-Morgan L, eds. Theories of Counseling and Psychotherapy - A Multicultural Perspective. Fifth Edit. Allyn & Bacon; 2002:456; pages xvii–xxiv.

Andrew: *That's just it. I am considering my gender identity; I have always identified myself as a gay male, but now I am not sure who I am. I can't tell my parents about my gender or sexuality. My parents are Mormon. I am not religious, but I pretend to be. My family has realized that some of my friends are queer, and their response to it is not good. I pretend to be something I'm not, but it has become extremely difficult, especially while dating. If I can't be myself sometimes, I feel like I am better off dead.*

The provider allows the patient to reflect on the most important elements of his cultural identity, and the elements of those he is currently considering. He is expressing how it is causing distress to his family and community and possibly contributing to his depression. He is noting that this process, including his fear of not belonging within his family or religious community, is exacerbating his depressive symptoms. He also feels as though he cannot be honest or open as he continues to contemplate his gender identity and sexual orientation. He feels unable to communicate his concerns, such that he experiences passive thoughts of death.

The provider can continue to use the CFI to further clarify the patient's psychosocial stressors and cultural features of the vulnerability before the treatment and can consider his case while using a framework, such as *RESPECTFUL*, to create a cultural formulation.

Case 1: Cultural formulation

Andrew is a 16-year-old boy from a religious, Mormon family of fourth-generation Irish immigrants with a history of depression and anxiety who presented after a suicide attempt, in the context of considering his gender identity and sexual orientation. Specifically, he feels he cannot communicate his cultural identity to his family, as he is concerned that he will not be accepted by them or by their greater religious community. In addition, he does not identify as religious but feels that he must pretend to fit in with his family and his community. Both his feeling unable to communicate about his identity and to pretend to fit in have increased his depression symptoms, such that he does not endorse a will to live, in part because he is not able to be true to himself in his family or community contexts.

Case 2: Christian

Our second case offers a reflection of a trainee's (child and adolescent psychiatry fellow [CAPF]) experience while completing consultation on a patient seen in the pediatric medical hospital. Christian is an 18-year-old African American young man with a history of cystic fibrosis (with subsequent hepatic failure) in addition to oppositional defiant disorder who was admitted to the pediatric floor in respiratory distress, thought to be because of a cystic fibrosis exacerbation. Psychiatry was consulted to rule out depression in the setting of a chronic medical illness as well as to evaluate for capacity as a result of treatment refusal.

After reviewing the chart and speaking to the primary team, the CAPF formed an idea of whom she expected Christian to be and began formulating a differential diagnosis. As Christian was admitted because of an exacerbation of his chronic medical illness, there could be some adjustment or depressive symptoms associated with both the acute exacerbation and the chronic medical condition. In addition, there could also be cultural identity issues with a teenager navigating and coping with living with a chronic medical illness with medical sequelae affecting his ability to live a "normal life" and potentially identity issues regarding his racial identity in the context of his specific chronic medical illness. He also has a history of oppositional defiant behavior, and his refusal may be because of inherent oppositionality, or now that he is 18, this may be his first time being asked to make his own decisions as an adult instead of his parents/guardians making those decisions. When the CAPF went to meet Christian, her perspective changed dramatically.

Christian was a young man of small stature who appeared younger than his stated age. He was sitting on his bed juggling texts from two different phones. After the CAPF introduced herself, he said "I have a tournament in 5 minutes; will this take long?" and pointed to his PlayStation. Thinking about his diagnosis of ODD, the CAPF encouraged him to play during the assessment, with hopes that he would continue talking instead of otherwise shutting down or refusing to engage in the interview if she had asked him to turn the game off.

The CAPF was able to use the CFI introduction "I would like to understand the problems that bring you here so that I can help you more effectively. I want to know about *your* experience and ideas. I will ask some questions about what is going on and how you are dealing with it. Please remember there are no right or wrong answers" to set the tone of the interview, making sure he knew she was hoping to understand his needs and ally with him on his care. In addition, they used questions about past help-seeking (CFI Question 12), self-coping (CFI question 11), and specifically barriers "Has anything prevented you from getting the help you need?" [CFI Question 13] to flesh out her cultural interview and formulation and liaison with Christian and the primary team.

At the end of the evaluation, Christian had no resemblance to a depressed teenager. He was motivated, future-oriented, and jovial during the interview and was able to convey his feeling about being misunderstood by his primary medical team. He described that his treatment refusal was because "the team not listening to me." He cited numerous side effects to medications as his reason for refusal of treatment. He reported that he would be more amenable if the team would provide options or interventions to counteract the side effects instead of "demanding" that he be compliant with care. He also asked if they could see him in the late morning instead of at 6AM because "I am not a morning person," and said he would better be able to understand and have a conversation with the team if he felt more awake.

On obtaining collateral by speaking to his mom, with Christian's permission, the CAPF also better understood the patient. Christian's mom echoed his sentiments and felt as though he had been misunderstood because of "how he looks. The team feels like he has an attitude, but they don't explain things or give him options or choices. All he wants is for them to listen and actually 'hear' him. Of course, he wants to live and be here, but he also wants to be heard." His mom denied any concerns for depression or safety and clearly expressed that he was, in fact, looking to take more ownership of his medical care.

After listening to Christian and his mom, the CAPF began to empathize and put herself in his shoes. Knowing that aggressive behaviors of the boys of African American ancestry are more likely to be seen as willful and more likely to be prescribed antipsychotics for emotional dysregulation, the CAPF could reflect on Christian's race and previous diagnosis of ODD.[18] With that diagnosis, a provider could easily walk into his room thinking, "this kid has an attitude," and subsequently act in a paternalistic manner, which may prove counterintuitive. Of note, research studies indicate that the number of African Americans diagnosed with ODD is disproportionately higher than other demographic groups.[29,30]

Instead, by using a cultural approach, the CAPF was able to understand Christian's perspective, which allowed him to feel safe enough and to be honest about his reasons for treatment refusal. The CAPF, in turn, was able to relay this information to the primary team, which ultimately changed their approach to communicating with Christian and his mother by partnering with him in his treatment going forward.

The approach to creating a cultural formulation is like "walking a mile in another's shoes"—it can be used to learn more about how patients feel, allowing providers to better engage them in treatment planning. The following Table illustrates how the CAPF was able to use the *ADDRESSING* framework to help create a cultural formulation (see **Table 3**).

Case 2: Cultural Formulation

Christian is an 18-year-old African American young man with a medical history of cystic fibrosis with subsequent hepatic failure and psychiatric history of the oppositional defiant disorder (ODD), who was admitted to the medical floor due to respiratory distress in the setting of a cystic fibrosis exacerbation. In the context of treatment refusal, remembering that there may be bias or assumptions about inherent temperament due to his diagnoses, including ODD, as well as his race, is crucial. Christian and his mother were concerned about implicit bias on behalf of his treatment providers, and Christian identified feeling judged prematurely and treated like a child when he was hoping, instead, to partner in his care. He did not feel that there was adequate communication with the treating team, including around risks, benefits, or side effects of treatments, which led him to feel less inclined to communicate with the team and to choose to use his electronics to distract himself from his symptoms. His mother was in agreement, as he indicated wanting treatment but also preferred to avoid certain side effects. This was further complicated by her inability to provide Christian with more emotional support, given she was a single mother and had to go to work because of their limited financial means and was not always present in the daytime when he was interacting with the primary medical team.

Case 3: Ayesha

Ayesha is a 15-year-old girl with a history of headaches, who has been referred to mental health care for anxiety. She and her family initially denied any anxiety or mood symptoms, but due to frequent headaches and an elevated score on a SCARED assessment[31,32] at her pediatrician's office, they were again referred for mental health treatment. Using the CFI, including the supplementary module for school-age children and adolescents,[9] the clinician explored that the family was from Pakistan, and although her parents were receptive to psychoeducation, they are concerned that other family members do not "believe" in mental health. Ayesha lives in a joint household with other family members, including grandparents, aunts, uncles, and some cousins. Some of whom on hearing about her headaches would compare her life with her less economically well-off family in Pakistan and call her "ungrateful." The Family are Sunni Muslims, and they emphasize the need for prayer and fasting to help with Ayesha's headaches and for her to focus on school instead of spending time with friends or on extracurricular activities. In a private interview, she reported moderate anxiety symptoms, including some social anxiety, and stated that she was struggling with aspects of her religious identity and also struggling to maintain friendships at school due to her limited ability to spend time with them due to lack of family permission and fear of inviting them over to her joint family household (**Table 5**).

Case 4: Lauren

Lauren is a 7-year-old Asian girl, adopted as an infant from Laos, raised by her Asian adoptive Christian family in an upper-middle-class suburban community. She is not connected to her biological parents. She presented with diffuse aches and pains associated with school avoidance and complex relational trauma by her father. Lauren had to leave her close friends after the second grade when her family decided to move from the Midwest to New Jersey in an attempt to get away from her father's parents who had been physically and emotionally abusive throughout her father's childhood as a result of their own mental health struggles. This move exacerbated her school avoidance as some peers have asked where she is from and why she is so shy and quiet. Owing to the trauma history, her father often managed Lauren's avoidance with emotional reactivity. Mom wondered if finding a clinician of similar cultural identity to Lauren would be best equipped to navigate these challenges associated with her adoption from an Asian country (**Table 6**).

SUMMARY AND FURTHER THOUGHTS

These are just a few example cases in which using the questions of the CFI as well as pre-existing frameworks can help clinicians navigate a more culturally informed understanding of their patients and families and how that enhances the overall evaluation process such that the provider can craft a richer assessment and formulation, as recommended in the OCF.

There are some concerns about using the CFI as a tool; for example, people report that lack of time is an issue with conducting the CFI; however, a study has shown it has only added an average of 11.4 minutes to the standard intake evaluation that clinicians are currently performing.[16] In addition, providers are neither expected to belong to nor to be experts in their patient's backgrounds,[33] but instead guide the patients through a narrative telling of their symptoms and experiences,[34] not only to build understanding but to also empathize with patients and families.[34] By affirming all cultural differences, all cultural identities are equally valued and, therefore, appreciated for their significant impact on our patients' understanding of themselves as well as society's understanding of our patients.[8]

Table 5
A cultural formulation using the CFI for Ayesha (case 3)

Four Domains of the CFI	Clinical Information
Cultural definition of the problem	• At first, Ayesha would say "headaches" but with probing, would describe symptoms of anxiety that she has trouble naming because of not feeling safe discussing mental health symptoms or treatment • She relays she can discuss her worries with teachers and her counselor at school, and she is also close to one friend at school who also understands her, but she has difficulty communicating with family
Cultural perceptions of cause, context and support	• Some family members think she is ungrateful for what she has compared with relatives "back home" [Pakistan], and her headaches are a punishment • She appreciates the support she feels at school but wishes she had a safe space for discussion at home and felt supported by her family • Her family are devout Muslims, and she feels guilty about exploring her religious identity
Cultural factors affecting self-coping and past help-seeking	• The Family has been a barrier to her receiving mental health treatment, and want her to pray and fast more and show more gratitude as a means to help heal her headaches and succeed in school • She has appreciated talking to the school guidance counselor but is afraid to seek further care due to fear of what her family and greater cultural and religious community might say
Cultural factors affecting current help-seeking	• After receiving psychoeducation, Ayesha would like to engage in therapy, preferably with a female provider • Parents are on board with therapy but prefer a Muslim, Pakistani provider whom they can relate to and would prefer to refer to this as "treatment for her headaches" and not as mental healthcare or therapy
Overall cultural assessment	Ayesha is a 15-year-old girl, born in the United States to parents who immigrated from Pakistan. She lives in a joint family system with three generations living in the same household, who presented with headaches. In a private interview, she endorses moderate anxiety and social anxiety symptoms that are likely impacting her headache frequency and intensity. Additional context reveals that she feels open to discussing this with a school counselor but has difficulty discussing this at home where her parents are on board, but other family members 'do not believe in mental health care' and instead want her to turn to religious practice, such as praying and fasting, to heal her symptoms. Her communication difficulties and feeling unsupported at home pose significant barriers to her being able to engage in treatment. The clinician should consider how to both engage with her in her individual cultural identity development while respecting and engaging family. They should engage Ayesha and her parents in psychoeducation and treatment planning, as well as other means of cultural consultation, including colleagues, and with Ayesha and parents' permission, community and religious leaders.

Data from American Psychiatric Association. Diagnostic and Statistical Manual of Mental Disorders, DSM-5. Fifth edition. American Psychiatric Publishing; 2013.

Table 6
A cultural formulation using the OCF for case 4 Lauren

Category	Clinical Information
Cultural identity of the individual	• An Asian girl born in Laos, raised by Asian American adoptive parents since infancy in an upper-middle-class suburban town
Cultural concepts of distress	• Lauren is exhibiting somatic manifestations of her strong feelings to possibly minimize psychopathology's impact on interpersonal relationships, as noted in Asian Americans • Lauren is expected to represent the "model minority"
Psychosocial stressors and cultural features of vulnerability and resilience	• Lauren might feel disconnected from her culture having been adopted, despite being adopted by Asian parents, as she is from a distinct Asian group with a less visible presence in America • Access to appropriate resources to address trauma is limited
Cultural features of the relationship between the individual and the clinician, treatment team, and institution	• Mental health stigma is a barrier to seeking help, particularly given the more holistic viewpoints Laurent's family might have, which can be thought to be inconsistent with the Western approach to mental health services • Finding a clinician of similar Asian American cultural identity may assist in the development of trust and Lauren's openness to seeking and remaining in treatment
Overall cultural assessment	Given cultural factors, such as adoption, intergenerational trauma, family relocation, and Lauren's developmental understanding of how these play in her life and her relationship with illness, Lauren's somatic symptoms are consistent with school avoidance in the setting of a generalized anxiety disorder perpetuated by strained relationships with her father and peers. A clinician with an openness to explore cultural identity with Lauren and family members, both as individuals and as a whole unit, while incorporating culturally aware resources, is recommended.

Data from American Psychiatric Association. Diagnostic and Statistical Manual of Mental Disorders, Fifth Edition, Text Revision. American Psychiatric Association; 2022.

In addition, the overarching goal is for clinicians to analyze their patient's symptoms from the patient's viewpoint and in the context of their situations and experience to craft a cultural formulation. We have reviewed and recommended different avenues to consider in different clinical scenarios and present numerous tools to use to create that cultural formulation. We recommend using those tools and collating that information into a more nuanced assessment that can assist the clinician and patient partner together to create a treatment plan, which also may require flexibility in how the tools were originally created. In that vein, not all the questions of the CFI must be asked at any one point in time. Incorporating the CFI is important to "place the experience of the patient front and center" and to allow the patient to tell their own story in their own construct, and there can be value in following the complete CFI.[35] However, there are also potential advantages to using it in pieces, including considering the length of the interview for children and families.[36] In addition, some questions may not be developmentally appropriate for certain children or adolescents, and, in fact, sometimes the information is best gathered from collateral sources including family, school, and community members.[33]

In the examples presented, a few questions from the CFI were able to begin conversations, and further evaluation (whether in future intake assessments or longitudinally in care) can be continued with more questions from the CFI or further questions expanding on the patient's and family's experience. Patients and providers should consider that discovering information to craft a cultural formulation is a dynamic process, which can be enriched by interdisciplinary case discussions among treatment providers and bring greater awareness to inform and enrich formulations and treatment plans, often bringing to light past trauma or current hurdles that affect care delivery.[10] Two additional frameworks, *ADDRESSING* and *RESPECTFUL,* were also shown to help collate information that could be gathered during an interview into a more nuanced, holistic assessment.

The authors call for future research to shed light on how best to document this nuanced information and how to respect patients and families while also documenting sensitive, clinically pertinent information. This is especially true in situations whereby the children or adolescents may not have disclosed information to their legal guardians or to other health care providers or other systems that can access the electronic medical record (EMR). We also hope for more research on how to longitudinally use tools such as the CFI with patients to continue to engage them and to continue the dynamic cultural formulation with each intake. In addition, we look forward to more research on clinician self-reflection in conducting a cultural interview, including considerations of how transference and counter transference can affect clinical decision-making.

CLINICS CARE POINTS

- Cultural assessment should be used in all encounters but can be especially helpful in difficult diagnostic assessments, limited engagement and adherence, or disagreement between clinician and patient
- Cultural formulation is a dynamic process and should continue as a clinician longitudinally works with a patient, including gathering information from appropriate collateral sources
- Use tools such as the Outline for Cultural Formulation and Cultural Formulation Interview, including its Supplementary Modules
- There are also frameworks in psychology literature, such as *ADDRESSING* and *RESPECTFUL,* to help guide clinicians in their cultural formulations
- Aim to be patient centered and allow the patient to narrate their own symptoms in their own experiential, cultural context
- Interdisciplinary case discussions can be helpful in crafting a more nuanced cultural formulation

DISCLOSURE

C.S. Al-Mateen has royalties from American Psychiatric Association Publishing and Springer Nature. The remaining authors of this article have no financial or other disclosures.

REFERENCES

1. American Psychiatric Association. Diagnostic and statistical manual of mental disorders. 4th edition. Washington, D.C.: American Psychiatric Association; 1994.
2. Angel RJ, Williams K. Cultural models of health and illness. In: Paniagua Freddy A, Yamada Ann Marie, editors. Handbook of multicultural mental health. San Diego: Academic Press; 2013. p. 49–68.
3. American Psychiatric Association. Diagnostic and statistical manual of mental disorders. 3rd edition. Washington, D.C.: American Psychiatric Association; 1980.
4. American Psychiatric Association. Diagnostic and statistical manual of mental health. 3rd edition, Revised. Washington, D.C.: American Psychiatric Association; 1987.
5. American Psychiatric Association. Diagnostic and statistical manual of mental disorders, DSM-5. 5th edition. Arlington, Virginia: American Psychiatric Publishing; 2013.
6. American Psychiatric Association. Diagnostic and statistical manual of mental disorders. 5th edition, Text revision. Washington, D.C.: American Psychiatric Association; 2022.
7. Aggarwal NK, Jarvis GE, Gómez-Carrillo A, et al. The Cultural Formulation Interview since DSM-5: prospects for training, research, and clinical practice. Transcultural Psychiatry 2020;57(4):496–514.
8. Jones KL, Jain P, Weintraub C, et al. DSM-5 outline for cultural formulation and cultural formulation interview: complex case examples. In: Parekh R, Al-Mateen CS, Lisotto MJ, Carter R Dakota, et al, editors. Cultural psychiatry with children, adolescents, and families. Washington, D.C.: American Psychiatric Association Publishing; 2021. p. 355–73.
9. American Psychiatric Association. Supplementary modules to the core cultural formulation interview. Diagnostic and statistical manual of mental disorders 5th edition, Text revision. 2022. Available at: https://www.psychiatry.org/File Library/Psychiatrists/Practice/DSM/DSM-5-TR/APA-DSM5TR-CulturalFormulationInterview SupplementaryModules.pdf. Accessed February 3, 2022.
10. Rousseau C, Johnson-Lafleur J, Papazian-Zohrabian G, et al. Interdisciplinary case discussions as a training modality to teach cultural formulation in child mental health. Transcultural Psychiatry 2020;57(4):581–93.
11. Pumariega AJ, Rothe E, Mian A, et al. Practice parameter for cultural competence in child and adolescent psychiatric practice. J Am Acad Child Adolesc Psychiatry 2013;52(10):1101–15.
12. Lewis-Fernández R, Aggarwal NK, Bäärnhielm S, et al. Culture and psychiatric evaluation: operationalizing cultural formulation for DSM-5. Psychiatry Interpersonal Biol Process 2014;77(2):130–54.
13. Yamada AM. Culture and mental health: an introduction and overview of foundations, concepts, and issues. In: Cuéllar I, Paniagua FA, editors. Handbook of multicultural mental health. San Diego: Academic Press; 2000. p. 3–24.
14. Arshad SH, Chua JD, Baker LP. Building up and breaking down: youth cultural identity development. JAACAP Connect 2021;8(1):21–3.

15. Sabogal F, Marín G, Otero-Sabogal R, et al. Hispanic familism and acculturation: what changes and what doesn't? Hispanic J Behav Sci 1987;9(4):397–412.

16. Sanchez AL, Jent J, Aggarwal NK, et al. Person-centered cultural assessment can improve child mental health service engagement and outcomes. J Clin Child Adolesc Psychol 2022;51(1):1–22.

17. Dana R. Asians and Asian Americans. In: Understanding cultural identity in intervention and assessment. 1998:141–73. Thousand Oaks, California. doi:10.4135/9781483328225.

18. U.S. Department of Health, Services H.. Mental health: culture, race, and ethnicity—a supplement to mental health: a report of the surgeon general. 2001. Available at: https://www-ncbi-nlm-nih-gov.proxy.library.vcu.edu/books/NBK44243/.

19. Shiang J, Kjellander C, Huang K, et al. Developing cultural competency in clinical practice: treatment considerations for Chinese cultural groups in the United States. Clin Psychol Sci Pract 1998;5(2):182–210.

20. Kisiel CL, Fehrenbach T, Conradi L, et al. Tailoring the Trauma-Informed Assessment to the developmental and sociocultural context of the child and family. In: Trauma-informed assessment with children and adolescents: strategies to support clinicians. Washington, D.C.: American Psychological Association; 2021. p. 57–83.

21. Soto A, Smith TB, Griner D, et al. Cultural multicultural competence: two meta-analytic reviews. J Clin Psychol 2018;74(11):1907–23.

22. Chin JL, Liem JH, Ham MDC, et al. Transference and empathy in Asian American Psychotherapy: cultural values and treatment needs. Westport, Connecticut: Praeger Publishers/Greenwood Publishing Group; 1993.

23. Hays Pamela A. The Starting Place - Knowing who you are. In: Connecting across cultures: the helper's toolkit. Thousand Oaks, CA: Sage Publications; 2012. p. 13–22.

24. D'Andrea M, Daniels J. Before you get started. In: Ivey AE, D'Andrea M, Ivey MB, et al, editors. Theories of counseling and psychotherapy - a multicultural perspective. 5th edition. Allyn & Bacon; 2002. p. 456, pages xvii-xxiv. Available at: https://www.sjsu.edu/counselored/docs/RESPECTFUL.pdf.

25. Smedley BD, Stith AY, Nelson AR. Unequal treatment: confronting racial and ethnic disparities in health care (with CD). Washington, D.C.: National Academies Press; 2003.

26. FitzGerald C, Hurst S. Implicit bias in healthcare professionals: a systematic review. BMC Med Ethics 2017;18(1):19.

27. Blair I, Steiner JF, Havranek EP. Unconscious (implicit) bias and health disparities: where do we go from here? Permanente J 2011;15(2):71–8.

28. Duckworth S. Power/Privilege Wheel. sylviaduckworth.com.

29. Feisthamel K, Schwartz R. Differences in mental health counselors' diagnoses based on client race: an investigation of adjustment, childhood, and substance-related disorders. J Ment Health Couns 2009;31(1):47–59.

30. Schwartz RC, Feisthamel KP. Disproportionate diagnosis of mental disorders among African American versus European American Cl. J Couns Development 2009;87(Summer 2009):295–301.

31. Birmaher B. Screen for child anxiety related disorders (SCARED). Available at: https://www.pediatricbipolar.pitt.edu/resources/instruments. Accessed April 2, 2022.

32. Birmaher B, Brent DA, Chiappetta L, et al. Psychometric properties of the screen for child anxiety related emotional disorders (SCARED): a replication study. J Am Acad Child Adolesc Psychiatry 1999;38(10):1230–6.

33. la Roche MJ, Bloom JB. Examining the effectiveness of the Cultural Formulation Interview with young children: a clinical illustration. Transcultural Psychiatry 2020; 57(4):515–24.

34. Aggarwal NK. The psychiatric cultural formulation: translating medical anthropology into clinical practice. J Psychiatr Pract 2012;18(2):73–85.

35. Lewis-Fernández R, Aggarwal NK, Kirmayer LJ. The cultural formulation interview: progress to date and future directions. Transcultural Psychiatry 2020; 57(4):487–96.

36. Rousseau C, Guzder J. Teaching cultural formulation. J Am Acad Child Adolesc Psychiatry 2015;54(8):611–2.

Dialog Across Cultures
Therapy for Diverse Families

Neha Sharma, DO[a],*, Margaret Cary, MD, MPH[b],
Nayla M. Khoury, MD, MPH[c], Khalid I. Afzal, MD[d],
Deepika Shaligram, MD[e], Rakin Hoq, MD[f], Erin L. Belfort, MD[g],
John Sargent, MD[a]

KEYWORDS

- Cultural humility • Family-based care • Acculturation • Mental health
- Cultural factors • Diverse families

KEY POINTS

- Culture defines the way families and clinicians understand mental health conditions.
- Families and clinicians of minority populations are negatively influenced by systemic racism, racial discrimination, social determinants of health, and potentially acculturative family distancing.
- Through family-based care, providers can mitigate impact of structural inequities and acculturative stress on youth and families of minority population.
- Cultural humility, curiosity, and respect are essential for successful family-based care.
- Family therapy-based strategies can help navigate situations where providers and families are misaligned in their goals, expectations, and values.

INTRODUCTION

The COVID-19 pandemic has highlighted health-care inequities and social injustices experienced by families of racial and cultural minorities.[1] Before the pandemic, up to 36% of children and youth in the United States experienced poor mental health.[2]

[a] Tufts University School of Medicine, Tufts Medical Center, 800 Washington Street #1007, Boston, MA 02111, USA; [b] Oregon Health Authority and Yellowhawk Tribal Health Center, Confederated Tribes of the Umatilla, 800 Northeast Oregon Street, Portland, OR 97232, USA; [c] Department of Psychiatry, SUNY Upstate Medical University, 713 Harrison Street, Syracuse, NY 13210, USA; [d] Department of Psychiatry and Behavioral Neuroscience, The University of Chicago, 5841 South Maryland Avenue, MC 3077, Chicago, IL 60457, USA; [e] Department of Psychiatry & Behavioral Sciences, Boston Children's Hospital/Harvard Medical School, 300 Longwood Avenue, Boston, MA 02115, USA; [f] NYU School of Medicine, Hassenfeld Children's Hospital at NYU Langone, 1 Park Avenue, 7th Floor, New York, NY 10016, USA; [g] Tufts University School of Medicine, Maine Medical Center, 66 Bramhall Street, Portland, ME 04102, USA
* Corresponding author.
E-mail address: nsharma@tuftsmedicalcenter.org

Child Adolesc Psychiatric Clin N Am 31 (2022) 603–614
https://doi.org/10.1016/j.chc.2022.05.002
1056-4993/22/© 2022 Elsevier Inc. All rights reserved.
childpsych.theclinics.com

Race and culture-based disparities in diagnosis and treatment are well established.[1] Because the medical community makes efforts to address these inequities, medical culture needs to align and speak a shared language of respect and understanding. More importantly, making behavioral health care accessible and welcoming for all youth and families who need it, helps mitigate negative impact of mental health on youth development.

Focusing exclusively on distress omits aspects of wellness. Seventy-five percent of children and youth in the United States report positive indicators of mental health.[2] Because culture often mediates protective factors, culturally attuned child and adolescent psychiatrist (CAP) better reinforce the strengths and supports that promote mental well-being. This article describes the best practices for culturally informed and inclusive child and adolescent psychiatric care with a family focus. Although written from the perspectives of CAPs, the clinical dynamics are common to all clinical interactions and the recommendations are universally relevant.

Orienting to the Dialog Across Cultures

Culture defines identities, roles, values, and norms. Most mental health disorders affecting children are not spontaneous or genetic but rather develop through a complex interplay of various cultures and relationships surrounding a child. For example, a child may present as reflection of the turmoil in family life, of being part of a school system that does not meet their social, emotional, and learning needs, of daily experiences of invalidation, and of different cultural expectations in their social environment. Furthermore, family and systems issues mediate all psychiatric disorders, even those with clear neurobiological causes, such as psychosis and attention-deficit hyperactivity disorder.[3,4] Culture also influences relational dynamics and guides decision-making. In every clinical interaction with a child, there are multiple cultures present, including the family's culture(s), the clinician's culture(s), and the culture(s) of clinical practice. Therefore, to provide a comprehensive assessment and treat children, CAPs must engage with families and understand with them the impact of the various cultures present.

Guidance for Successful Family Engagement

Providers: dialog with self

Psychiatric practice demands engaging in life-long learning of understanding our blind spots, explicit and implicit biases, positions of power, presumptions of responsibility, and ways that we perpetuate dominant cultural norms. Self-reflection, language and behavior change, and taking responsibility for correcting missteps fosters transparency, collaboration, and acknowledgment of historical and ongoing oppression. These are cornerstones of trauma-informed practice.[5] Learning from others, through reading published works and participating in discussions, workshops, and trainings, helps deepen understanding and reinforce learning.[6,7]

For white CAPs in the United States, whose racial identity is the default and norm against which others are judged, some of the efforts to understand internalized racial superiority may be new and unsettling. For minority CAPs, this study may uncover ways that certain privileges and racial oppression have been internalized, as well as harms accumulated. The health of all of us depends on the healing of each of us. "There are no safety nets, no shortcuts, and no easier routes."[6] When the clinician's nuanced understanding of their whole self is present, it invites families to share their whole selves.[8]

Dialogs and the Practice of Cultural Humility

There is inherent power and privilege that comes with being a CAP, which requires recognition and responsibility. Clinicians must meet families where they are and aim with them where they dream to be, while avoiding imposing our expectations.[9] The hidden curriculum in medical education and practice includes valuing competency over humility, a tradition of patriarchal treatment.[10] Thus, one needs to take the step of unlearning these assumptions to foster partnership and to better support children and families. Although the medical model assumes assessment and diagnosis are work done by the clinician, cultural humility and person-centered care includes prioritizing collaboration and allowing families to define their concerns, set their own goals, and guide treatment plans. Cultural humility is a stance that is person oriented, includes reflection and self-evaluation, and is also structurally aware, recognizing and working to correct power differentials as they show up in clinical practice.[11] There is a higher likelihood of missteps in treatment when cultural humility is not practiced. Missteps that occur too early or are too great may threaten the therapeutic alliance and the goal of engaging the family. Reflecting and learning from examples of early aborted treatments are important growth opportunities. Although starting the interview primarily with the child may be effective in some settings to help the child feel comfortable, in other settings, the parents may feel left out, distrustful of the process or may benefit from initial interventions aimed at partnering and aligning.

An example of alliance missteps includes the work of 2 nonindigenous CAPs working with a young indigenous man, who was brought to care by his mother at the request of the school for behavioral concerns and a question of exposure to violence. In the middle of the first interview, the mother abruptly ended the session, noting "my son isn't comfortable with these questions." The questions had been directed mainly at the child and involved asking him to share about himself. He began sharing his passion for a horror film, which had been part of the school's concerns. Initial reflections as to the reasons for this discomfort included considering the impact of the mother's trauma history and history with Child Protective Services (CPS), which may have affected her view of the providers in this clinic. Further reflection on the CAPs' lack of understanding of this mother's values, her potential ambivalence with regards to seeking treatment, and her experience of being criticized by the clinicians, CPS, and school, highlights a critical need to hear families and understand their life experiences. Introductions that include clinicians' intentions may be an olive branch for many families amid numerous negative interactions with systems.

Dialog that Engages a Family Holistically

Families seek the support of CAPs in many contexts. Contextual understanding is critical to family engagement to effectively work with children and adolescents, no matter the cultural background. The presenting problem is created, maintained, and sustained within the family system context and, thus the treatment is best addressed in the family system context. To create a welcoming space to discuss difficult circumstances that families have experienced, it may be beneficial to start from the family's experience. **Box 1** identifies ways to engage families holistically.

It is worthwhile to spend time early in treatment getting to know each family member outside of the context of the presenting problem. Starting from a place of strengths and hopes for a better future, we acknowledge that each person is more than their problems. *Share something about you that is unrelated to our meeting today.* When identifying the positives in a family, the CAP recognizes their competence and highlights what they are good at or care about.[12]

Box 1
Skills for engaging with families and working through challenges

Awareness of your bias and blind spots

Welcome and seek understanding of the culture of the family

Learn from mistakes, ruptures, and impasses

Explore how the family's cultures and intersectionalities affect the problem and their goals for resolution with curiosity and humility

Validate injustices and exclusions

Collaborate with the family to reframe the problem to a shared achievable goal

Understand the context of engagement

Assess family vital signs

The CAP may want to ask the family about their journey to the present moment. This maybe an immigration journey, response to the experience of discrimination, response to the experience of feeling different, and their response to the challenges of stigma and exclusion. Such dialog begins the relationship of respect with the appreciation of resilience and struggle experienced by the family.

As the conversation moves toward the primary reason to seek care, CAPs must take the responsibility for setting the frame for a successful treatment. Often CAPs assume that families know how the treatment works and what the likely outcome will be of the engagement. For example, a family mandated to treatment by CPS or the legal system may enter treatment with different hopes, fears, and expectations than one self-referred or referred by a trusted provider. Similar to many parents from marginalized groups, immigrant parents can feel disenfranchised, shamed, blamed, or fearful when the school, the state, or another authoritative agency mandates an evaluation for their child. Thus, their expectation of the treatment is likely to be different. Aligning with the parents demonstrates respect for their expertise as parents and can create the foundation to move toward an understanding. It is an understanding of the different perspectives (of child, parents, CAP, and other systems) on mental illness, the meaning all parties involved make of the illness and its impact.

Careful validation and reframing are the required skill when families seek treatment where the youth is the identified patient, as a reflection of the family turmoil. Similarly, providers must focus on the larger picture of seeing families within their systems when multiple systemic issues are involved. For example, when a family may present as quite distressed and disorganized due to social and structural determinants of health and intergenerational trauma, in addition to cultural factors that may be at odds with the medical and mental health systems.

A CAP's ability to assess the family contextually depends on cultural and intersectional factors relevant to a family, and the ability to take a culturally humble stance. Furthermore, exploring the ideas and values of each family from a nonassuming and curious stance helps us avoid assumptions or judgments about a family based on our idea of "sameness" or "difference," especially, when working with diverse families. Additional factors that can add complexity to a family include preimmigration trauma, acculturative family distancing (AFD), trauma related to being different from the immediate community, generational racism, and the relationships between the cultures in the room. Exploring the intersectionality of the family's identity, particularly around aspects of marginalization, prejudice, and oppression (racial/ethnic, gender/sexuality, religious minority, and so forth) can be an important part of the healing process for families. For example, *how does a family whose culture and values prioritize autonomy or privacy interact with a CAP whose medical culture may prioritize risk reduction or safety?*

Family vital signs, conceptualized as the emotional climate, family flexibility, connectedness, parental relationship quality and authority style may all be impacted by cultural and structural factors.[13] *How did this family arrive at treatment with us? Who is most willing in the family to be in treatment? Who is least willing? What are their hopes of treatment? What are their prior experiences with other 'helpers' or 'systems'?*

Families from oppressed groups or those from communities with historical trauma such as genocide or slavery may present with a great distrust of the medical and mental health system. Engagement in such justified fear of harm contexts requires recognition that trust must be earned. It may be helpful to explicitly invite the family to teach the clinician what will be necessary to build trust. *"Sometimes the medical system or other systems mistreat people. I wonder if that is true for your family and what I can do to make this experience go better."* To build trust, starting the family conversation with the father figure may make sense for families of strongly patriarchal cultures, whereas starting with elders, if present, may be more appropriate for other families. *"What do you like to be called?"* conveys respect for a patient's autonomy and preferred language. *"Who should we hear from first?"* may also convey a CAP's value of hearing all voices but giving the family preference about how to begin. Additionally, making explicit statements conveying respect to a family for simply showing up can be validating. Acknowledging the range of possible emotions present including shame and fear may help to normalize a family's experience.

One goal of family interventions may be to engage the family in conversations about themselves.[12] When working with immigrant and refugee families, these conversations may be challenged by both generational and cultural gaps specifically because of acculturative stress. Acculturative stress is stress that is experienced by immigrant families when acclimating to the mainstream culture.[14] A family may present with youth engaging in self-harm due to breakdowns in communication and cultural value differences, such as, individuation, separation, gender roles, dating and relationships, career goals, educational goals, the meaning of success, the definition of happiness, and so forth. This breakdown in communication and values between immigrant parents and children is referred to as AFD. AFD is a risk factor for adolescent mental health issues.[15] Often, by the time AFD challenges come to a CAP's attention, "parent-child relationships have become negatively charged, disrespect is predominant, and the family is filled with hopelessness, mutual misunderstanding and hurt. To make matters worse, these problems have often been developing and progressing for some time when the family seeks help, leaving family members fixed in their opinions and with little expectations of change."[14] Families of minority cultures, races, or ethnicities who have lived in their country for generations also contend with acculturation stresses and conflicts, although they may have become acclimated to the degree that is explicitly asking about these stresses is necessary to surface them.[16]

CONDUCTING A CHALLENGING DIALOG

When preparing for the meeting with the family, it is useful to consider few structural components. These include seating arrangements—*who sits close to who, which way are they facing, where the clinician sits*, and so forth. It is important to be mindful of who is in the room and who is not. *Why is a family member missing? What is the impact* of their absence? What is their impact at home? Additionally, the CAP must prepare a plan about how to make sure that everyone has a chance to speak. What are the rules around active listening and speaking that need to be explicitly defined? What are the rules around language of respect versus punitive language?

The "Speaker–Listener Technique" is a powerful tool to make conversations clear and safe.[17] See **Table 1** for rules to consider. The task for the clinician is to facilitate discussion while avoiding problem-solving or seeking solutions. The speaker is encouraged to use the "I" statements such as *"I feel...,"* *"I saw that...."* After active listening, paraphrasing is helpful: *"What I hear you saying is . . .,"* *"Sounds like . . .,"* *"If I understand you right . . . ."*

Because difficult conversations will be part of any appointment, it is helpful to consider *how different family members support each other and how they maintain a courageous space. How can one ask for a break if one is not feeling safe in the appointment? What should be done to re-engage after such a break? What is the plan if physical safety becomes an issue? Moreover, finally, what should be expected after the appointment? What should happen in-between sessions?*[18]

THE PROCESS OF WORKING WITH FAMILIES

Families often come to treatment unsure of how to deal with their child. For example, when parents are frustrated with their adolescent for attempting suicide and needing hospitalization, one can reframe by saying: *"It seems that worries about your child, and having to miss work is very overwhelming, is that right? Moreover, yet, here you are in the emergency room for your child's wellbeing. I sense a strong bond between you and your child even if it is difficult to experience it at times."* Turning the attention to moments when family members offer love and support can bridge distance that has emerged and reinforce a positive feedback loop that diminishes the distress associated with the illness or the problem. Highlighting the strengths of the family reinforces the hope that propels healing.[12,19] Identifying the cultural factors and ethnic social capital that are protective and health promoting may validate the connections that are prioritized for family members as well.[19]

Once perspectives are shared, the CAP and family work together to synthesize the problem using each person's perspective in a validating fashion. This process also helps address stigma that may be held by the family, cultural factors affecting acceptance of the challenges, and parents' values. Synthesizing the problem also helps the family prioritize goals and assess which goals are achievable and which needs to be modified. To expand the cultural impact further, Sharma and Sargent (2021) describe that families from different cultures can have different reactions to the reality of this difference (ie, child's challenges). The person experiencing the difference can be seen as "other" and not a full member of the family collective. This can be a source of shame and embarrassment for the family, or seen as a sign of poor parenting. It can feel to the family as a challenge to their sense of community and to belonging. Part of setting the agenda for therapy will always be to understand the family's sense of the difference and their willingness to live with it. Family therapy may promote accommodation to difference with the expectation that with the increased knowledge and comfort with the difference the family becomes less distressed. Knowing the family's way of understanding the difference and honoring their language when describing the situation are a part of the keys for successful treatment.[14]

Aligning around description of the problem and its acceptance is a challenging process. It cannot be done without integrity, curiosity, and respect on the part of the provider.[14] Ultimately, the CAP's goal is to help families negotiate and accept differences

Table 1
Speaker–listener technique

General Rules	Speaker has the floor	Wait for your turn to speak	Respect everyone
Rules for the speaker	Use "I" and speak only for self	Focus on expressing thoughts and feelings	Be brief
Rules for the listener	Confirm/paraphrase what was heard	Ask clarifying questions when it is your turn to speak	Focus on the speaker's message

such that there is better prognosis for the youth's mental health. A striking example of this is how a family acceptance has been noted to improve the parent–child relationship and mental health outcomes of lesbian, gay, bisexual, transgender and queer or questioning youth (LGBTQ) youth.[20] Please see the article titled 'Clinical Considerations in working with LGBTQ+ Youth' for more details.

Once the problem has been defined, the goal is to gather information because it relates to the problem and the relationship between the problem and the family members. Often, at this stage, it may help to personify or externalize the problem as a separate entity, which helps with having a difficult conversation without blaming an individual. For example, a parent may identify their 7-year-old's clingy behavior, difficulty with transition, and inability to sleep independently as the problem. This minority child with anxiety can be identified as the problem by the other parent. By externalizing the anxiety driving the behavior, and calling it by another name such as *"monster," "fear,"* or *"worries,"* it may be easier to discuss *how the "worries" cause change in behavior of the child, how the "worries" may recruit a parent into agreeing with it, and how the "worries" exclude the other parent from the unit.*

The circular interview is another strategy that is used to gather information about factors that sustain the problem in the family system. These are a series of questions that identify connections among behaviors, beliefs, feelings, meanings, and relationships as they manifest among family members. An example of circular questions is demonstrated with the case here: An African American adolescent woman being raised by her grandmother and presenting with suicidal ideation may have a difficult time identifying a parent figure who she can talk to openly about these thoughts, particularly if there is ambivalence in the family about the grandmother's role, or where caregiving duties may be a source of responsibility and pride/strength, or, the family culture holds a significant amount of mental health stigma or shame.[21]

Circular questions may help them appreciate each other's point of view: *Is your grandmother aware of the kind of thoughts you've had? How would your grandmother react if you were to talk openly? What would she worry about? What does your grandmother think of your struggles? And to the grandmother: 'what must it be like for her to not have her mom around to turn to for these kinds of struggles? Is she right to feel like a burden? What are your hopes for her … if it's not the role of a grandmother to hear about these kinds of thoughts, whose role is it? What are the sources of support in your family and community?*

At the end of every appointment, it is a good practice to reflect on the process— *what was positive about this appointment? What would you do differently? What are the changes you would want to make in your life? What are the things that you are satisfied with that need to be maintained?* Such reflections and feedback provide more information for future sessions and can inspire changes that family may want to try between sessions. A collaborative contract to attempt a change in family pattern can be a family eating dinner together, using different language to communicate frustration, changing the role of the disciplinarian. Learning how these changes go, whether positive or negative, or the reasons or barriers to trying them brings additional useful information to understand the family and their relationship to the problem (**Table 2**).

Dialog to Repair Ruptures

Challenging family dynamics, difficulty understanding the family context, and family's ambivalence can often make the CAP feel "stuck." Assessing each family member's stance on the problem in this process is important. Family's denial of the problem or control over the situation is a set-up for failure based on unrealistic expectations of the clinician role in the treatment. Helping to reframe the problem such that the whole family sees the relational context of the problem and are willing to work with us in a collaborative way on improving the problem are crucial steps toward engagement and a successful treatment.[22]

Working Through a Family's Ambivalence

Family's ambivalence toward treatment can be overt and verbal (*"I don't think this will work." "It is the school's problem." "This is how we do things."*- with more cultural elements the conversation) or subconscious (*"I am trying to help my kid to go to school but, I don't think that school is the right fit."*). Navigating ambivalence requires the clinician to label the ambivalence and allow for it. When the ambivalence is reenacted in the room, support the family members to support the ambivalent member. Remind the family members of the ultimate goal and focus on change needed while also allowing for an option to change the family goal if one chooses to be adherent to the ambivalence. Working through ambivalence requires patience and ability to allow for 2 opposing ideas to coexist while accepting that this dynamic sustains the problem.

Working Through Communication Challenges

Family communication is how verbal and nonverbal information is exchanged among family members.[23] Facilitating conversations becomes the primary target of family engagement and intervention in situations where conflicts are related to communication issues. Fear of consequence or perceived vulnerability could drive difficulty in conversations, especially when the theme signals safety concerns. In such situations, protective instincts may trigger avoidance, overprotectiveness, or noncollaborative problem solving, all of which do not address the root issue. The family's cultural and ethnic background plays a crucial role in navigating difficult conversations. Thus, CAPs need to follow the principle of active listening by paying close attention to both verbal and nonverbal communication. Requesting clarifications frequently assists in avoiding assumptions. The CAP's role of fostering a discrete connection with each family member while maintaining a semblance of understanding and comfort helps to promote conversations in such situations.

Difficult conversations vary according to the family's communication style, cultural background, and problem-solving skills. Every family has its own communication style that varies depending on the setting, the culture, and the purpose of the conversation.[23] Different styles of conversation between parents and youth can exacerbate the generational gap and contribute to AFD. This occurs especially when the youth are more familiar with the Western European approach of directness, which can be experienced as disrespectful in many minority cultures. This view of direct communication is western-centric and culturally problematic. There are many examples of indirect communication, which is also effective, such as the role of humor in many

Table 2
Family therapy process and outcome goals for each task

Task	Joining and Engagement	Defining Problem	Information Gathering	Redefining the Problem	Reflection on the Process and Contracting
Process goal	Welcoming, understanding the culture of the family, establishing a shared sense of the problem	Better understanding the culture of the family, better defined sense of the problem, ensuring a collaborative team	Continuing to learn the family's unique culture and ways of functioning, recognizing movement toward the shared goals	Reframing the problem, appreciating any losses associated with progress, addressing ruptures	Ensuring the family's satisfaction with the treatment, movement toward termination by practicing strategies at home environment
Outcome goal	Engaged family who commits to the future meeting and has a shared sense of the problem	Deepened connection between the cultural elements and the shared sense of the problem	Identified patterns that sustain and maintain the problem and how it impacts the family members	Revised view of the problem and the role each person plays and renewed interpersonal trust	Family establishes renewed form of rules and commitment by which to resolve current and future problems

cultures as a way to help families navigate difficult scenarios. The clinician's role is to identify the hidden messages in conversation styles and intervene to facilitate an uninterrupted flow while refraining from placing judgment due to the bias of their style, upbringing, and culture.

Working Through Structural Challenges

Structural challenges, such as the logistics of having all or relevant family members attend the meeting, the logistics of transportation and management of other commitments, and access to care, can be barriers to working with families. The COVID-19 pandemic has advanced the acceptance and utility for telemedicine significantly. One should be aware of the impact of telemedicine, positive or negative, in their community. Langarizadeh and colleagues (2017) noted that it allows for improved attendance, increased convenience for some people, and improved access to care, particularly in rural communities with access to reliably robust Internet service.[24] Telemedicine creates an opportunity to engage with families in ways that allows for family members to attend sessions even if they are not cohabitating. Although there are many benefits of telemedicine, it has its limitations, from Internet connectivity to registering nonverbal cues and less flexible interaction during the session.

Beside practical considerations that are necessary for all sessions, in-person or remote, such as seating arrangements, who is in what room, how they support each other, a safety plan during the session, how to ask for a break, and what to expect after the sessions, there are some unique aspects to be mindful for practice of telemedicine.[18] To be specific, the clinician must be familiar with the platform to assist the families with troubleshooting if necessary, consider how many devices are needed to have all members visible, have a plan for connectivity issues, and for the lack of privacy. These barriers must be evaluated before deciding whether telemedicine is the appropriate modality for the family.

Working Through Systemic or Cultural Challenges

When at an impasse in clinical care or uncertain of which concerns to follow, reorienting to familial, cultural, and other systemic impacts can be effective. For example, when the clinical recommendations are ineffective, it may be because the clinician is solving a problem that is not shared by all. A CAP's goal is not always culturally relevant to or a priority for the family. Different aspects of diagnosis and treatment may carry more or less stigma for each family member. Consider raising the question of *"how each family member defines the presenting problem,"* *"who expects who to change,"* or *"how everyone will know that problem has been resolved."* Listen for influences of cultural factors and life experiences. Retelling stories and renegotiating a shared understanding may encourage curiosity that leads to the discovery of a path forward.[12,14]

Involving an important member of the extended family or community may restart stalled progress. Including the perspective of more people can facilitate understanding and connection to the supports that are instrumental for healing and health. Adding more people may entail consulting with others, making culturally relevant adaptations to a treatment, inviting others to a clinical appointment, or asking those present to bring in the perspective of others important in their life. *"If your grandmother were here, what would she say to each of you?"* Additional people to consider include additional family members, youth or parent peers, cultural navigators, traditional healers, and religious leaders. It may be helpful to inquire about the angels, ghosts, visitors, spirits, or vampire bites that may have been influencing the family.[8,12]

SUMMARY

CAPs work at the intersections of families, cultures, and systems, which affect engagement in care, assessment, and treatment planning. Welcoming youth and their families to share about themselves, their culture, community, faith, social histories, ethnic and racial identities, gender, and sexuality works to foster understanding, strengthen therapeutic alignment, clarify diagnosis, reinforce strengths and supports, guide treatment recommendations, and promote healing. Acknowledging intersectional relationships among identities and communities, as well as relationships with other systems the child and family interact with, clarifies the experiences that shape stressors, distress, opportunities, and access to resources. Providing the most inclusive and comprehensive child psychiatric treatment also requires the CAP's understanding of one's own culture, biases, and internalized beliefs to counter harm, promote connection, make repairs, learn, and authentically foster sharing. There are several practical strategies that CAPs can apply to practice cultural humility, to join families, to facilitate difficult conversations and to work through misalignment to help families of all backgrounds to have conversations together, identify their strengths and work toward their goals. A family and cultural frame widens the lens and broaden the scope of what is possible for all individuals involved in otherwise tenuous or seemingly treatment resistant clinical cases.

CLINICS CARE PEARLS

- Cultural humility is the person-centered approach that limits implicit bias and allows child and adolescent psychiatrists to understand the family's values, goals, and perspective.

- Validation, reframing, contextual understanding for the reason of the meeting, and assessing the family vital signs are skills that help engage family holistically.

- When the provider and the family are not aligned, focusing on joining the family, redefining the problem, gathering the appropriate information and then, reflecting on the process can be helpful.

DISCLOSURE

The above authors have no disclosures.

REFERENCES

1. Protecting youth mental health: US surgeon general advisory. 2021. Available at: https://www.hhs.gov/sites/default/files/surgeon-general-youth-mental-health-advisory.pdf. Accessed March 2022.
2. Bitsko RH, Claussen AH, Lichstein J, et al. Mental health surveillance among children — United States, 2013–2019. MMWR Suppl 2022;71(Suppl-2):1–42.
3. Sharma N, Sargent J. Overview of the evidence base for family interventions in child psychiatry. Child Adolesc Psychiatr Clin N Am 2015;24(3):471–85.
4. Onwumere J, Bebbington P, Kuipers E. Family interventions in early psychosis: specificity and effectiveness. Epidemiol Psychiatr Sci 2011;20(2):113–9.
5. Substance Abuse and Mental Health Services Administration. SAMHSA's concept of trauma and guidance for a trauma-informed approach. HHS Publication No. (SMA) 14-4884. Rockville (MD): Substance Abuse and Mental Health Services Administration; 2014.

6. Saad LF. Me and white supremacy: combat racism, change the world, and become a good ancestor. Naperville (IL): Sourcebooks; 2020.
7. Kendi IX. How to be an antiracist. New York: One World; 2019.
8. Duran E. Healing the soul wound: counseling with American Indians and other native peoples. 2nd edition. New York: Teacher's College Press; 2019.
9. Ginwright S. Trauma-informed care and the future of healing. [Keynote address] 2019 the Northwest children's Foundation Community Forum, Seattle (WA).
10. Brooks KC. A piece of my mind. A silent curriculum. JAMA 2015;313(19): 1909–10.
11. Tervalon M, Murray-García J. Cultural humility versus cultural competence: a critical distinction in defining physician training outcomes in multicultural education. J Health Care Poor Underserved 1998;9(2):117–25.
12. Combrinck-Graham L. On being a family systems thinker: a psychiatrist's personal odyssey. Fam Proc 2014;53(3).
13. Wood BL, Woods SB, Sengupta S, et al. The biobehavioral family model: an evidence-based approach to biopsychosocial research, residency training, and patient care. Front Psych 2021;12. https://doi.org/10.3389/fpsyt.2021.725045.
14. Sharma N, Sargent J. Family therapy with diverse families. In: Ranna P, Al-Mateen CS, Lisotto MJ, et al, editors. Cultural psychiatry in child and adolescent psychiatry. Washington (DC): American Psychiatry Association Publishing; 2021. p. 151–63.
15. Kane JC, Johnson RM, Iwamoto DK, et al. Pathways linking intergenerational cultural dissonance and alcohol use among Asian American youth: the role of family conflict, parental involvement, and peer behavior. J Ethn Subst Abuse 2018;18: 613–33.
16. Jones J, Begay K, Nakagawa Y, et al. Multicultural counseling competence training: adding value with multicultural consultation. J Ed Psych Consultation 2016;26(3):241–65.
17. Markman H, Stanley S, Blumberg SL. Talking safely without fighting. Speaker Listener Tech. In: Fighting for your marriage: positive steps for a loving and lasting relationship. 3rd edition. San Francisco (CA): Jossey-Bass; 1994. p. 106–33.
18. Levy S, Mason S, Russon J, et al. Attachment-based family therapy in the age of telehealth and COVID-19. J Marital Fam Ther 2021;47(2):440–54.
19. Pearrow M, Sander J, Jones J. Comparing communities: the cultural characteristics of ethnic social capital. Educ Urban Soc 2019;51(6):739–55.
20. Ryan C, Russell ST, Huebner D, et al. Family acceptance in adolescence and the health of lgbt young adults. J Child Adolesc Psychiatr Nurs 2010;23(4):205–13.
21. Weaver A, Greeno CG, Fusco R, et al. Not just one, it's both of Us": low-income mothers' perceptions of structural family therapy delivered in a Semi-rural Community Mental Health Center. Community Ment Health J 2019;55:1152–64.
22. Madsen W. Collaborative therapy with multi-stressed families. 2nd edition. New York: The Guilford Press; 2007.
23. Epstein N, Bishop D, Baldwin L. (1982) The McMaster Model of Family Functioning: a view of the normal family. In F. Walsh (ed.) Normal Family Processes (pp. 15–141). New York: Guilford Press. 138–160.
24. Langarizadeh M, Tabatabaei MS, Tavakol K, et al. Telemental health care, an effective alternative to conventional mental care: a systematic review. Acta Inform Med 2017;25(4):240–6.

Religion and Spirituality
Why and How to Address It in Clinical Practice

Richard F. Camino-Gaztambide, MD, MA[a],*,
Lisa R. Fortuna, MD, MPH, MDiv[b], Margaret L. Stuber, MD[c]

KEYWORDS

- Religion and spirituality • Attachment • Moral foundation theory • Forgiveness
- LGBTQ+ • Immigrant families • Trauma

KEY POINTS

- Religious beliefs, rituals, and spiritual practices can strengthen family bonds, serve as inspiration and comfort in times of difficulty, trauma, or loss, and create psychological stress when there is familial conflict.
- There is evidence that early attachment styles can influence children and adolescents' concept of God.
- Moral foundation theory provides a useful explanatory model to understand a family's conception of morality and religious beliefs.
- The integration of religious beliefs and spiritual practices can be important to adolescent development along with a sense of cultural and ethnic identity.
- Forgiveness, an important concept and practice in many religious and spiritual worldviews, can be a source of strength and resilience for children and adolescents.

INTRODUCTION

Religion and spirituality (R/S) have been influential in societies' history, daily life, and identity in the past and in today's society. From a sociological perspective, R/S contributes to family development and organization, influences culture, and often contributes to forming opinions, beliefs, and concepts about oneself, family, society, and the world.[1] In addition, R/S help shape individual's, families', and communities' ethical and moral understanding, thus influencing their behavior. This review article aims to provide the clinician with tools to understand, assess, and provide interventions that consider the patients' and their families' R/S. Although a recent review of the topic focused on general aspects of the R/S[2], we are unaware of reviews that integrate attachment, moral foundation theory (MFT), and forgiveness. This review will integrate these additional features into our understanding of the role of R/S into the delivery of

[a] Medical College of Georgia, Augusta University, 997 Street, Sebastian Way, Augusta, GA 30912, USA; [b] University of California, San Francisco; [c] University of California, Los Angeles
* Corresponding author.
E-mail address: rcamino@augusta.edu

Child Adolesc Psychiatric Clin N Am 31 (2022) 615–630
https://doi.org/10.1016/j.chc.2022.05.007
1056-4993/22/© 2022 Elsevier Inc. All rights reserved.

mental health. Clarifying statement: The use of the word God is not an ontological statement, meaning that we do not state the nature or existence of God or deities. All statements referring to God or deities describe or explain relationships and their impact on beliefs, emotions, actions, and the clinical significance of those relationships.

In this article, we will present:

1. Definitions of R/S
2. The connection between religion/spirituality and attachment
3. Religion/spirituality and MFT.
4. Religion/spirituality and LBGTQ+ identity
5. Approaching religion/spirituality with immigrant families
6. Trauma and religion/spirituality
7. Clinical considerations of forgiveness
8. Provide specific assessment tools for clinical practice

DEFINITION OF RELIGION AND SPIRITUALITY

From the Latin *religionis*, religion means religation or binding together with a higher reality.[3] Religion, in general, presents a greater emphasis than spirituality on the institutional, dogmatic, ritual, and moral aspects of beliefs.[4] The sociologist Christian Smith defines religion as a cultural complex of prescribed practices, based on the premise and nature of the existence of superhuman powers, whether personal or impersonal, that helps its practitioners to communicate, and align with those powers in the hope of achieving human benefits and avoiding negative consequences.[1] For Smith, these powers or forces are not human creations and do not depend on human activity for their existence or production. In this definition, the omission of God or gods or deities makes it possible to include multiple religions without a deity but with beliefs and practices to access power beyond that of human beings.

Spirituality comes from the Latin *spiritus*, equivalent to the Greek term *pneuma*, and the Hebrew *ruah*, meaning wind, breath. Floristan defines spirituality as a reflection of religious wisdom, experience with the Absolute or the ultimate and profound values that transcend the human being.[5] Spirituality does not depend on a religious component, and many atheists or agnostic practitioners see themselves as spiritual. An instance can be found in the practice of the 12 Steps of Alcoholics Anonymous modified as the "12 Agnostic Steps" in the description of steps 11 and 12:

11. Sought through meditation to improve our spiritual awareness and our understanding of the AA way of life and to discover the power to carry out that way of life.
12. Having had a spiritual awakening as a result of these steps, we tried to carry this message to alcoholics, and to practice these principles in all our affairs.[6]

These definitions are consistent with people who consider themselves religious and spiritual, with those spiritual but not religious, or vice versa, or neither religious nor spiritual. It is essential to clarify the distinction between religion as a social institution and religion as viewed and practiced by the individual. Each person may have idiosyncratic differences in interpretation and practice of faith.[1] Religious belief, rituals, and spiritual practices can strengthen the family, promote a healthy relationship among its members, and serve as inspiration and comfort in times of difficulty or loss.[7] The acquisition and transmission of values and religious beliefs may be from family members of previous generations. Bengtson, Putney, and Harris conducted longitudinal research that followed 4 generations of families for nearly 50 years.[8]

The study (n > 3500) included interviews with grandparents, parents, grandchildren, and great-grandchildren, which showed families' significant influence on subsequent generations.

Before going further, we need to be mindful that there are individual differences in how people view and practice their faith traditions. A wise aphorism states: Like all of us, like some of us, like none of us.[9] This is quite applicable to religious practice and faith. Although religious beliefs can be an organizing set of principles for identity development, coping, common practices, and connections to others, these beliefs' ultimate expression and meaning is also individual and, thus, worthy of clinical inquiry.

Religion/Spirituality and Attachment

Attachment theory is a theory of relationships, allowing the study of the relationship of children and adolescents with God through the lens of attachment. For Bowlby, "attachment behavior is conceived as any form of behavior that results in a person attaining or retaining proximity to some other differentiated and preferred individual, who is usually conceived as stronger and/or wiser. While especially evident during early childhood, attachment behavior is held to characterize human beings from the cradle to the grave."[10] Ainsworth described attachment in the context of affectionate bonds. "An 'attachment' is an affectional bond, and hence attachment figures are never wholly interchangeable with or replaceable by another, even though there be another to whom one is also attached."[11]

Granquist considers that attachment to God complies with 3 general aspects of attachment theory: God as a safe haven, God as a secure base, and God as an attachment figure perceived to be stronger and wiser.[12] *Safe haven* implies activation of attachment behaviors on frightening situations, illness or injury, or perceived separation. For example, the believer or practitioner turns to prayer, meditation, or a ritual or activity perceived to protect in the face of danger. *A secure base* provides the confidence and sense of security to explore. The qualities of a secure base are expressed through the believers' sense of confidence, allowing them to explore the unknown, even in the face of danger. Finally, God is overwhelmingly viewed as stronger and wiser than humans are in most religions.[13]

Attachment to God or deities is consistent with children, adolescents, and young adults' attachment styles with their parents.[14,15] There seems to be a correlation between avoidant attachment with parents, and images of a distant and impersonal God, and anger toward God. Anxious parental attachment styles are associated with moral and religious or spiritual struggle.[16] In contrast, secure attachment to God correlates with less psychological and emotional distress in Christian, Muslim, and Jewish adult populations.[13]

Religion/Spirituality and Moral Foundation Theory

Most child psychiatrists are familiar with moral developmental theories of Piaget, Kohlberg (based on cognitive development), Gilligan (moral judgment of care), and Turiel (moral domains based on welfare, justice, and rights). However, MFT uses insights from evolutionary psychology, attachment, and basic emotions found in other species, such as fear, sadness, anger, disgust, and joy, to provide the underpinnings of morality within evolutionary theory.[17] MFT states that our moral decisions are based on intuitions, or deep feelings or emotions, more than intellectual or cognitive reflections.[18] Moral intuitions are understood as primarily emotionally based rather than an intellectual or cognitive reflection. Therefore, the initial moral response "in this view, is more a product of the gut than the head."[18] Moreover, some MFT researchers state that intellectual reasoning tends to justify the moral response more than it challenges it. This statement does not mean that moral intuitions are fixed but that this first response tends to have a powerful effect on the person's moral response.

There are 2 broad categories of moral intuitions(**Table 1**): first, individualizing foundations, and second, binding foundations. *Individualizing foundations* are termed because of their emphasis on welfare (care) and fairness toward others.[19,20] Evolutionary psychologists have found evidence of behaviors that display care, fairness, and altruism in several mammal species.[21-23] Individualizing foundations are also consistent with attachment theory and explain reactions of empathy when perceiving suffering or joy, even from strangers. However, *binding foundations* are those qualities that bind people into roles, duties, and mutual obligations toward family, community, and society in general. From an evolutionary perspective, the binding foundation's function focuses on the welfare of the group and community in contrast to the individual. Individualizing foundations have 2 essential elements: welfare and fairness. Binding foundations have 3 distinct features: *ingroup/loyalty* (allegiance, constancy, conformity, and self-sacrifice), *authority/respect* (social order, adherence to class structure, respect, obedience, and role fulfillment), and *purity/sanctity* (chastity, wholesomeness, control of desires, and avoidance of physical and spiritual contamination).[24] There is evidence that the emotion of disgust can be a response to violations of purity/sanctity, be that of foods or behaviors.[25] Although it seems reasonable to think that ingroup/loyalty and authority/respect are essential for group maintenance, the purity/sanctity aspects of binding foundations are less obvious. Many species, including humans, have an instinct or emotion of disgust that helps avoid eating toxic foods and contamination with pathogens.[26,27] From a social perspective, disgust has been associated with "distasteful behaviors"[28] and may contribute to the concept of purity, which helps maintain group homogeneity and differentiate insiders from outsiders.[29]

Moral Foundations

Table 1.

Clinical Applications of Moral Foundation Theory

Sammy's vignette (**Box 1**) helps illustrate some MFT concepts. Sammy's angst, depressive symptoms, and shame and guilt can be seen as his moral response to binding foundations. By having romantic homosexual or same sex feelings, he questions his loyalty, nonconforming feelings, threat to authority, and disrespect to his elders, traditions and role in the family. His feelings and behavior also clearly violate the purity/sanctity foundations of his family's beliefs. Binding foundations explains the challenge that Sammy is going through and helps us understand his family's response. Irrespective of the clinician's worldview, MFT helps to acknowledge the family's moral dilemma.[12] Studies looking at MFT have found that conservatives

Table 1		
In Moral Foundation Theory divides moral behavior in 2 categories: 1. *individualizing*, focused on individual welfare and fairness, and 2. *binding*, focused on group loyalty, authority, and purity		
Individualizing Foundations		**Binding Foundations**
Care		Ingroup/loyalty
Fairness		Authority/respect
		Purity/sanctity

> **Box 1**
> **Example: "Sammy"**
>
> Sammy's mom, Melinda, was hoping to find a Christian therapist that could help Sammy with his problems while respecting their family's values. Both Sammy and his mom were concerned about his academic performance. He was diagnosed with ADHD and had long-standing reading and math learning disabilities. One teacher had mentioned that he might have dyslexia. He struggled with self-esteem, and he worried that he was a disappointment to his family. More importantly, he recently "came out" as "maybe gay" to his sister because he realized that he had romantic feelings for a boy in his class. His sister was shocked by this disclosure, and she told their parents. The family attended a conservative, Christian Evangelical Church, where Sammy had always felt loved and accepted. Sammy considered himself religious and ever since he was a small child, he had sensed a close and loving relationship with God. When Melinda found out about his disclosure, she was saddened. Her first thought was that he would go to hell due to his sexuality and that the family would be separated from him in the afterlife for all eternity. In her mind, she was losing her son. His dad did not talk about "it" and became very emotionally distant and inaccessible to Sammy. Sammy became increasingly depressed and isolated from his family. Then one day at church several members of the congregation shared testimonials about being healed by Jesus. One of them, who was known as having "suffered from homosexual sin," held up a sign that read: *Once Broken, Now Healed and Made Whole*. This a reference to scripture: Be in faith that God saved you and you have been healed and made whole (Ephesians 2:8–9). Sammy was distressed by his growing awareness of his sexuality and the resulting destructiveness it was having on all of his relationships. He wondered if he was forever separated from God and his family. Was he broken? What shame would he cause his family if others found out?

seemed to give equal importance to individualizing and binding foundations. However, liberals tend to give preference to individualizing foundations over binding ones. Thus, liberals tend to be more inclusive and individually oriented, and conservatives give greater importance to binding or group cohesion and conformity to authority, loyalty, and purity.

Sammy's parents seem to give greater importance to binding foundations of morality, with the effect of distressing and producing harm (clearly not intentional) to their son.[13] The first clinical impulse may be to advocate that Sammy's parents accept his sexual identity. That may take longer or never fully come to fruition. The first step is to help the family lean into their collectivist values, the familial binding aspects of love and attachment.[30] By acknowledging the importance of their religious and group values, the clinician can then also focus on the individualizing virtues of care and welfare of their son. This includes educating the family about their son's increased risk of depression and even suicide, if left to feel rejection by his family, and the ensuing guilt and shame.

Research suggests that religion may reduce suicidality by providing a supportive community, influencing beliefs about suicide as sinful, instilling hope in times of stress[31] and by reducing other associated risk factors such as substance use disorders.[32] However, religious institutions in the United States are not always supportive of LGBTQ + identities. In those situations, the risk to supportive bonds can have serious consequences. Studies of LGBTQ + youth have found that parental religious beliefs about homosexuality leading to rejection are associated with double the risk of attempting suicide in the past year.[33,34]

Addressing a patient/family when religious worldviews conflict is a complex challenge for the patient and the therapist. Beliefs regarding sexuality is one important area where conflicts within families can occur. More broadly, a clinician whose guiding principles tend to be more strongly oriented toward fairness and "heavily endorse individualizing foundations (eg, harm–care) could also benefit from reflecting on what it is like for clients who use binding foundations such as ingroup/loyalty and purity/sanctity in their moral thought processes."

In working with Sammy, and youth like him, and across faiths, integration of religious identity with other aspects of identity (gender, ethnicity, sexuality, community membership) is important, as is supporting healthy relationships with family and/or community. Sammy tried to reconcile his sexual identity with his faith and strived to be the "good" and loved son who makes his family proud. How to support family interconnectedness, bonding and love was important to explore in his therapy. What did his family need in order to be close again? A primary focus was to avoid family rejection, which is associated with a high risk for poor mental health, substance abuse and suicidality, including for minoritized youth. Ryan and colleagues,[34] through the Family Acceptance Project, have demonstrated that family understanding of the risks of rejection to mental health and risk behaviors is important. Families can learn to lean into faith and/or cultural values of family-centeredness and turn toward caring and acceptance of their child as the priority (Ryan, 2010). Family acceptance predicts greater self-esteem, social support, and general health status. It also protects against depression, substance abuse, and suicidal ideation and risk behaviors for LGBTQ + youth.[33,35]

Ryan and colleagues,[34,35] suggest several family actions or behaviors that clinicians can encourage in order to protect youth mental health when religious belief in families poses a risk for LGBTQ + youth. This means moving beyond actions that are rejecting to behaviors that demonstrate acceptance, love and caring for the well-being of the youth. Examples include engaging with LGBTQ + affirming communities of faith, accepting the youth's friends, advocating for the youth when they are discriminated against or mistreated by others. Studies have found that for Black youth who identify as LGBTQ+, being part of a faith community can be protective against poor mental health even if their religious tradition is not specifically affirming of their sexuality or gender identity.[36] This suggests the importance of social support and inclusion in family, culture, and faith for racially minoritized youth and young adults.

When a religious community rejects a child or adolescent, the clinician may consider not only the attachment relationship that has been lost with the community but also the potential loss of attachment to their deity and faith, and the resulting feeling of abandonment, guilt, and shame that such a rejection can create. In a review article, Cherniak and colleagues[13] reported, "secure attachment to God is inversely related to psychological distress and emotional problems" in studies that included Christian, Muslim, and Jewish populations.[9] The implications for risk of mental illness, substance use disorders, and suicidality is important to evaluate and address clinically and through social supports.[32] Secure attachment to God "predicted mental health above and beyond intrinsic religiosity, social support, or interpersonal attachment styles."[9] Another study found that secure God attachment could be associated with positive affect via emotion-focused coping that can include such things as hope and feeling protected.[37]

Approaching Religion/Spirituality with Immigrant Families

The traditional model for understanding the role of R/S in the lives of immigrants to the United States emphasizes the importance of these for cultural continuity and the psychological benefits of religious faith for resilience following the trauma of immigration.[31,38,39] The church/synagogue/temple/mosque and the community of faith can be a place of comfort in times of trouble. From the viewpoint of considering religiosity as part of culture, youth identity forms through connections with others, including a faith community with specific practices, expectations, and perspective for meaning-making. For that reason, R/S, along with other cultural practices, can be an important aspect of the acculturation process of immigrant youth. Youth who are able to integrate their culture of origin (including religious belief and faith group membership) with a new and evolving cultural identity in the host country are more likely to have good mental health as compared to youth who completely assimilate to the host country and lose the benefits of their cultural and religious identity.[38] Immigrant youth whose identity and acculturation process are in conflict with that of their family of origin can be at risk for mental illness, due to family conflict, isolation, and internal psychological distress.[31,34,40,41]

Children of immigrants with elevated risk for mental health problems are more likely to be undocumented immigrants, refugees, or unaccompanied minors, primarily due to high rates of trauma exposure.[38,42,43] Migrating for these youth implies a high level of stress prior to, during, and after migration that may destabilize the immigrants' mental health. The sense of spiritual fulfillment provided by feelings of faith, religiosity, and transcendence beyond ordinary material life could mitigate the stress and benefit mental health. [39,44] However, persons with mental illness might seem dangerous or out of control, and this can result in rejection and ostracism. Religious coping, such as prayer and faith in God, can be protective. Attendance at church might help to meet a need for mental health support and coping. However, religious causal attributions for illness (ie, a result of lack of faith, not praying, the acts of demons on an individual, and sinful behaviors of parents) may also lead to distress.[45]

Equally important is the socioeconomic role of churches, synagogues, temples, and mosques in American society. The creation of an Immigrant church, temple, or mosque often provides ethnic communities with refuge from the hostility and discrimination from the broader society as well as opportunities for economic mobility and social recognition. Youth may or may not continue these connections but it is important to understand the role of the faith community, faith, and religion in resilience, social support and identity formation. The interaction between religiosity, acculturation and relationship, trauma and risk behaviors is complex. As youth enter adolescence and young adulthood, they may make decisions related to whether they will retain religious practices, beliefs and/or how they will integrate these into adulthood, potentially differently than their parents and with adaptations to their current cultural contexts and identity.[42] Clinicians can explore how youth do or do not consider their religious beliefs in decision-making and behaviors, or for coping with trauma.[44,46]

Trauma and Religion/Spirituality

Victims of traumatic events can rely on their faith for coping.[37] Religiosity can help mitigate the effects of trauma and could even lead to posttraumatic growth.[47–49] Alternatively, youth who experience retraumatization may develop a highly ambivalent relationship to God and all religiosity.[39] They may choose to blame God for not having protected them, for having left them to feel alone, or for having been indifferent to them.[43,48] They may even turn their wrath on God, as the source of cruelty.

Example: "Martin"

Martin is a 15-year-old immigrant unaccompanied youth from Central America. He often came into therapy sessions with a notebook filled with lyrics of songs he had written to share with his therapist. His songs memorialized experiences of violence and traumatic loss. Many of the themes in his songs included references to God, sometimes as a protector and sometimes as cruel and abandoning. When asked about these themes, Martin shared that his faith in God is central to him, although he sometimes questions why God allowed bad things to happen to him. Nonetheless, he often prays because his grandmother taught him to do so. He finds prayer helpful. When he prays he is able to let go of his worries about his family back in his country of origin, and place their safety in God's protective hands. This is an important coping strategy for him. He is sad about leaving his family, knowing the struggles and dangers they face and that they did not have enough food. Martin believes there must be a reason God has kept him alive. If God protects and favors the lowly and the oppressed, then his purpose should be to serve the vulnerable and oppressed. Although conflicted, he found that his faith offered some agency through prayer and sense of purpose (**Box 2**).

More research is needed about the role of religion/spiritualty in traumatized children and adolescents. However, depending on their beliefs, youth who have experienced trauma may benefit from adding a spiritual dimension to their recovery. A brief assessment of the impact of trauma on spirituality and vice versa can be helpful.[45] Possible questions include: Are you affiliated with a religious or spiritual community? Are religion and/or spirituality important in your family?

1. Do you see yourself as a religious or spiritual person? If so, in what way?
2. Has the (traumatic) event affected your religious activity or your faith? If so, in what ways?
3. Has your religion or spirituality been involved in the way you have coped with this (traumatic) event? If so, in what way?

Providers interested in assessing these issues with youth more systematically can use a brief measure of multiple domains of R/S that was created by the National Institutes of Health to identify those domains of religiousness/spirituality that are most likely to impact health.[50] Clinicians can explore how youth do or do not consider their religious beliefs in decision-making and behaviors, or for coping with trauma.[44,46] Although developed primarily for adults, this measure has been used in research with adolescents.[51,52] For younger children, themes about relationship to God, or that reflect whether they see themselves as "bad" or "good" can emerge in drawings and play, can indicate cognitive themes that perpetuate distress and can be a focus of

---

Box 2
Example: Martin

The example of Martin (Box 2) illustrates the ambivalent and complex relationship with faith that can exist for a youth who has experienced trauma. Some youth may feel abandoned by God. Schaefer and colleagues[46] highlight the importance of examining cognitions related to religious coping by asking questions about how faith, spirituality, or religiosity help when youth are distressed rather than assessing general religiosity (ie, are you religious?). They found that only positive religious coping was associated with adaptive outcomes. They suggest bolstering protective factors, including religious coping if important (ie, family support, positive thinking, gratitude, and positive religious coping skills) among youth exposed to childhood physical and sexual victimization and other traumatic experiences. Another study, Cotton[42] examined spirituality in youth as measured by religious well-being ("I believe that God loves/cares about me") and existential well-being ("Life doesn't have much meaning"). Religiosity was assessed with questions about youth's belief in God/higher power and importance of religion. Youth with higher levels of spiritual well-being, especially existential well-being, had fewer depressive symptoms and fewer risk-taking behaviors. In contrast, individuals who experience spiritual struggle may experience persistent posttraumatic stress symptoms. Spiritual themes may serve as a positive cognitive coping mechanism for many trauma victims and may have relevance for cognitive therapy for PTSD.[44]

CBT and/or play therapy. Religiosity can influence traumatic stress symptoms through cognitions about divine punishment, guilt, and shame.[43,49]

Forgiveness

Forgiveness is often associated with R/S. Most religions advocate for some form of forgiveness as an essential tenet of their faith. Nevertheless, what Forgiveness constitutes and under what circumstances it is indicated are diverse and dependent on the faith tradition and culture. Although an in-depth understanding of forgiveness in world religions is beyond our scope, clinicians will find it valuable to have a basic understanding of some commonalities and differences in this important concept. In Islam, for instance, "in contrast to the unconditional and absolute concept of Forgiveness in other traditions, such as Christianity, Islam does not expect a person to forgive before justice, or punitive measures are made possible or implemented. However, both the Qur'an and Hadith encourage believers to forgive because it reflects a higher virtue."[53] Buddhism views forgiveness as a means to dispel negative thoughts and emotions. "Forgiveness frees the offended from harboring thoughts of anger, ill will, and malice. It frees the offender from harboring thoughts of resentment and retaliation and enables reflection on the self and the wrong committed, followed by regret and a determination for change to occur. The result for both is self-purification and reconciliation."[54] In the Hindu tradition, "Forgiveness is thus a central tenet of Hindu spirituality; it has been defined as mental strength in the face of offenses; it implies lack of emotional upset or impassivity and tolerance under difficult circumstances. Lack of Forgiveness, negative feelings, and unresolved anger can be expected to spill over into future births, as, through Karma (law of cause and effect) individuals face consequences of their actions in subsequent reincarnations."[55] In Christianity, the New Testament in the gospel of Matthew 18:21-22 provides, what is for many the epitome of the Christian view of Forgiveness: "Then Peter came and said to him, 'Lord, if another member of the church sins against me, how often I should forgive them? As many as seven times?' Jesus said to him, 'Not seven times, but I tell you, seventy times seven.'"[56] Christianity, in general, views Forgiveness as an act and attitude given unconditionally.

FORGIVENESS IN A CLINICAL SETTING

We will define forgiveness as a volitional and intentional "process (or the result of a process) that involves a change in emotion and attitude regarding an offender."[57] The process of forgiveness includes addressing the strong emotional aspects that the injury brought about to the patient. Some of these emotions include shame, guilt, a sense of unfairness and injustice, anger, and the urge for retribution. Forgiveness focuses on the internal process of the victim or injured person and should not be confused with reconciliation, settlement, or compromise (**Fig. 1**). Forgiveness does not require and differs from reconciliation or justification of the offender. When appropriate, civil or criminal justice endeavors can be pursued. The goal of forgiveness is "to help people overcome resentment, bitterness, and even hatred toward people who have treated them unfairly and at times cruelly. Therefore, condoning, excusing, tolerating, commuting punishment, reconciliation, or forgetting, are not a necessary component of Forgiveness."[58]

A meta-analysis published by Baskin and Enright,[59] analyzed 9 studies (n = 330) that compared forgiveness intervention (specifically, process-based intervention) versus control groups in adolescents and transitional-aged adults. They found that process-based forgiveness intervention resulted in significant emotional health

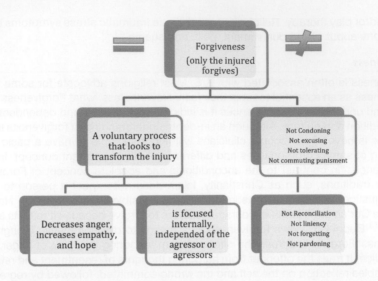

Fig. 1. Forgiveness: what is and what is not and desired results from the process.

benefits, including increased self-esteem, decreased anger, increased empathy and hope, and an improved attitude toward parents.[59]

What is and what is not forgiveness (**Fig. 1**).

International Studies on Forgiveness Interventions

A study done in South Korea examined 24 female adolescents from a middle school and 24 female adolescents in a correctional facility who were identified as "aggressive victims." Aggressive victims were defined as "adolescents who act aggressively toward others and who are victims of others' aggression."[60] The study compared the outcomes of interventions using Enright's Forgiveness Process Model to a Skill-streaming Program and a no-treatment group. They found that those participating in the forgiveness program presented significant decreases in anger, hostile attribution, aggression, delinquency, and increased empathy and overall grades compared with the no-treatment group.[60] In India, a study with 124 university students at Karnatak University in Darwha, Toussaint, and colleagues conducted a manualized REACH Forgiveness psychoeducational program. Participants included 55 men and 69 women, with the religious affiliations distribution of 89% Hindu, 15% Muslim, 5.4% Christian, and 1.08% Jain.[61] Inclusion criteria for the study included having experienced "a hurtful experience that was still bothering them, creating anger, resentment, bitterness, hate, feelings of wanting to hurt the person back, anxiety, hostility." Additionally, the participants were willing to consider Forgiveness and discuss the painful experience in a group setting to be able to participate. This study found improvements, compared to controls, in relationship quality, empathy, and negative mood across 1-, 3-, 6-, and 12-month follow-up assessments."[61]

Bullying and Forgiveness

Research on forgiveness provides supporting evidence on the benefits to mental health on children and adolescents victims of bullying, abuse, and trauma. Quintana-Orts and Rey[62] assessed whether Forgiveness had any moderating effects on traditional and cyberbullying in a group of 1044 early adolescents (females = 527,

Table 2	
General structures of Enright's and Worthington's forgiveness model	
Forgiveness Process Model **Enright**	**REACH** **Worthington**
Uncovering phase	Recall the hurt
Decision phase	Empathize with the one who committed the hurt
Work phase	Offer the Altruistic gift of forgiveness
Deepening or outcome phase	Make a Commitment to forgive;
	Hold on to forgiveness

mean age = 13.09 years; SD = 0.77). They found that adolescents who reported higher levels of forgiveness also reported significantly higher levels of life satisfaction and lower suicide risk, compared with those who reported lower levels of forgiveness.[62]

Therapeutic Models

We will briefly present 2 therapeutic approaches to forgiveness (Table 2), primarily studied in adults, by Enright[58] and Worthington.[63–65] There are some differences between the approaches and some similarities. Both approaches emphasize the need to recognize the hurt and suffering and the right to feel anger and/or a sense of injustice. The table below shows that both approaches start with this acknowledgment (uncovering phase/recall the hurt). Both stress to recognize the injustice, the feelings of anger, shame, and desire for retribution, and how these emotions continue to affect their sense of well-being. Not all forgiveness therapy needs to end in forgiveness but the process can be therapeutic (**Table 2**).

Enright and Worthington approach to forgiveness in clinical settings.

SUMMARY

R/S are a vital part of the daily lives of a significant portion of individuals and families we serve. For many, R/S shapes their moral values, belief systems, family, and community traditions and provides a sense of meaning and belonging. Exploring how patients' belief system and emotional connection affects their lives can provide an invaluable tool to understand and promote healthy changes in their lives. Research on the clinical aspects of R/S is growing exponentially, not only for understanding but also for providing appropriate clinical intervention. R/S can be a source of strength, support, and resilience; however, it can be an important factor in causing shame, trauma, and a sense of loss and despair. With the present influx of immigrants worldwide, R/S is an essential aspect of millions of people's lives, making it relevant the need to talk, learn, research, and know how to provide evidenced-based and ethically sound interventions.

CLINICAL TAKEAWAYS

- An assessment of religiosity and spirituality can be helpful and informative in the clinical setting. Religion/spirituality is an important component of cultural identity and is passed down across generations. However, the specifics of religion/spirituality are unique to each family and cannot be assumoked to be the same as others from their culture.

- Moral foundation theory can be useful for clinicians in mediating conflict between parents and children/adolescents about behaviors and values by understanding the emphasis each place on individualizing versus binding foundations.

- Immigrants and minoritized youth can be caught between their religious and spiritual beliefs and those of their parents or faith community, with serious psychiatric consequences.

- Religion and spirituality can help cope with and find meaning after traumatic events.

- Forgiveness is valued in many faith traditions. Therefore, interventions that help individuals who have been wronged to process the feelings of hurt, shame, and wish for retribution can be helpful, even if complete forgiveness is not achieved.

DISCLOSURE

Authors have no disclosure.

REFERENCES

1. Smith C. Religion: what it is, how it works, and why it matters. Princeton, NJ: Princeton University Press; 2017.
2. Dell ML, Sheppard J. Religion and spirituality in child and adolescent cultural psychiatry. In: Parekh R, Al-Mateen CS, Lisotto MJ, et al, editors. Cultural psychiatry with children, adolescents, and families. American Psychiatric Association Publishing; 2021. p. 129–49. https://doi.org/10.1176/appi.books.9781615373710.
3. Velasco JM. Religion (fenomelogia y ciencias de las religiones). In: Tamayo JJ, editor. Nuevo Diccionario de Teologia. Madrid, España: Editorial Trotta, S.A.; 2005. p. 777–89.
4. Quintero N. Espiritualidad salud y bienestar: su importancia en la calidad de vida. In: Rivera Miranda LMY, Rodriguez Gomez JR, editors. Investigaciones eclesiales. San Juan, Puerto Rico: Publicaciones Puertorriqueñas; 2005. p. 1–23.
5. Floristan C. Espiritualidad. In: Tamayo JJ, editor. Nuevo Diccionario de Teologia. Madrid, España: Editorial Trotta, S.A.; 2005. p. 312–20.
6. Agnostics AA. Available at: http://www.aaagnostics.org/agnostic12steps.html. Accessed January 12, 2022.
7. Walsh F. Religion and spirituality: a family systems perspective in clinical practice. In: Walsh F, editor. Spiritual resources in family therapy. New York: The Guilford Press; 2009. p. 3–30.
8. Bengtson VL, Putney NM, Harris S. Families and faith: how religion is passed down across generations. Oxford University Press; 2013. https://doi.org/10.1093/acprof:oso/9780199948659.001.0001.
9. Lartey EY. In Living color: an intercultural approach to pastoral care and counseling. 2nd edition. Jessica Kingsley Publishers; 2003. p. P. 34.
10. Bretherton I. The origins of attachment theory: John Bowlby and Mary Ainsworth. Dev Psychol 1992;28(5):759–75.
11. Granqvist P. Attachment in religion and spirituality: a wider view. New York: The Guilford Press; 2020.
12. Granqvist P. Attachment, culture, and gene-culture co-evolution: expanding the evolutionary toolbox of attachment theory. Attach Hum Dev 2021;23(1):90–113.
13. Cherniak AD, Mikulincer M, Shaver PR, et al. Attachment theory and religion. Curr Opin Psychol 2021;40:126–30.
14. Abu-Raiya H, Exline JJ, Pargament KI, Agbaria Q. Prevalence, predictors, and implications of religious/spiritual struggles among muslims. J Sci Study Relig

2015;54(4):631–48. Available at: https://staff.najah.edu/media/published_research/2017/11/10/JSSR_2016_RS_STRUGGLES_MUSLIMS.pdf. Accessed February 9, 2019.

15. Abu-Raiya H, Pargament KI, Krause N. Religion as problem, religion as solution: religious buffers of the links between religious/spiritual struggles and well-being/mental health. Qual Life Res 2016;25(5):1265–74.

16. Zarzycka B. Parental attachment styles and religious and spiritual struggle: a mediating effect of god image 2018;40(5):575–93. https://doi.org/10.1177/0192513X18813186.

17. Vozzola EC. Moral Development : Theory and Applications. New York: Routledge; 2014. Available at: https://www.ncbi.nlm.nih.gov/nlmcatalog/101652751.

18. Graham J, Haidt J, Koleva S, et al. Moral foundations theory: the pragmatic validity of moral pluralism. In: Advances in experimental social psychology, 47. Academic Press Inc.; 2013. p. 55–130. https://doi.org/10.1016/B978-0-12-407236-7.00002-4.

19. Graham J, Haidt J, Koleva S, et al. Moral foundations theory. In: Advances in experimental social psychology, 47. Academic Press; 2013. p. 55–130. https://doi.org/10.1016/B978-0-12-407236-7.00002-4.

20. Graham J, Nosek BA, Haidt J, et al. Mapping the moral domain. J Pers Soc Psychol 2011;101(2):366–85.

21. de Waal FBM. The antiquity of empathy. Science (New York, NY) 2012;336(6083):874–6.

22. de Waal FBM. How animals do business. Philosophical Trans R Soc B: Biol Sci 2021;376(1819). https://doi.org/10.1098/rstb.2019.0663.

23. de Waal F, Sherblom SA. Bottom-up morality: the basis of human morality in our primate nature. J Moral Educ 2018;47(2):248–58.

24. Simpson A. Moral foundations theory. In: Zeigler-Hill v, Shackelford TK, editors. Encyclopedia of personality and individual differences. Springer International Publishing; 2017. p. 1–11. https://doi.org/10.1007/978-3-319-28099-8_1253-1.

25. Liuzza MT, Olofsson JK, Cancino-Montecinos S, et al. Body odor disgust sensitivity predicts moral harshness toward moral violations of purity. Front Psychol 2019;10(MAR):458.

26. Del Giudice M. The Evolutionary Context of Personality Development. In: McAdams D, Shiner RL, Tackett JL, editors. Handbook of Personality Development. New York: Guiford Press; 2019. p. 20–39.

27. del Giudice M. Evolutionary Psychopathology: A Unified Approach. Oxford: Oxford University Press; 2018. https://doi.org/10.1093/med-psych/9780190246846.001.0001.

28. Shariff AF, Tracy JL. What are emotion expressions for? Curr Dir Psychol Sci 2011;20(6):395–9.

29. Monroe AE, Plant EA. The dark side of morality: prioritizing sanctity over care motivates denial of mind and prejudice toward sexual outgroups. J Exp Psychol Gen 2018;148(2):342–60. https://doi.org/10.1037/xge0000537.supp.

30. Lai HY. Regarding "Family acceptance in adolescence and the health of LGBT young adults. J Child Adolesc Psychiatr Nurs 2011;24(3). https://doi.org/10.1111/j.1744-6171.2011.00297.x.

31. Fortuna LR, Álvarez K, Ramos Ortiz Z, et al. Mental health, migration stressors and suicidal ideation among Latino immigrants in Spain and the United States. Eur Psychiatry 2016;36. https://doi.org/10.1016/j.eurpsy.2016.03.001.

32. Porche Mv, Fortuna LR, Wachholtz A, et al. Distal and proximal religiosity as protective factors for adolescent and emerging adult alcohol use. Religions 2015; 6(2). https://doi.org/10.3390/rel6020365.

33. Ryan C, Huebner D, Diaz RM, et al. Family rejection as a predictor of negative health outcomes in white and latino lesbian, gay, and bisexual young adults. In: Pediatric collections: LGBTQ+: support and care (Part 2: health concerns and disparities). 2021. https://doi.org/10.1542/9781610025409-family.

34. Ryan C, Huebner D, Diaz RM, et al. Family rejection as a predictor of negative health outcomes in white and latino lesbian, gay, and bisexual young adults. Pediatrics 2009;123(1). https://doi.org/10.1542/peds.2007-3524.

35. Ryan C, Russell ST, Huebner D, et al. Family acceptance in adolescence and the health of LGBT young adults. J Child Adolesc Psychiatr Nurs 2010;23(4). https://doi.org/10.1111/j.1744-6171.2010.00246.x.

36. Quinn K, Dickson-Gomez J, Kelly JA. The role of the Black Church in the lives of young Black men who have sex with men. Cult Health Sex 2016;18(5). https://doi.org/10.1080/13691058.2015.1091509.

37. Bryant-Davis T, Ellis MU, Burke-Maynard E, et al. Religiosity, spirituality, and trauma recovery in the lives of children and adolescents. Prof Psychol Res Pr 2012;43(4). https://doi.org/10.1037/a0029282.

38. Wu Q, Ge T, Emond A, et al. Acculturation, resilience, and the mental health of migrant youth: a cross-country comparative study. Public Health 2018;162. https://doi.org/10.1016/j.puhe.2018.05.006.

39. Dale S, Daniel JH. Spirituality/religion as a healing pathway for survivors of sexual violence. In: Surviving sexual violence: a guide to recovery and empowerment. 2011.

40. Ryan C, Perelman L, Arcarons A. Role of families in promoting risk and well-being for LGBT (Lesbian,Gay, Bisexual, and Transgender) youth. 10th Congress of the European Federation of Sexology Sexology Past, Present and Future: Celebrating a Century of the Multidisciplinary Science of Sex, EFS 2010 Porto Portugal. 2010;19. Available at: https://www.sciencedirect.com/journal/sexologies/vol/19/suppl/S1.

41. Gibbs JJ, Goldbach J. Religious conflict, sexual identity, and suicidal behaviors among LGBT young adults. Arch Suicide Res 2015;19(4). https://doi.org/10.1080/13811118.2015.1004476.

42. Cotton S, Larkin E, Hoopes A, et al. The impact of adolescent spirituality on depressive symptoms and health risk behaviors. J Adolesc Health 2005;36(6). https://doi.org/10.1016/j.jadohealth.2004.07.017.

43. Wortmann JH, Park CL, Edmondson D. Trauma and PTSD symptoms: does spiritual struggle mediate the link? Psychol Trauma Theor Res Pract Policy 2011;3(4). https://doi.org/10.1037/a0021413.

44. Whitmire CH. The role of spirituality in self-care for counselors working with trauma. ProQuest Dissertations and Theses; 2014. https://www.semanticscholar.org/paper/The-role-of-spirituality-in-self-care-for-working-Whitmire/87945247c850dc8885b2af6d873f28f97ac44deb.

45. Lloyd CEM, et al. Contending with Spiritual Reductionism: Demons, Shame, and Dividualizing Experiences Among Evangelical Christians with Mental Distress. Journal of Religion and Health 2021;60(4):2702–27. https://doi.org/10.1007/s10943-021-01268-9.

46. Schaefer LM, Howell KH, Schwartz LE, et al. A concurrent examination of protective factors associated with resilience and posttraumatic growth following

childhood victimization. Child Abuse Negl 2018;85. https://doi.org/10.1016/j.chiabu.2018.08.019.

47. Dew RE, Daniel SS, Goldston DB, et al. Religion, spirituality, and depression in adolescent psychiatric outpatients. J Nerv Ment Dis 2008;196(3). https://doi.org/10.1097/NMD.0b013e3181663002.

48. Zhang H, Hook JN, van Tongeren DR, et al. The role of spiritual fortitude in meaning and mental health symptoms following a natural disaster. Psychol Religion Spirituality 2021. https://doi.org/10.1037/rel0000420.

49. McCormick WH, Carroll TD, Sims BM, et al. Adverse childhood experiences, religious/spiritual struggles, and mental health symptoms: examination of mediation models. Ment Health Religion Cult 2017;20(10). https://doi.org/10.1080/13674676.2018.1440544.

50. Masters KS. Brief multidimensional measure of religiousness/spirituality (BMMRS). In: Encyclopedia of behavioral medicine. 2020. https://doi.org/10.1007/978-3-030-39903-0_1577.

51. Underwood LG. Daily Spiritual Experiences in Multidimensional Measurement of Religiousness/Spirituality for Use in Health Research: A Report of the Fetzer Institute:National Institute on Aging Working Group.; 1999. Kalamazoo, MI

52. Johnstone B, McCormack G, Yoon DP, et al. Convergent/divergent validity of the brief multidimensional measure of religiousness/spirituality: empirical support for emotional connectedness as a "spiritual" construct. J Relig Health 2012;51(2). https://doi.org/10.1007/s10943-011-9538-9.

53.. Abu-Nimer M, Nasser I. Forgiveness in The Arab and Islamic Contexts. Journal of Religious Ethics 2013;41(3):474–94. https://doi.org/10.1111/jore.12025.

54. Bishop DH. Forgiveness in religious thought. Stud Comp Religion 1968;2(1). www.studiesincomparativereligion.com.   [Accessed   18   January   2022]. Accessed.

55. Tripathi A, Mullet E. Conceptualizations of forgiveness and forgivingness among Hindus. Int J Psychol Religion 2010;20(4):255–66. https://doi.org/10.1080/10508619.2010.507694.

56. Metzger B, editor. Holy bible: new revised standard version with apocrypha. Oxford University Press; 1989.

57. Bullock M. Forgiveness–definitions and overview. Forgiveness: a sampling of research results. Published online 2008:4-7.

58. Enright RD, Fitzgibbons RP. Forgiveness therapy: An empirical guide for resolving anger and restoring hope. Washington: American Psychological Association; 2015.

59. Baskin TW, Enright RD. Intervention studies on forgiveness: a meta-analysis. J Couns Dev 2004;82(1):79–90.

60. Park JH, Enright RD, Essex MJ, et al. Forgiveness intervention for female South Korean adolescent aggressive victims. J Appl Dev Psychol 2013;34(6):268–76.

61. Toussaint L, Worthington EL, Cheadle A, et al. Efficacy of the REACH forgiveness intervention in Indian college students. Front Psychol 2020;11:671.

62. Quintana-Orts C, Rey L. Forgiveness, depression, and suicidal behavior in adolescents: gender differences in this relationship. J Genet Psychol 2018;179(2):85–9.

63. Worthington EL, Sandage SJ. Forgiveness and spirituality in psychotherapy: a relational Approach. American Psychological Association; 2016. https://doi.org/10.1037/14712-000.

64. Worthington EL, Lin Y, Ho MY. Adapting an evidence-based intervention to REACH Forgiveness for different religions and spiritualities. Asian J Psychiatry 2012;5(2):183–5.

65. Nation JA, Wertheim EH, Worthington EL. Evaluation of an online self-help version of the REACH forgiveness program: outcomes and predictors of persistence in a community sample. J Clin Psychol 2018;74(6):819–38.

FURTHER READINGS

Dell ML, Sheppard J. Religion and Spirituality in Child and Adolescent Cultural Psychiatry. In: Parekh R, Al-Mateen CS, Lisotto MJ, et al, editors. Cultural Psychiatry With Children, Adolescents, and Families. Washington, D.C: American Psychiatric Association Publishing; 2021. p. 129–49. https://doi.org/10.1176/appi.books.9781615373710.

Koenig HB. Spirituality in Patient Care-Why, How, When, and What. Third Edition. West Conshohocken, PA: Templeton Press; 2013.

Romig CA, Holeman VT, Sauerheber JD. Using Moral Foundations Theory to Enhance Multicultural Competency. Couns Values 2018;63(2):180–93. https://doi.org/10.1002/CVJ.12087.

Neng Lin, W., Enright, R., & Klatt, J. (2011). Forgiveness as character education for children and adolescents. Journal of Moral Education, 40(2), 237–253. https://doi.org/10.1080/03057240.2011.568106

Promoting Resiliency and Eliminating Disparities—Best Practices when Working with Child Welfare Involved Youth of Color

Wynne Morgan, MD[a,*], Kristie V. Schultz, PhD[b],
Afifa Adiba, MD[c,d], W. David Lohr, MD[b]

KEYWORDS

- Child welfare • Racial disparities • Inequity • Foster care

KEY POINTS

- The US child welfare system continues to have racial disproportionality and inequities that present barriers to the best outcomes for children and families of color.
- Racial and ethnic disparities exist at the entry points into child welfare and expand at each subsequent step in the child welfare decision-making process.
- Efforts to guide best practices must consider the causative factors of disparities, which include implicit biases in caregivers and workers, systemic factors associated with poverty, and structural racism.
- Special populations, such as lesbian, gay, bisexual, transgender, queer or questioning, intersex, asexual or ally+ youth, unaccompanied children, and those in the juvenile justice system will face additional disparities in achieving optimal outcomes.

INTRODUCTION

The child welfare system in the United States is designed to ensure the safety, permanency, and well-being of the children and families it serves. Yet, the US Child Welfare System has a long history of disproportionality among children and families of color that impact outcome disparities across multiple domains, and the experiences of racial and ethnic minorities interfacing with this system of care are diverse. For the

[a] Division of Child & Adolescent Psychiatry, Department of Psychiatry, UMass Chan Medical School, 55 Lake Avenue North, Worcester MA 01655, USA; [b] Department of Pediatrics, University of Louisville School of Medicine, 200 East Chestnut Street, Louisville, KY 40202, USA; [c] Adolescent Mood Disorder Unit, Sheppard Pratt Health System, Towson, MD, USA; [d] Yale Child Study Center, Yale School of Medicine, New Haven, CT, USA
* Corresponding Author
E-mail address: Wynne.morgan@umassmemorial.org

Child Adolesc Psychiatric Clin N Am 31 (2022) 631–648
https://doi.org/10.1016/j.chc.2022.06.011
1056-4993/22/© 2022 Elsevier Inc. All rights reserved.

child psychiatrist working with these families, it is key to understand how minority populations may be impacted differently by child welfare involvement and how to advocate effectively to ensure appropriate care.

In the United States, it is not uncommon for children and families to interact with the child welfare system. In the fiscal year 2019, there were 4.4 million referrals to child protective services (CPS) involving the alleged maltreatment of 7.9 million children. Of these referrals, 2.4 million required CPS response and investigation, impacting 3.5 million children.[1] At any given moment there is just under half a million youth in state custody or foster care. The most common reason for youth to come into the foster care system is neglect followed by physical abuse, sexual abuse, and abandonment. The average age of youth in foster care is about 7 years and children spend on average 16 months in care. Youth generally have multiple placements during their time in the child welfare system. The most common out-of-home placement for youth in foster care is with a nonrelative at 46% of youth nationally, followed by kinship placement at 32%. About 10% of youth are in a congregate care placement. Trends do show increased placements with kin and decreased placements in group homes and institutions over the past decade.[2] The most common reason for exiting the child welfare system is reunification with a parent or primary caretaker, but data has shown an increased rate of adoption and guardianship as outcomes for permanency. Annually, about 26% of youth are adopted out of foster care. Despite efforts for permanency, just under 10% of youth age out of foster care annually. Most states offer support called extended foster care up until age 21 but the quality of services offered by states varies. Even with these supports, youth aging out of care face multiple challenges transitioning to adulthood and independence, and most youth will return to their family of origin in some capacity.[3]

Racial disproportionality within the child welfare system has been an identified concern for some time. The term disproportionality is used to describe the overrepresentation and under-representation of a racial or ethnic group compared with the total population while disparities are unequal outcomes between ethnic and racial groups. Black and American Indian (AI)/Native Alaskan are two groups that are overrepresented in the child welfare system. Black children make up 14% of the child population nationally and 23% of the foster care population. AI/Native Alaskans make up 1% of the child population but 2% of the foster care population.[4] The disproportionality in racial and ethnic groups varies by geographic location. Data from the National Council of Family Court Judges identify the overrepresentation of black youth in the child welfare system in 46 out of 50 states with disproportionality ratios ranging from 1.1 to 3.5.[5] Asian/Pacific Islander and Latinx children are often not highlighted in the disproportionality data when in fact these two groups have their own important experiences that need a closer look. Latinx children are less likely to encounter the child welfare system and are underrepresented in national data, but there are disparities within this population, including overrepresentation in some parts of the country and under-representation in other parts.[6] Asian/Pacific Islanders are often under-represented as well in child welfare data but this group represents 20 or more ethnic groups with individual histories, values, traditions, and languages, indicating a need to assess subgroups to understand the impact of the child welfare system on Asian/Pacific Islanders.[7]

IMPACT OF LEGISLATION AND POLICY ON RACIAL INEQUITIES IN CHILD WELFARE

The disproportionality and disparities in child welfare are perpetuated in part by structural racism that developed out of historical and cultural factors, allowing these inequities to grow. To better understand the drivers that have contributed to these injustices, it is important to look back at the federal and state laws, programs, and policies that helped to shape our child welfare system in the United States and may have contributed to the current racial divides.

The Jim Crow laws that enforced a separate but equal society greatly impacted the care of orphaned Black children who were not permitted to be cared for by white-only institutions. This created a dual-track system of care for close to 100 years that unfairly benefited white children who were orphaned. The Jim Crow laws also penetrated the early child welfare policies and created a system of inequity that greatly discriminated against Black families. Early child welfare legislation, such as the Social Security Act of 1935, created programs that provided aid to families who were in "suitable homes," often excluding Black families from these aid programs. A more formalized federal child welfare system developed with the Child Abuse Prevention Treatment Act of 1974, which created a funding source for child welfare services but also created practices that were fraught with avenues for biases and discrimination leading to disparities in outcomes of maltreatment reporting. Rates of all youth coming into the child welfare system continued to rise into the mid-1980s that were driven also in part by economic instability, the War on Drugs, and high rates of female incarcerations, all of which disproportionately impacted Black families.[8] The Adoption and Safe Families Act (ASFA) of 1997 sought to establish permeance for children in foster care by requiring states to proceed with the termination of parental rights (TPR) when youth have been in care for 15 months. This disproportionately impacted children of color and families with diverse ethnic backgrounds because families often did not have access to the services they needed to help with reunification. The ASFA ignored the unique needs of children of color and has been criticized for fueling racial disproportionality, especially for Black children.[4]

The Multi-Ethnic Placement Act (MEPA) enacted in 1994 (Public Law 103–382) sought to address the disparities related to adoption rates between white and minority children by prohibiting states from delaying or denying adoption and foster care placements based on race or ethnicity. MEPA also required states to recruit prospective adoptive and foster care families from different racial and ethnic backgrounds to reflect the diversity of children needing placement. Assessments of the impact of MEPA note an increase in the number of white and Hispanic adoptions but for Black youth, the only permanency increase seen was exiting foster care to guardianship.[9]

The historical experiences of AI and Native Alaskan children and families with the federal government and the US child welfare system are troubling and important for providers working with these families to acknowledge. Tribal communities were subject to an Indian Boarding School policy for over 100 years that removed thousands of children from their families, impacting multiple generations, and decimating their cultures, which finally ended in the 1960s.[10] The Congress passed the Indian Child Welfare Act (ICWA) in 1978 in response to the disproportionate rates that AI and Native Alaskan children were being removed and placed into foster care. The investigation that prompted this legislation highlighted the devastating impact the removal of children from homes has had on the Indian tribes and their culture. Upward of 35% of all AI children were in out-of-home placements at the time. The ICWA outlines that all states must provide "active efforts" to prevent the break-up of families to address the shockingly high rates of out-of-home placements. This "active effort" clause is still key as rates of AI and Native Alaskan removal remain disproportionate.[11]

Family First Prevention Services Act of 2018 offers the promise of increasing family unity by allowing for redirection of federal funds to pay for services that can keep children from being placed into foster care, but requirements for the Western-style evidence studies may overlook traditional Native AI programs. Native Americans have noted they were not involved in the development of guidelines and note it is difficult to meet costly standards developed by non-Native American infrastructure. So far, one program "Family Spirit" has been rated as promising, but many other programs may not be accepted by the Clearing House. Guidelines on cultural adaptations are needed to approve prevention programs targeting Native Americans.[12]

Historical policies have also impacted child welfare involvement for minority groups that are under-represented, as seen in Asian American/Pacific Islander populations. The Chinese Exclusion Act of 1882, which limited the immigration of Chinese persons, was not fully overturned until the Civil Rights Movement in 1965. Our country also has a challenging history of forcibly removing men, women, and children of Japanese descent from their communities and placing them in internment camps during World War II. Racist governmental policies have in part made it challenging for Asian minority subgroups to trust and accept government service and likely factor into the disproportionality seen in national child welfare data, among other factors.[7]

Recent discriminatory policies by the federal government still impact our most vulnerable families, as seen in the Trump-era policies that targeted the Latinx communities. In 2018, the Trump administration's "zero tolerance" policy at the border led to the creation of the family separation policy, where children were forcibly removed from their adult caregivers at the US border. This caused significant trauma and harm to those families directly impacted, but also caused distrust within the Latinx communities of government services, likely further contributing to the disproportionalities seen in Latinx child welfare data as being an under-represented population along with perpetuating racism against the Latinx communities.[13]

FACTORS THAT CONTRIBUTE TO DISPARITIES IN CHILD WELFARE DECISION-MAKING

Child welfare systems have procedures and policies they follow to meet their mission of protecting children and families. These procedures lead to successive steps in how a child and family engage these systems. Providers and stakeholders may recognize and report child abuse or unhealthy neglectful environments. These reports are triaged and screened to determine the imminence of risk and danger to a child. If a report is accepted, then case workers engage in a period of investigation and monitoring. If sufficient risk is present, then a child may be removed and placed in a safe living situation. This can include other family members, fictive kin, or directly into foster homes, and is called out-of-home care (OOHC). Next, there may be a phase of case planning where parents may work on a case plan detailing needed steps for reunification. There are guidelines for how long this period lasts, and courts are often involved in evaluating ongoing parental capacity for safe parenting. A decision ultimately is made to reunify the child with the family or seek permanency in the form of adoption or independent living for older youth. It is all too common for many children to wait years for adoption and so some children transition out of the child welfare system as they turn 18, a term referred to as "aging out."

Each of these steps moving through the child welfare system requires evaluation of the individual family and child to decide the permanency goal. When working with child welfare-involved youth and families, providers should understand where disparities enter the child welfare decision-making process. Evidence suggests bias exists at each stage of child welfare decision-making[14] and increasing disparity along racial lines occurs at each successive decision point whether reporting for abuse/neglect, referral for investigation, reunification services, out-of-home placement, and TPR or transitions out of the child welfare system. At each decision point, race is a significant factor.[15]

Although racial/ethnic disproportionality has been seen at the front end of child welfare by evidence of altered rates of referral and investigation/substantiation/placement into care, it is also seen that children of color have long OOHC time, receive fewer services, and are less likely to reunify than white children.[16]

Theories have been developed to explain these disparities and to guide interventions to reach equity. There may be implicit biases in providers and personnel that influence decisions to report suspected abuse, accept cases for investigation, and determine risks for safety. Systemic factors and racism built into the infrastructure of child welfare systems may limit the availability of prevention or reunification services. Around it all, multiple children and family risk factors are present that affect race disproportionately, such as poverty and access to care.[16] For example, child maltreatment and removals are highly correlated with poverty, which is disproportionately represented among Black and Native American children.[17]

Substance use problems, including the opioid epidemic, have ravaged many states, leading to overdoses and deaths, and it is a driving force in many children under the age of 5 entering foster care. The national prevalence of parental substance use disorders (SUD) in the child welfare system has been estimated to be as high as 26% and regional/state estimates may be higher.[18] The SUD epidemic interacts with social vulnerabilities, including adverse childhood experiences (ACEs) and racism, such that those with more risk factors are more at risk.[19] SUD is considered a brain disease that can respond to medical and psychosocial treatment.[20] But like most health conditions, racial and socioeconomic disparities act to mediate and amplify risk factors at each stage of involvement. Since the 1980s and the War on Drugs, the criminalization of SUD has led to unequal application of justice along racial and ethnic lines.[21] The numbers and proportion of children entering the foster care system have increased dramatically from 14.5% in 2000 to 36.3% in 2017 and with regional variations.[22] Currently, states having criminally focused SUD policies have more disparate outcomes in referrals, removals, and lack of reunifications.[23]

PROTECTIVE CONCERNS: ABUSE REPORTING OR "FILING"

There are disparities in the demographics of victimization. For Federal Fiscal Year (FFY) 2020, the overall victim rate was 8.4 victims per 1000 children, with children younger than 1-year-old having the highest rates of victimization. AI or Alaska Native (AN) children have the highest rate of victimization at 15.5 per 1000 children of the same race or ethnicity, and Black children have the second highest rate at 13.2 per 1000 children of the same race or ethnicity. For nearly all race categories there was a decrease of victims in the last 6 months of FFY 2020 except victims of AI/AN descent had an increase of 1.4% for FFY 2020.[24] Disparities are also reported for Asian and Pacific Islander children, but rates vary by country of maternal origin, indicating the need to look closer at subgroups within this category of racial identification.[25]

Minority children and Black children have higher rates of reporting and substantiation of abuse. Minority children at least 12 months old with accidental injuries were three times more likely than their white counterparts to be reported for suspected abuse.[26] Also, cases of abuse and neglect for Black children are reported and substantiated at about twice the rate for white children.[27]

There may be bias in how providers respond to allegations or concerns of abuse. Medical providers are more likely to test peripartum urine drug screen for Black, Indigenous, and People of Color patients than for white patients. It has been proposed that there exists an implicit bias in reporting among medical providers and workers within child-serving systems.[28] However, Drake has proposed racial bias in reporting is not a large factor to explain the disparate demographics in reporting, and substantiation is due to underlying risk factors that are much more common and disproportionate in Black families and those of color. For example, evidence for racial disproportionality in reporting was seen after controlling for poverty.[27,29] Reducing disproportionality in underlying risk factors affecting Black families is a needed public health approach.

Latinx children and families are less likely to encounter the US child welfare system despite significant socioeconomic risk and slightly higher rates of child maltreatment compared to whites. The reason for this paradox is complex but one key factor is linked to disparities in maltreatment reporting. Latinx children experience pervasive disparities in accessing health care across the continuum of health care services from having access to health insurance to completing subspecialty appointments.[30,31] These challenges in accessing health care likely contribute to the differences in identification and subsequent reporting of maltreatment to CPS. Research also shows that Latinx children are more likely to be reported by the educational system but less likely to be reported by social services workers, parents, friends, or neighbors.[32]

OPEN CASES/REFERRALS FOR INVESTIGATIONS

Reported cases may be investigated and substantiated for concerns of risk to the child. Racial and ethnic disparities are found here as well. Administrative data shows a disproportionate number of referrals accepted for investigation among Black and Native American children.[14] And in Canada, Black children were more likely than white children to be investigated but not more likely to substantiate, transfer to ongoing services, or place out of the home.[33]

It has been shown that AN/AI children in Alaska have higher rates of contact with CPS, higher rates of substantiated maltreatment, higher rates of child removal, and placement into OOHC.[34] This study found CPS contact before age 5 years was higher for AN/AI children compared with non-Native children (40.1% vs 15.8%) and greater CPS contact was seen in each age interval for AN/AI children. Possible explanations for the increased rate include institutional bias, detection bias, poverty, SUD, and intergenerational and collective trauma. For the 20% of AN/AI children that had continuous CPS contact, maternal substance use was the largest individual risk factor.

Latinx children have lower rates of substantiated maltreatment reports by CPS when compared with the national average and similar rates to white children.[32,35]

HOME REMOVALS/YOUTH IN CUSTODY

Race, risk, and income predict decisions to remove children from their biological homes.[36] Not surprisingly, such data has led to concerns of bias among families served by child welfare systems. A focus group study reveals a fear of cultural bias in caseworkers and the court system by respondents.[37] Multiple studies have shown African American children are removed from homes and placed in foster care at 2 to 3 times the rate of white children. Six themes involving poverty, trauma, and other family and child factors were identified by African American parents along with suggestions to improve cultural and trauma-informed competence of the child welfare service functions.[17]

The influence of parental drug use on removals is striking. From 2008 to 2017 the rate of parental drug use increased by 71% in the general population and across all racial/ethnic groups. Opioid overdose deaths have increased by 143% in non-Hispanic whites and Native Americans. Native American children had the highest and fastest growth rate of parental drug use entries into child welfare systems and had the highest disproportionality in foster care entries.[38] In fact, consuming drugs during pregnancy as evidenced by a positive urine drug screen is considered child abuse in at least 19 states in the United States, and women can lose custody of newborns even without confirmation.[39]

REUNIFICATION

Racial and ethnic disparities lead to disproportionate data in reunifications as well. Many reports have documented that Black children and their families are less likely to receive alternative services like in-home services and less likely to reunify with their families.[40] In addition to cumulative ACE exposure, a child's race was significantly associated with a probability of reunification, as nonwhite children were 21% less likely to reunify than white children and race did not predict substantiation but was influenced by caseworker perceived risk.[41] Native American children and families also are less likely to obtain reunification. Data from the 2017 Adoption and Foster Care Analysis and Reporting System (AFCARS) showed Native American children aged 0 to 5 had lower odds of reunification than white children (AOR = 0.87, P < .001), while Hispanic children had higher odds of reunification (AOR = 1.08, P < .001).[42]

Children removed due to SUD are less likely to reunify than older children,[43] and engagement in substance use treatment is less common in Black, Hispanic, and Native American persons.[44] Foster care infants who live in states with criminal justice-related prenatal substance abuse policies have a lower chance of reunification with a parent, specifically non-Hispanic Black children have an OR = 0.87 chance of reunification compared to non-Hispanic white children in a state without such policies.[23]

OUT-OF-HOME PLACEMENTS AND TERMINATION OF PARENTAL RIGHTS

Close to one-third of all children in the foster care system are waiting on adoption as a permanency goal.[24] These children are in OOHC and reside in foster homes, residential treatment facilities (congregate care), hospitals, and so forth. It has been shown that Black children are more likely to disrupt foster home placements and enter group homes.[45] Also, Black children historically are less likely to be adopted than white children meaning longer time in the child welfare system.[46]

Sattler and Font demonstrated that over 2% of adoptive placements and 7% of guardianship placements were dissolved. Compared with white and Hispanic children, Black children had a higher risk of guardianship, but not adoption, or dissolution.[47] AFCARS evaluates the prevalence of TPR and finds that nearly 3.0% of AI/NA and 1.5% of AA children will experience TPR, nationally about 1% of children in the United States will have TPR. There are large variations between states and racial/ethnic variables are important.[48] Parental incarceration may represent a tipping point for TPR as parental incarceration has similar breakdowns by racial risk. Once an investigation has begun AI/NA children are more likely to have TPR than white or Black children.[48]

Tribal child welfare agency leaders feel foster care programs should be managed by the tribes to keep children in their families and/or communities and maintain connections to tribal culture. Such inputs could lead to longer reunification time frames before TPR.[49] In two states, Kentucky and Arizona, parental rights may be terminated by exposure of infants to opioids at the time of birth unless the birth mother is involved in a substance abuse treatment program.[50]

ADOPTION FROM THE CHILD WELFARE SYSTEM

When children in foster care are legally adopted, parental rights have first been terminated, and custody is transferred from the state to the adoptive parents, creating a
permanent home in which to facilitate a sense of security and stability.[51,52] Of the children exiting foster care in the United States in 2020, 25% were adopted. The average
age of children adopted was 6.5 years, while the average age of children waiting for
adoption was 7.9 years. The majority (54%) of children were adopted by a foster
parent, while 35% were adopted by a relative.[24] Most of the children who are adopted
remain with their adoptive families,[51] but some children may have more difficulty with
adjusting to their new environments, such as older children or children with previous
exposure to trauma or current externalizing behavioral difficulties.[52] Thus, adoptive
families may need additional support to provide for their adopted children, both at
the time of adoption and beyond, into adolescent years for example.[51,53]

TRANSRACIAL ADOPTION

Transracial adoption remains a controversial topic in adoption care. The primary
concern about transracial adoption is whether the adopted parents can help the children to build their racial identity. It is not uncommon to see in transracial adoption that
adopted parents often struggle with teaching their children about the birth culture,
tradition, and history and creating the necessary skills children require to survive in
this racially unequal world.

Recommendation for transracial adoption:
1. Encouraging families to have a conversation about race with the children at an
   earlier age. The conversation should be developmentally appropriate.
2. Adoptive parents need to acknowledge that the cultural identity and racial identity might differ in transracial adoptees.
3. Adoptive parents need to develop cultural competency. According to Vonk, parents need to understand three aspects of cultural competency: racial awareness,
   survival skills, and multicultural family planning (**Box 1**).[54]

TRANSITIONS TO PERMANENCY

Legal permanency is defined through family reunification, adoption, guardianship, or
other planned permanent living arrangement. In 2018, about 7.5% of youth "aged
out" without permanency and this group features more Black and Hispanic individuals.
These youth are at higher risk for homelessness, have poor health care access, lack of
education, early pregnancy, physical and mental health issues, low employment, and
criminal justice involvement.[56,57] Machine learning methods were used to identify
youth at higher risk of not exiting to permanency by age 18. Black youth and those
with missing race information had the highest rate of exiting without permanency.
Youth at risk of exiting without permanency had patterns associated with poorer outcomes. These findings may allow proactive interventions to augment support specific
to the youth's cultural background.[57] Garcia and colleagues studied how well child-
serving systems of care prepare racially diverse youth in foster care to do well in adulthood. These results can guide efforts to improve functioning in these youth as they
leave the foster care system. Placement stability, having youth live with a family at
the time of exit, having access to mental health services, preparation to leave care,
and satisfaction with a foster family was among the factors predicting better
outcomes.[58]

Box 1		
In transracial adoption, parents should be encouraged to learn self-awareness[55]		
Self-Awareness	**Survival Skills**	**Multiracial Family Planning**
• Understanding the impact of race, ethnicity, and culture in people beliefs and values • Be aware of "our own feelings of cultural superiority" • Acknowledging within the family that racial prejudice, biases, and discrimination do exist and the "white benefits" might not extend to the minority adopted children	• Acknowledge and understand the needs of preparing the children to fight against racism • Encouraged discussion about race and racism within family members • Prepare children with answer for racially insensitive comment and teach them not to tolerate racially biased remarks • Not to ignore or minimize racial difference among child and family	• It is important to understand that if transracial adoptees are only surrounded by the parent's racial group, they find it hard to identify or develop pride in their own race or culture of birth. • Making opportunities to learn about their birth culture • Encouraging to learn about other cultures and tradition along with their own racial culture • For a religious family, parents should have open communication and conversation about religion in the family. • Taking the children to a place of worship where they might find people from their ethnicity which will give them the opportunity to know the people from their culture, find a mentor.

SPECIAL POPULATIONS
LGBTQ + Youth

Lesbian, gay, bisexual, transgender, queer or questioning (LGBTQ) youth are overrepresented in the foster care system.[59] Their overall reason for presenting to foster care may not differ much from those in the general, but familial rejection due to the child's identity or expression of identity may further lead the child to enter foster care or placements outside of the home.[59,60] Further, the foster care system is not properly equipped to meet all of the needs of LGBTQ youth, thus exposing them to further discrimination in foster care placements.[60] In fact, LGBTQ youth are more likely to experience homelessness, placement in group homes rather than residential homes, and movement to new placements than non-LGBTQ youth.[61,62] As a result of unstable placements, they experience higher emotional distress, poorer school functioning, and more concerns related to substance abuse and mental health.[59,63]

LGBTQ youth would clearly benefit from legislation to protect them from further discrimination when entering the foster care system. In regard to related legislation, however, there are no national laws in effect that dictate what is or is not discrimination for LGBTQ in the foster care system. State legislation varies widely, in that some states have laws in place to protect youth in foster care from discrimination based on sexual orientation and gender identity, other states have laws in place just related to sexual orientation, and the remaining states have no legislation to protect LGBTQ youth in foster care.[60]

UNACCOMPANIED CHILDREN

In the United States, unaccompanied children are often presented from Mexico or Central America, at times fleeing violence or unsafe living environments. Unaccompanied children are often processed by US Customs and Border Protection but then transferred to the Office of Refugee Resettlement in Health and Human Services. Children could be immediately deported, qualify for various forms of relief (such as asylum or visas), or enter into legal proceedings, but without a government-appointed lawyer.[64] Unfortunately, there is no distinction between adults and children in immigration legal proceedings, leaving children to defend their need to remain in the United States.[65]

When children flee their original country, they encounter trauma from separation, the passage to the United States, and potential harms along the way; further, they are at risk for re-traumatization by the government processes that they subsequently encounter. Given the large number of unaccompanied minors presenting to the United States and facing decisions on their future, a human rights crisis has formed.[66] As many as 35% of unaccompanied children are ultimately placed in long-term foster care placements. They face difficulties with acculturation in a new country and coping with the uncertainty of their legal status. Furthermore, they need culturally competent placements, as well as trauma-informed treatment for prior trauma and mental health concerns, both during their placements and beyond.[67]

JUVENILE JUSTICE

Youth in foster care who also are involved in the foster care system are known as crossover youth, creating a phenomenon known as the foster care to prison pipeline.[60,68] Estimates of crossover youth vary by study, but often span estimated ranges, such as from 7% to 24%, indicating a noticeable portion of youth in foster care who go on to become involved with the juvenile justice system.[69] At highest risk of involvement in the juvenile justice system are individuals who have been placed in congregate or groups settings, or had an older age at first involvement with the foster care system; in addition, African American males were at higher risk, noting a complex intersection and overall systemic concern.[69] Crossover youth are more likely to have a history of abuse, encounter problems in educational settings, and have more substance use and mental health concerns.[60] Further, looking beyond youth, adults who are incarcerated are more likely to have been in foster care, signaling this pipeline exists well beyond the end of a foster care placement.[70]

BEST PRACTICE INTERVENTIONS

Efforts to guide best practice interventions, including those listed later, follow factors proposed to explain disparities in outcomes for children and families of color.[16]

Training Regarding Implicit Biases in Child Welfare Personnel

Health care providers and those working with children in the child welfare system need to be vigilant in detecting their own racial biases and seeking training or experiences to address their biases. The ways clinicians and child welfare workers read various clinical and demographic factors, such as racial/ethnic identity, poverty, and addresses are inherently influenced by their own lived experiences, training, and ongoing exposures. Organizations can work to become antiracists by institutional efforts to identify and change racist patterns.[14] These can lead to organized efforts to evaluate and understand experiences of discrimination and racial stressors in those served.

Such practices could include routine, universal, verbal screening for SUD of every pregnant patient, which is an objective approach that minimizes any provider bias as current practices for screening for substance use during pregnancy disproportionately impact women of color and need to be informed by racial equity.[28] Medical providers are encouraged to be thoughtful and consider the social context when reporting and base concerns on evidence only to be internally consistent.[40]

Child- and Family-Level Risk Factors that Affect Race Disproportionately: Poverty

The disproportionate exposure to risk factors, such as poverty faced by Black children, has been felt to explain much of the racially disparate outcomes in child welfare.[27] Efforts to improve these underlying societal factors are important to policymakers charged with improving population health outcomes. Child psychiatrists and child welfare workers must consider how social determinants of health place an inequitable burden on racial and ethnic groups leading to additional adverse exposures in childhood.

Access to substance abuse treatment for all racial/ethnic groups is needed because maternal substance abuse may be the factor with the biggest impact on the trajectory of a child's child welfare involvement.[34] States also need to evaluate punitive prenatal drug abuse policies that define drug use during pregnancy as abuse and their disparate impact on racial/ethnic groups.[38]

System Factors and Structural Racism—Availability of Prevention Services

Child welfare systems have been charged to build an antiracism framework.[71] Child welfare policies and judicial practices need to be examined in light of potential racial bias to identify and eliminate interventions that unfairly penalize children and families of color, especially those involving substance abuse issues.[42] To address these issues the Breakthrough Series Collaborative framework was developed by the Casey Family Programs to reduce disproportionality and disparate outcomes for children and families of color in the child welfare system. It addressed all three theories of cause to create more positive outcomes through the QI process of plan, do, study, and act.[46] One example of this work is the King County Coalition on Racial Disproportionality, which focused on children in care longer than 2 years and developed programs to fight disproportionality and increase awareness within the community. The program collected data on the problem, and targeted strategies for change, including collaborative teams of child welfare workers, and permanence champions. The effort has resulted in legislation requiring statewide analysis of disproportionality and increased local awareness, including more court-appointed special advocates workers of native descent.[72]

In addition, Wisconsin developed the Wisconsin ICWA as a collaborative approach to achieve better outcomes for Indian children in the state. These services address the historical disproportionality of removals of Indian children to placements outside their homes. Joint development of the program occurred with tribal representatives, with ongoing stakeholder education and advocacy. Targeted areas include improved (1) regulations, policies, and practices, (2) better working relationships between tribes and child welfare, (3) improved knowledge and sensitivity of providers and agencies, and (4) improved identification of Indian children.[73]

Advocates have called for child welfare systems to build networks of Black foster parents and those of color to support a child's ability for skill building, role play, and processing of racial disparities and discrimination. In some cases, children in OOHC with congruent ethnicity with the families have improved behavioral outcomes.[74]

DISPARITIES IN PSYCHOTROPIC MEDICATION

Children in foster care have complex mental health needs and so have high rates of mental health diagnoses and service utilization, including the use of psychotropic medications.[75] Rates of psychotropic medications for children in foster care are estimated to be thrice greater than for children in the general population and seems driven by child characteristics rather than mental health need.[76,77] Given the lack of evidence for efficacy and growing concerns for adverse effects it is important to consider racial and ethnic disparities in the use of psychotropic medications for children in foster care.

Studies of psychotropic medication use in children show that African-American children with Medicaid have lower rates of medication use when compared with white children.[78] Similarly, studies looking at children in the public service sector, including those in child welfare, showed less medication use in African-American and Latino children compared with white children,[79] and fewer expenditures on psychotropic medication.[80,81]

Other studies, however, show increased usage. A study of the use of psychotropic medication in children entering foster homes showed African American children were more likely (AOR = 5.4) than Latino children to have prescribed stimulants and atypical antipsychotics (AOR = 5.1).[82] Children who are Black and of other races have also been found to have higher odds of concomitant antipsychotic treatment.[83] These results indicate ethnic children may not receive standard of care treatments for some mental health disorders. Limited evidence is available, so more research is needed.

SUMMARY

As practicing child and adolescent psychiatrists, knowledge about the racial disproportionality and disparities in the child welfare system is important so that the treatment of the children and families served considers the families' identity, values, and culture. Understanding the complexities of the child welfare system process helps the provider to better advocate and inform best practices and decrease unconscious biases that so often perpetuate racism in our society. Psychiatrists can also help to advocate for state and federal legislation that is inclusive of all families from all racial identities and provides avenues for culturally appropriate, trauma-informed mental health services. Racial disparities are still a large challenge for the child welfare system. More research into the disproportionality and subsequent disparities among race and ethnicity in the child welfare system is needed for all cultural minorities, not just Black and AI/Native Alaskan populations. This research should investigate subgroups of the racial and ethnic category as well to help better understand and then subsequently address these disparities. Program development that is culturally and trauma-informed is key to serving this population. These programs need to meet the families where they are and help prevent home removals. Programs that can integrate cultural responsiveness while still addressing the impact of trauma are key for youth and families in child welfare as these two factors are often intertwined. Areas of need include specialized substance use treatment for new mothers with a focus on the infant–mother dyad relationship creating culturally informed family stabilization that understands the values of AI/Native Alaskan peoples and many more. As child psychiatrists, it is imperative to use our voices and expertise to fight against laws and policies that promote racism and discrimination.

CLINICS CARE POINTS

- Racial disproportionality within the child welfare system has been identified as an identified concern. Black and American Indian/Native Alaskan youth are two groups that are overrepresented in the child welfare system, while Asian/Pacific Islander and Latinx youth are underrepresented.

- Significant disparities impact Black and American Indian/Alaska Native youth and families at each step of the child welfare system, including higher rates of abuse reporting, substantiation, and longer lengths of stay in the system when compared with white youth.

- Each cultural and ethnic group has unique experiences with the child welfare system that need further research, particularly Asian/Pacific Islander and Latinx groups.

- Child welfare legislations, policies, and programs should be inclusive of all racial and ethnic groups and work to identify and eliminate interventions that unfairly penalize children and families of color.

- Best practices for addressing and eliminating these disparities include, but are not limited to, requiring implicit bias training for all professionals working with children's welfare involved youth and families; investigating and changing societal factors that perpetuate poverty; and fostering an antiracist culture within child welfare to combat structural racism.

- Programs to support child welfare youth and families need to address both cultural preferences as well as the impact of trauma on child development and caregiver relationships.

- Child welfare involved youth are at risk for inappropriate use of psychotropic medication, and preliminary data suggests disparities in psychotropic use for youth of color in foster care.

DISCLOSURE

Dr W.D. Lohr has received funding from the Kentucky Department of Medicaid through a State-University Partnership award and Norton's Healthcare. He is currently serving as a medical director for the Department for Community Based Services in the Kentucky Cabinet for Health and Family Services.

REFERENCES

1. U.S. Department of Health & Human Services, Administration for Children and Families, Administration on Children, Youth and Families, Children's Bureau. Child Maltreatment 2019: Summary of Key Findings .. In: Numbers and trends. Child Welfare Information Gateway; 2021. Available from. https://www.acf.hhs.gov/cb/research-data-technology/statistics-research/child-maltreatment.
2. U.S. Department of Health and Human Services Administration for Children and Families Administration on Children, Youth and Families Children's Bureau. Foster Care Statistics, Numbers and Trends. March 2021.https://www.childwelfare.gov/pubs/factsheets/foster/
3. Morgan W, Lee T, Van Deusen T. Supporting connections: a focus on the mental health needs and best practices for youth in out-of-home care transitioning to adulthood. In: Chan V, Derenne J, editors. Transition-age youth mental health care: bridging the gap between pediatric and adult psychiatric care. Cham: Springer International Publishing; 2021. p. 439–58.
4. U.S. Department of Health and Human Services. Administration for Children and Families, Children's Bureau. *Child welfare practice to address racial disproportionality and disparity.* Child Welfare Information Gateway; 2021. https://www.childwelfare.gov/pubs/issue-briefs/racial-disproportionality/.

5. Ganasarajah S, Siegel G, Sickmund M. Disproportionality rates for children of color in foster care. In: Seigel G, editor. Technical assistance bulletin. Nevada: National Council of Juvenile and Family Court Judges; 2017. p. 1–74.
6. Davidson R, Morrissey M, Beck C. The Hispanic Experience of the Child Welfare System FAMILY COURT REVIEW April 2019;57(2):201–16.
7. Fong R, Petronella G. In: Dettlaff A, editor. Underrepresented populations in the child welfare system: asian American and native Hawaiian/pacific islander populations. Switzerland: Springer: Child Maltreatment: Contemporary Issues in Reseach and Policy; 2021. p. 125–40.
8. Pryce J, Yelick A. Racial disproportionality and disparities among african american children in the child welfare system. In: Dettlaff A, editor. Racial Disproportionality and disparities in the child welfare system. Switzerland: Springer: Child Maltreatment: Contemporary Issues in Research and Policy; 2021. p. 45–61.
9. Kalisher A, Radel L, Madden E. The multiethnic placement act 25 Years later. In: Gosciak J, editor. Trends in adoption and transracial adoption. Washington, D.C.: U.S. Department fo Health and Human Services: Office of the Assistant Secretary for Planning and Evaluation; 2020. p. 1–22.
10. US indian boarding school history. Available at: https://boardingschoolhealing.org/education/us-indian-boarding-school-history/.
11. Hartway L, Korthase A. The Indian child welfare act and active efforts: past and present. In: Korthase A, editor. Reno, NV: National Council of Juvenile and Family Court Judges; 2020. https://www.ncjfcj.org/wp-content/uploads/2021/02/NCJFCJ_ICWA_Active_Efforts_Final.pdf.
12. Connolly C. Path to Federal Foster Care Prevention Funds Overlooks Tribal Programs, Experts Say, in The Imprint. Youth and Family News 2022;. https://imprintnews.org/child-welfare-2/tribal-practices-overlooked-family-first/62641.
13. Johnson-Motoyama M, Phillips R, Beer O. Racial disproportionality and disparities among Latinx children. In: Dettalaff A, editor. Racial disproportionality and disparities in the child welfare system. Switzerland: Springer: Contemporary Issues in Research and Policy; 2021. p. 69–98.
14. Harris MSaH. Wanda, Decision points in child welfare: An action researchmodel to address disproportionality. Child Youth Serv Rev 2008;30:199–215.
15. Hill RB. Synthesis of research on disproportionality in child welfare: an update. 2006. Available at: https://www.cssp.org/reform/child-welfare/other-resources/synthesis-of-research-on-disproportionality-robert-hill.pdf.
16. Osterling KL, D'Andrade A, Austin MJ. Understanding and addressing racial/ethnic disproportionality in the front end of the child welfare system. J Evid Based Soc Work 2008;5(1–2):9–30.
17. Kokaliari ED, Roy AW, Taylor J. African American perspectives on racial disparities in child removals. Child Abuse Negl 2019;90:139–48.
18. Seay K. How many families in child welfare services are affected by parental substance use disorders? a common question that remains unanswered. Child Welfare 2015;94(4):19–51.
19. Amaro H, Sanchez M, Bautista T, et al. Social vulnerabilities for substance use: STRESSORS, socially toxic environments, and discrimination and racism. Neuropharmacology 2021;188:108518.
20. Douaihy AB, Kelly TM, Sullivan C. Medications for substance use disorders. Soc Work Public Health 2013;28(3–4):264–78.
21. Fornili KS. Racialized mass incarceration and the war on drugs: a critical race theory appraisal. J Addict Nurs 2018;29(1):65–72.

22. Meinhofer A, Anglero-Diaz Y. Trends in foster care entry among children removed from their homes because of parental drug use, 2000 to 2017. JAMA Pediatr 2019;173(9):881–3.

23. Sanmartin MX, Ali MM, Lynch S. Association between State-level criminal justice-focused prenatal substance use policies in the US and substance use-related foster care admissions and family reunification. JAMA Pediatr 2020;174(8):782–8.

24. U.S. Department of Health and Human Services. Administration for Children and Families, Administrationon Children, Youth and Families, Children's Bureau. The AFCARS Report 2020. Oct 2021;. https://www.acf.hhs.gov/sites/default/files/documents/cb/afcarsreport28.pdf.

25. Finno-Velasquez M, Palmer L, Prindle J, et al. A birth cohort study of Asian and Pacific Islander children reported for abuse or neglect by maternal nativity and ethnic origin. Child Abuse Negl 2017;72:54–65.

26. Lane WG, Rubin D, Christian C, et al. Racial differences in the evaluation of pediatric fractures for physical abuse. JAMA 2002;288(13):1603–9.

27. Drake B, Jolley J, Fluke J, et al. Racial bias in child protection? A comparison of competing explanations using national data. Pediatrics 2011;127(3):471–8.

28. Kravitz E, Suh M, Russell M, et al. Screening for substance use disorders during pregnancy: a decision at the intersection of racial and reproductive justice. Am J Perinatol 2021;0.1055/s-0041-1739433. https://doi.org/10.1055/s-0041-1739433.

29. Drake B, Lee SM, Jonson-Reid M. Race and child maltreatment reporting: are Blacks overrepresented? Child Youth Serv Rev 2009;31(3):309–16.

30. Larson K, Cull W, Racine A, et al. Trends in access to health care services for US children: 2000-2014. Pediatrics 2016;138(6).

31. Zablotsky B, Black L, Maenner M, et al. Prevalence and trends of developmental disabilities among children in the United States: 2009-2017. Pediatrics 2019; 144(4).

32. Graham LM, Lanier P, Johnson-Motoyama M. National profile of Latino/Latina children reported to the child welfare system for sexual abuse. Child Youth Serv Rev 2016;66:18–27.

33. King B, Fallon B, Boyd R, et al. Factors associated with racial differences in child welfare investigative decision-making in Ontario, Canada. Child Abuse Negl 2017;73:89–105.

34. Austin AE, Gottfredson NC, Zolotor AJ, et al. Trajectories of child protective services contact among Alaska Native/American Indian and non-Native children. Child Abuse Negl 2019;95:104044.

35. Dakil SR, Cox M, Lin H, et al. Racial and ethnic disparities in physical abuse reporting and child protective services interventions in the United States. J Natl Med Assoc 2011;103(9–10):926–31.

36. Rivaux SL, James J, Wittenstrom K, et al. The intersection of race, poverty and risk: understanding the decision to provide services to clients and to remove children. Child Welfare 2008;87(2):151–68.

37. Detlaff AJ, Rycraft JR. Factors contributing to disproportionality in the child welfare system: views from the legal community. Social Work 2010;55(3):213–24.

38. Meinhofer A, Onuoha E, Angleró-Díaz Y, et al. Parental drug use and racial and ethnic disproportionality in the U.S. foster care system. Child Youth Serv Rev 2020;118.

39. Price HR, Collier AC, Wright TE. Screening pregnant women and their neonates for illicit drug use: consideration of the integrated technical, medical, ethical, legal, and social issues. Front Pharmacol 2018;9:961.

40. Berkman E, Brown E, Scott M, et al. Racism in child welfare: ethical consider-ations of harm. Bioethics 2022;36(3):298–304.
41. Liming KW, Brook J, Akin B. Cumulative adverse childhood experiences among children in foster care and the association with reunification: a survival analysis. Child Abuse Negl 2021;113:104899.
42. LaBrenz CA, Findley E, Graaf G, et al. Racial/ethnic disproportionality in reunifi-cation across U.S. child welfare systems. Child Abuse Negl 2021;114:104894.
43. Lloyd M, Akin B, Brook J. Parental drug use and permanency for young children in foster care: a competing risks analysis of reunification, guardianship, and adoption. Child Youth Serv Rev 2017;77:177–87.
44. Saloner B, Le Cook B. Blacks and hispanics are less likely than whites to com-plete addiction treatment, largely due to socioeconomic factors. Health Aff (Mill-wood) 2013;32(1):135–45.
45. Wulczyn F, Gibbons R, Snowden L, et al. Poverty, social disadvantage, and the Black-White placement gap. Child Youth Serv Rev 2013;3:65–74.
46. Miller OA, Ward KJ. Emerging strategies for reducing racial disproportionality and disparate outcomes in child welfare: the results of a national breakthrough series collaborative. Child Welfare 2008;87(2):211–40.
47. Sattler KMP, Font SA. Predictors of adoption and guardianship dissolution: the role of race, age, and gender among children in foster care. Child Maltreat 2021;26(2):216–27.
48. Wildeman C, Edwards FR, Wakefield S. The Cumulative prevalence of termination of parental rights for U.S. children, 2000-2016. Child Maltreat 2020;25(1):32–42.
49. Leake R, Potter C, Lucero N, et al. Findings from a national needs assessment of American Indian/Alaska native child welfare programs. Child Welfare 2012;91(3):47–63.
50. Kelly J. Two states near plans to terminate parental rights at birth in some drug cases. The imprint - youth and family news. 2018. Available at: https://imprintnews.org/substance-abuse/two-states-near-plans-terminate-parental-rights-birth-drug-cases/30417.
51. Rolock N, Pérez A, White K, et al. From foster care to adoption and guardianship: a twenty-first century challenge. Child Adolesc Social Work J 2018;35:11–20.
52. White KR. Placement discontinuity for older children and adolescents who exit foster care through adoption or guardianship: a systematic review. Child Adolesc Social Work J 2016;33(4):377–94.
53. Rolock N, White KR. Post-permanency discontinuity: a longitudinal examination of outcomes for foster youth after adoption or guardianship. Child Youth Serv Rev 2016;70:419–27.
54. Vonk ME. Cultural competence for transracial adoptive parents. Soc Work 2001;46(3):246–55.
55. Johnson PR, Shireman JF, Watson KW. Transracial adoption and the development of Black identity at age eight. Child Welfare: J Pol Pract Program 1987;66(1):45–55.
56. Eastman A, Putnam-Hornstein E, Magruder J, et al. Characteristics of youth re-maining in foster care through age 19: a pre- and post-policy cohort analysis of California data. Journal of Public Child Welfare; 2016. p. 1–17.
57. Ahn E, Gil Y, Putnam-Hornstein E. Predicting youth at high risk of aging out of fos-ter care using machine learning methods. Child Abuse Negl 2021;117:105059.
58. Garcia AR, Pecora PJ, Aisenberg E. Institutional predictors of developmental out-comes among racially diverse foster care alumni. Am J Orthopsychiatry 2012;82(4):573–84.

59. Wilson, Bianca DM, Kastanis, Angeliki A. Sexual and gender minority disproportionality and disparities in child welfare: A population-based study. Children and Youth Services Review, 58, issue C 2015;11–7.

60. Herz D, Ryan J, Bilchik S. Challenges facing crossover youth: an examination of juvenile-justic decision making and recidivism. Fam Court Rev 2010;48:305–21.

61. Wilson BDM, Kastanis AA. Sexual and gender minority disproportionality and disparities in child welfare: a population-based study. Child Youth Serv Rev 2015; 58:11–7.

62. Jacobs J, Freundlich M. Achieving permanency for LGBTQ youth. Child Welfare 2006;85(2):299–316.

63. Baams L, Wilson BDM, Russell ST. LGBTQ youth in unstable housing and foster care. Pediatrics 2019;143(3).

64. A guide to children arriving at the border: laws, policies, and responses. 2015. Available at: https://www.americanimmigrationcouncil.org/sites/default/files/research/a_guide_to_children_arriving_at_the_border_and_the_laws_and_policies_governing_our_response.pdf.

65. Staz M, Heidbrink L. A better "best interests": Immigration policy in comparative context. In: HL, editor. Law & policy. Law & Policy; 2019. p. 365–86.

66. Ataiants J, Cohen C, Riley AH, et al. Unaccompanied children at the United States border, a human rights crisis that can be addressed with policy change. J Immigr Minor Health 2018;20(4):1000–10.

67. Crea TM, Evans K, Lopez A, et al. Unaccompanied immigrant children in long term foster care: identifying needs and best practices from a child welfare perspective. Child Youth Serv Rev 2018;92:56–64.

68. Goetz S. *From removal to incarceration: how the modern child welfare system and its unintended consequences catalyzed the foster care-to-prison pipeline.* U. M d . L.J. R ace R elig. G ender & C lass 2020;20:289–305.

69. Cutuli JJ, George R, Coulton C, et al. From foster care to juvenile justice: exploring characteristics of youth in three cities. Child Youth Serv Rev 2016;67: 84–94.

70. Yi Y, Wildeman C. Can foster care interventions diminish justice system inequality? Future Child 2018;28(1):37–58.

71. Dettlaff AJ, Boyd R. Racial disproportionality and disparities in the child welfare system: why do they exist, and what can be done to address them? ANNALS Am Acad Polit Social Sci 2020;692(1):253–74.

72. Clark P, Buchanan J, Legters L. Taking action on racial disproportionality in the child welfare system. Child Welfare 2008;87(2):319–34.

73. Porter LL, Zink PP, Gebhardt AR, et al. Best outcomes for Indian children. Child Welfare 2012;91(3):135–56.

74. Jewell J, Brown D, Smith G, et al. Examining the influence of caregiver ethnicity on youth placed in out of home care: ethnicity matters – for some. Child Youth Serv Rev 2010;32(10):1278–84.

75. dosReis S, Zito JM, Safer DJ, et al. Mental health services for youths in foster care and disabled youths. Am J Public Health 2001;91(7):1094–9.

76. Raghavan R, Zima B, Andersen R, et al. Psychotropic medication use in a national probability sample of children in the child welfare system. J Child Adolesc Psychopharmacol 2005;15(1):97–106.

77. Raghavan R, Inoue M, Ettner S, et al. A preliminary analysis of the receipt of mental health services consistent with national standards among children in the child welfare system. Am J Public Health 2010;100(4):742–9.

78. Zito JM, Safer DJ, dosReis S, et al. Racial disparity in psychotropic medications prescribed for youths with Medicaid insurance in Maryland. J Am Acad Child Adolesc Psychiatry 1998;37(2):179–84.
79. Leslie LK, Weckerly J, Landsverk J, et al. Racial/ethnic differences in the use of psychotropic medication in high-risk children and adolescents. J Am Acad Child Adolesc Psychiatry 2003;42(12):1433–42.
80. Raghavan R, Brown D, Thompson H, et al. Medicaid expenditures on psychotropic medications for children in the child welfare system. J Child Adolesc Psychopharmacol 2012;22(3):182–9.
81. Raghavan R, Brown D, Allaire B, et al. Medicaid expenditures on psychotropic medications for maltreated children: a study of 36 States. Psychiatr Serv 2014; 65(12):1445–51.
82. Linares LO, Martinez-Martin N, Castellanos FX. Stimulant and atypical antipsychotic medications for children placed in foster homes. PLoS One 2013;8(1): e54152.
83. Dosreis S, Yoon Y, Rubin D, et al. Antipsychotic treatment among youth in foster care. Pediatrics 2011;128(6):e1459–66.

Considering "Spheres of Influence" in the Care of Lesbian, Gay, Bisexual Transgender, and Queer-Identified Youth

Jonathon W. Wanta, MD[a],*, George Gianakakos, MD[a],
Erin Belfort, MD[b], Aron Janssen, MD[a]

KEYWORDS

- LGBTQ • Mental health • Transgender • Spheres of influence • Pediatrics

KEY POINTS

- Although commonly confused, biological sex, gender, and sexual orientation are distinct and independent entities with each playing uniquely important roles throughout a child's development.
- Gender-affirming care for transgender and gender nonbinary youth is individualized to each person and may consist of medical and nonmedical interventions.
- The Spheres of Influence is a useful framework for mental health professionals working with LGBTQ youth to systematically identify the various contextual levels at which to target clinical services and advocacy in pursuit of more equitable care.

INTRODUCTION

Based on a recent large, national sample, almost 2 million youth ages 13 to 17 years (9.5%) identified as lesbian, gay, bisexual, and/or transgender (LGBT).[1] While a helpful starting point, even the largest survey studies only begin to capture the true diversity of the LGBTQ (LGBT + queer-identified) community. In no other time has there been such a significant cultural shift in how society (and youth in particular) conceptualizes gender and sexuality. Clinical education and research on more traditional or familiar LGBTQ identities are sparse to begin with, and youth are constantly expanding beyond what many of us studied in medical school or postgraduate training. Although

[a] Pritzker Department of Psychiatry and Behavioral Health, Ann and Robert H. Lurie Children's Hospital of Chicago, 225 East Chicago Avenue, Box 10, Chicago, IL 60611, USA; [b] Maine Medical Center and Tufts University School of Medicine, 66 Bramhall Street, Portland, ME 04102, USA
* Corresponding author.
E-mail address: jwanta@luriechildrens.org

Child Adolesc Psychiatric Clin N Am 31 (2022) 649–664
https://doi.org/10.1016/j.chc.2022.05.008
1056-4993/22/© 2022 Elsevier Inc. All rights reserved.

childpsych.theclinics.com

these shifts can be intimidating and harrowing for providers, they also provide an opportunity for cultural humility, education, and building meaningful connection and understanding with patients who often believe stigmatized by the health care profession and society at large.

The goal of this article is to establish for the mental health provider a foundation on which to build their clinical knowledge and practice. We present the "Spheres of Influence," adapted from discourse in international policy making, to guide the clinician during clinical encounters and encourage a holistic approach at every social level our patients encounter. At each level, we consider the current evidence base as well as the highest yield and most relevant debates a provider is likely to confront in the care of LGBTQ youth. We aim to provide the latest trends, advances, and discourses to empower the clinician in choosing and advocating for sound, evidence-based treatment of their LGBTQ patients.

DISCUSSION
Gender and Sex Development

From a doctor's classic delivery room pronouncement that "It is a girl!" to the rising popularity of "gender reveal" parties on the Internet, society has long been fascinated with the concept of biological sex and gender. Traditionally, sex is assigned at birth as either "male" or "female" and is determined by two concepts: phenotypic sex and/or genotypic sex. Phenotypic sex is commonly determined by an individual's internal and external genitalia in addition to sex characteristics influenced by prenatal hormone exposure. Genotypic sex is defined by an individual's genotype—the collection of genes located on their chromosomes. Of the 23 pairs of human chromosomes, the sex chromosomes X and Y are often considered the most important in determining sex, with an "XX" pair typically resulting in a female and an "XY" pair typically resulting in a male.

Discoveries in the mid-twentieth century added to the complexity of sex determination. Karyotypes performed on individuals with similar constellations of symptoms were found to possess differing combinations of sex chromosomes. People with Klinefelter and Turner syndromes, for example, have XXY or just X chromosomes, respectively, a distinct break from the traditional genotypic binary.[2] Further, additional genes outside of the sex chromosomes have been discovered that can play a role in regulating protein synthesis and altering an individual's phenotypic presentation.[3] For millions, phenotypic and/or genotypic sex may fall outside the traditional "male" or "female" binary.

Often confused with biological sex, but considered distinctly different for a multitude of reasons, is gender, a complex construct consisting of three separate components. The first is the relationship one has with their body, comprising the genetic, hormonal, and structural processes described above, as well as the experience and meaning of these processes for each individual. The second is gender identity, further described below, which is simply defined as one's sense of self on the spectrum of maleness, femaleness, or some combination of the two. Words to describe these concepts vary in definition based on norms present within the individual's society.[4] The third is gender role or the socially and culturally informed behaviors, dress, and attitudes that are broadly normative for a person based on their assumed gender. Although it seems that society defines what is generally meant by "maleness" or "femaleness," trends change over time and across cultures.

One's environment, both prenatally and postnatally, plays a smaller role in determining an individual's gender identity than once thought. From as young as 3 month old, female infants showed preferences for toys traditionally associated with girls over those associated with boys, choosing dolls over toy cars or balls. To control for societal influence, the same experiment was performed on female green vervet monkeys, only to reveal a similar trend among our primate cousins. Human "XX" females born with congenital adrenal hyperplasia, a genetic condition resulting in moderately high levels of androgen beginning in early gestation and continuing through prenatal life, often identify as girls throughout their lives. This is despite varying degrees of virilization at birth and behaviors and preferences similar to their male peers throughout development. These observations, in addition to many others, support the idea that gender identities have more or less coalesced before we are even born, even if the understanding of these identities do not develop until later in life.[5]

Many theories have attempted to explain the progression of gender development in humans. What is generally agreed on is that awareness of gender identity typically develops by 2 years of age when children begin to identify themselves as either a "boy" or a "girl." At this age, children are likely to have fairly concrete ideas about gender. For example, a child may identify a male child who has long hair as a girl, believing that "only girls have long hair. Within a few years, around the ages of 4 or 5 years, children are able to sort toys, clothing, tools, and appliances based on their stereotypical association with either traditional gender. By the time they are 6 or 7 years, children have developed some form of rudimentary "gender constancy" and are often able to determine whether a person is a "man" or a "woman" regardless of the person's job, clothes, or haircut.[5,6]

Sexual Orientation Development

Human beings seem programmed for sexual exploration from birth. Even within 24 hours of being born, male infants may achieve erection, and female infants may show vaginal lubrication. Babies under 3 years of age have been observed fondling their genitals with rhythmic movements seeming to imitate adult masturbation. Self-directed sexual play typically occurs between the ages of 6 and 9 years, although this takes on a more clandestine nature as children become more aware of societal norms. Adolescents have reported their first experience of sexual attraction occurring between 10 and 12 years, with sexual fantasies developing soon after. An interest in sex and sexual exploration increases between the ages of 13 and 19 years, corresponding with puberty and the development of secondary sex characteristics. Many males start masturbating between the ages of 13 and 15 years, with females initiating self-stimulatory behavior over a broader range of ages. Sexual orientation, broadly defined as one's inherent and "enduring pattern of emotional, romantic, and/or sexual attractions to other genders," typically starts to develop around this time as well.[4,7]

Sexual Orientation and Gender Development in LGBTQ Youth

Despite many similarities during sexual maturation between sexual- and gender-minority youths and their heterosexual peers, there are also distinct differences that will be briefly introduced. Studies have emphasized four "milestones" through which nonheterosexual subjects progress during development of their sexual identities: first same-sex attractions, first same-sex sexual contact, first self-labeling as nonheterosexual, and first disclosure of a nonheterosexual identity to others or "coming out." Among the study's population, significant differences were noted particularly along gendered lines. Adolescent males met all the aforementioned milestones before their female counterparts except for disclosure to others. Both groups identified the same-sex attraction occurring between the ages of 8 and 9 years. Men typically pursued sex before identifying themselves as gay, whereas the opposite was true for women. The average age of disclosure was around 18 years, although we suspect temporal trends may differ.[8]

As was mentioned earlier, gender is a complex consolidation of one's relationship to their body, their gender identity, and the gender roles expected of them in their society. For some youth, being labeled as either a "man" or a "woman" does not adequately describe their sense of self. Natal males identifying as women or natal females identifying as men have been traditionally labeled as "transgender" individuals. Recently, more attention has been brought to the potential existence of multiple genders beyond the traditional binary, a concept that has existed in multiple cultures across the globe. This would include genders such as "nonbinary," "pan-, poly-, or omni-gendered," or "gender fluid" among many others. All the aforementioned identities are often described as "gender nonconforming," "gender diverse," or "gender creative." Transgender and gender nonbinary (TGNB) individuals may undergo some form of transition in line with their gender as discussed further below.

Almost all the data currently available on gender development focus on gender-conforming youth. What has been observed in gender-diverse children, like in their gender-normative peers, is the ability to label their natal sex around the age of 2 years. However, TGNB children may show distress as they come to realize that the gender assigned at birth is not the gender with which they identify. These youth may show a strong dislike for their gendered anatomy, demonstrate a strong preference for toys or play of their identified gender, or show a strong preference for peers of the same identified gender, for example.[9,10] While limited, the studies we do have show that not all youth who endorse a gender-diverse identity in childhood will maintain that identity into adulthood, a phenomenon referred to as desistence. Some predictors of gender identity persistence have been identified. For example, clinicians have noted an important distinction in "being" (the child saying they are X gender) versus "wishing" (the child merely stating they *want* or *wish to be* X gender).[9,11] Further research is warranted.

Typically, individuals who develop gender nonconforming identities in adolescence or adulthood are more likely to persist in their gender identities over time. One possible consideration is the role adolescence plays in the crystallization of one's gender identity through response to shifting hormone levels and accompanying development of secondary sexual characteristics. Additionally, with frontal lobe and cognitive development in adolescence comes further insight and awareness into one's sexual orientation and identity.[12]

A notable development that has garnered some recent attention and rebuke describes the "rapid onset" of gender dysphoria (ROGD) in adolescents where there were no preceding signs or clues to parents. Although supporters of this hypothesis point to social influence, parental conflict, and maladaptive coping mechanism as potential etiologies, the critics note the considerably flawed study design and poor evidence.[13] They cite the ROGD study's reliance on parent surveys to develop the theory, recommending analyses of data collected from clinical and community sources to obtain a more complete picture of what is currently being observed.[14]

Gender-Affirming Care for Transgender and Gender Nonbinary Youth

Clinicians caring for TGNB youth should familiarize themselves with the World Professional Association for Transgender Health (WPATH) Standards of Care (SOC), currently in its 7th version. Succinctly, the WPATH SOC was developed to guide providers of TGNB individuals "with safe and effective pathways to achieving lasting personal comfort with their gendered selves to maximize their overall health, psychological well-being, and self-fulfillment."[15]

Gender-affirming care for TGNB youth can be conceptualized into several different categories depending on the youth's age and gender journey. It should be noted that these categories are not necessarily linear or mandatory steps, and every youth's gender journey is unique and valid. Not all TGNB youth will experience dysphoria, and not all TGNB youth necessitate referral to specialists working in gender-affirming care.

Most commonly, TGNB youth may choose to undergo a social transition as a first step in their journey. Social transition encompasses a wide swath of changes a youth may adopt to bring their social identity into closer alignment with their gender identity. The youth may choose a name that better reflects their gender identity (instead of their name assigned at birth or "dead name"), use pronouns consistent with their gender identity, and wear their hair or clothing in a way that is more consistent with their gender identity. These outwardly visible cues about gender are referred to as one's gender expression or gender role. Children and families might choose to take a step-wise approach to social transition with various affirming interventions at different times and in different settings. Social transition is "fully reversible" in that there are no negative medical outcomes for youth who choose to socially transition and then transition to an entirely different gender or choose to return to the gender consistent with their sex assigned at birth.

Some youth may choose to undergo a medical transition, which is using pharmacologic agents, to bring their physical bodies closer into accordance with their gender identity. Medical transition may include puberty suppression and/or gender-affirming hormones, depending on the age and pubertal stage of the youth.

Gonadotropin-releasing hormone (GnRH) agonists are the preferred medical intervention for puberty suppression, commonly referred to as "puberty blockers." GnRH agonists can be used as early as Tanner stage II, the onset of puberty, to arrest or delay natal puberty. Puberty suppression serves two main functions. First, puberty can be exquisitely distressing for TGNB youth. For example, breast development in a transgender male can exacerbate gender dysphoria or place the youth at risk for bullying. Second, puberty suppression may effectively give the youth and their family more time to consider subsequent gender-affirming medical interventions that carry more risk and permanent sequelae. An older adolescent is likely to have more developed executive functioning skills to weigh important pros and cons of further interventions compared with a young adolescent just beginning their gender journey.[16] Puberty blockers, well studied for years in certain disorders of sex development, are considered "fully reversible" in that long-term risks of such an intervention are considered low for those who wish to discontinue treatment; natal puberty resumes once the intervention is removed.[15] At the same time, youth who start gender-affirming hormones immediately after puberty blockers are at risk for infertility in adulthood. It is therefore prudent to begin counseling youth and their families on future sexual and reproductive health implications from the start.

The second type of medical transition includes gender-affirming hormone therapy, specifically exogenous androgen therapy for transgender males and estrogen therapy (with or without antiandrogens) for transgender females. As opposed to the GnRH agonists described above that suppress puberty of the sex assigned at birth, the androgen and estrogen therapy essentially induces the pubertal changes aligned with one's gender identity. Whereas puberty suppression is fully reversible once stopped, gender-affirming hormones are "partially reversible" in that there are both reversible and irreversible changes if/once discontinued.[15] For example, estrogen therapy may lead to permanent breast growth if estrogens are discontinued, but changes to fat distribution are likely to be lost over time if exogenous estrogen is discontinued. Some youth may elect to explore fertility preservation options before starting gender-affirming hormones due to future risk for infertility.

Finally, some TGNB individuals may choose to undergo irreversible surgical interventions to align their physical body with their gender identity. Gender-affirming surgical interventions may include breast/chest surgery, genital surgery, liposuction/lipofilling, and various other esthetic procedures. With the exception of chest masculinization surgery, irreversible surgical interventions are reserved for individuals reaching the legal age of majority and thus are out of the scope of this article.[15]

Although the potential adverse outcomes of gender-affirming medical or surgical interventions are commonly cited, it is vital to emphasize that withholding care is not a "neutral option" and is potentially harmful.[15] Risks of withholding treatment include increased risk for adverse mental health outcomes, suicide, exposure to trauma, and youth seeking out medical interventions illicitly without proper medical supervision.[17] The clinician must carefully navigate risks and benefits of treatment versus withholding treatment in collaboration with the youth and their family.

Note on Conversion Therapy

It is worth noting that "conversion" or "reparative" therapies that aim to change an individual's sexual orientation or gender identity have been explicitly discouraged by the American Academy of Child and Adolescent Psychiatry, American Psychiatric Association, American Academy of Pediatrics, and others. Such practices have no evidence base for efficacy and, conversely, have negative long-term consequences on mental health. Clinicians should instead encourage developmentally appropriate exploration of sexual orientation and gender identity without any predetermined outcome.[18]

SPHERES OF INFLUENCE

The term "spheres of influence" was first adapted from international policymaking to the health care arena in 2020 to address health care's ethical commitment to social determinants of health.[19] DeCamp and colleagues argue that individuals (clinicians) and institutions (health care organizations) have "spheres of influence" or domains in which they exert influence extending from the bedside to the community. In one iteration, Karches and colleagues[20] argue that clinicians have a "professional duty" to advocate on behalf of their patients within their purview, for example, using their medical expertise to advocate for policy around climate change as it relates to the well-being of their patients. Here, we apply the spheres of influence approach systematically to identify and direct mental health professionals working with LGBTQ youth to the various levels at which they might execute their expertise and advocacy in pursuit of more equitable care.

Individual Sphere

Our first sphere, and the sphere within which most clinicians will believe most comfortable operating, is the individual level. Our medical model is best situated to intervene on this level, although clinicians should be careful not to focus treatment interventions entirely at the individual level when interventions on other levels may be more suitable. The provision of gender-affirming care, and helping youth make complex medical decisions, necessitates working also within the context of the family, school, and community, which we will discuss in later sections.

Studies of LGBTQ adults have consistently demonstrated increased risk for psychopathology when compared with heterosexual cisgender controls. Although robust data on LGBTQ youth are generally sparser, there have been several studies suggesting an increased risk for the development of depression, anxiety, and suicidal ideation or attempts.[21–23] Large cross-sectional studies have demonstrated lifetime suicide attempt prevalence around 20% for LGB adults and 40% for transgender adults,[24] although there is notably less prospective data on youth.

It is worth noting that LGBTQ youth represent a vast and heterogenous population. Subgroup analyses point to higher risks for suicide in transgender, gender nonbinary, bisexual, and pansexual individuals.[25] The intersectionality of LGBTQ identity with certain at-risk minority ethnic or racial groups may further exacerbate risk. The results of one study suggested that Black/African American and Hispanic/Latinx LGBTQ youth had an increased risk for suicide attempts when compared with White LGBTQ youth, demonstrating the need for comprehensive assessment and care that is culturally informed.[25]

The Minority Stress Model in its adaptations for sexual and gender minority individuals was proposed to help explain the observed mental health disparities in the LGBTQ population. Simply put, the theory posits that mental health disparities arise from external and internal factors grounded in stigma and prejudice.[26,27] Transgender youth, for example, experience on average higher rates of physical violence/threat, sexual assault, and bullying owing to their minority status, examples of "external stressors."[28] Although discussed within other spheres, it is important to note that other external factors such as discrimination, family rejection, and homelessness can all significantly contribute to individual psychopathology and suicide risk.[25] With repeated exposure, external factors can become internalized and further propagate minority stress and adverse outcomes. Lived or observed experiences of victimization and discrimination may support expectations of rejection, need for concealment, and internalized homophobia or transphobia which can manifest as depression, anxiety, or suicidality.[26,27] Where discrimination and stigma are strong, as exposure to minority stress-related factors increases, there is expected to be greater disparity in mental health outcomes.[25]

What Is the Intervention?

First and foremost, the clinician working with LGBTQ youth can better the mental health of their patients by identifying and treating underlying mental health conditions. Regardless of contributing factors, the clinician should aim to deliver evidence-based care using the full spectrum of their pharmacologic and non-pharmacologic interventions.

Clinicians must also be mindful of the minority stress theory when treating an LGBTQ youth in their office. The clinician working with LGBTQ youth can work to identify external and internal factors negatively impacting a patient's lived experience. At the same time, the clinician can work toward building pride in the patient's community and facilitate connection with peers to mitigate risk and promote resilience. The clinician can help the LGBTQ youth cope with stigma through supportive psychotherapy techniques or evidence-based adaptations of cognitive behavioral therapy.[29]

For TGNB youth seeking gender-affirming medical care, mental health providers find themselves in the role of collaborative path pavers.[30] Providers in this role have an obligation to advocate for timely access to care while balancing and navigating psychosocial hurdles. Of note, WPATH SOC requires that mental health comorbidities be "reasonably controlled" before proceeding with gender transition; there is no absolute contraindication to pursuing gender-affirming care.

There is some evidence that initiation of gender-affirming care may temporarily exacerbate underlying mental health conditions, requiring careful monitoring and support early in a patient's medically-supervised gender journey.[31] However, there is a growing body of evidence that gender-affirming care is likely to decrease long-term risk for severe psychopathology or adverse mental health outcomes.[31,32] One unblinded prospective cohort study demonstrated a statistically significant 60% decrease in depression based on Patient Health Questionnaire-9 (PHQ-9) and a 73% in suicidality.[31] Another retrospective study of over 20,000 transgender adults demonstrated the lower odds of lifetime suicidal ideation for those who wanted and had received pubertal suppression as adolescents compared with those who did not have access.[33]

The access to care seems to mitigate adverse mental health outcomes is particularly concerning given a wave of anti-LGBTQ legislation that has recently arisen. One recent editorial identified 8 states that have passed anti-transgender laws and another 29 states that have attempted to pass similar laws that are inconsistent with current evidence-based SOC. The authors assert that such discriminatory measures may further exacerbate mental health disparities, increase stigma, and thwart access to potentially life-saving interventions.[34]

Finally, there is much we do not know about LGBTQ youth and their risk for psychopathology. There remains research to be done to further elucidate other risk and resilience factors within the LGBTQ population or how our interventions mitigate risk over time. Some co-occurrences, such as autism spectrum disorder, do not clearly fit within the minority stress theory, yet there seems to be a positive bidirectional association.[35] Although several hypotheses have been posited, further research is warranted.

Home Sphere

The home sphere encompasses a child's supports, which may include parents, guardians, siblings, extended family, and more. Especially during their childhood years, youth are likely to spend the most time within the home sphere and to take the most direction from it. Thus, evaluating and supporting LGBTQ youth within the home sphere are essential for the child psychiatrist.

Youth are disclosing their sexual orientation or gender identity to friends or family ("coming out") at younger ages, and, in general, there is more societal acceptance.[36] Younger age of coming out may be met with more criticism and skepticism by parents, and conflict may arise within the home around issues of religion, culture, politics, and other closely held belief systems that are seemingly at odds with the youth's orientation or identity.

Studies consistently show that LGBTQ youths who experience family rejection are at increased risk for depression, anxiety, suicide attempts, and substance abuse.[37,38] One such study found a three and a half times increased lifetime risk of a suicide attempt in transgender and gender nonconforming adults with a history of family rejection; more significant rejection was associated with a higher risk for a lifetime attempt.[39]

At the same time, family acceptance and support can be an incredibly powerful protective factor for LGBTQ youth. Research has consistently demonstrated that family acceptance is associated with long-term positive mental health outcomes such as self-esteem and is protective against adverse mental health outcomes such as depression and suicidality.[40] Transgender youth who are supported in their gender identity and social transition show depression rates on par with their cisgender peers and only mildly elevated rates of anxiety.[32]

What Is the Intervention?

When challenges arise in the family sphere, the child psychiatrist should aim to create a safe environment to explore differences in perspective on gender and gender identity with the patient and their parent. Generally, we assume that parents are doing the best they can with the skills and knowledge they have and the parents are acting in their child's best interest. The goal, then, is to help the patient and family align on some shared goal—commonly, the youth's well-being—and to help the patient identify adaptive or maladaptive patterns in the current relationships that are supporting or not supporting that goal. Parents of transgender youth can create an affirming environment in which their child can explore gender comfortably as they grow into their developing identity. Over time, the psychiatrist can help the family move toward increasing validation, communication, and affirming language such as using the youth's identified name and pronouns.

Oftentimes families may be misinformed or have questions, lending the psychiatrist to take on the role of educator. Psychoeducation using tools such as The Gender Unicorn (**Fig. 1**) can also help ensure that everyone is using a shared language.[41] Families can be directed to resources such as American Academy of Child and Adolescent Psychiatry (AACAP) Gender and Sexuality Resources for information on LGBTQ youth and gender/sexuality development. Organizations such as the Family Acceptance Project have developed research-driven interventions to help families learn how to best support their LGBTQ child. Organizations such as PFLAG can be helpful for parents to learn, process, or grieve with other parents and away from their youth with the goal of strengthening the family sphere and fostering resilience in their child.

School Sphere

Although the home remains the first and most immediate sphere of influence for many youth, the school sphere plays a key role in not only their cognitive development but also their socialization and understanding of cultural expectations and societal norms.[42] For LGBTQ youth, classes and extracurricular activities have historically come into conflict with their lived experiences and self-understanding which can have global, negative consequences on well-being, and academic achievement.[43,44] Recent studies have shown, however, that extracurricular activities and support groups with sympathetic peers and understanding teachers can counteract these deleterious elements and, in fact, have a protective effect on the health and happiness of LGBTQ students.[45-47] When these factors are in place, students have reported decreased levels of stress, exhibited increased academic performance, and missed fewer days of school.[28,48]

Homeschooling was often seen as the exception to this traditional educational model, with about 3% of American children receiving home instruction and varied levels of extracurricular socialization in 2016.[49] Some LGBTQ youth may pursue nontraditional schooling as a means to avoid social stigma, peer pressure, and shaming endemic to many public schools.[50,51] The outbreak of COVID-19 in early 2020 forced education systems across the globe to adopt "virtual" or "remote" curricula to continue providing services to children under lockdowns.[49] At the peak of pandemic isolation, almost 93% of American students reported receiving instruction remotely, with various levels of success.[52] Preliminary studies suggest that lack of access to social supports and adequate therapeutic resources during quarantine took a disproportionate toll on the mental health of already vulnerable minority populations with LGBTQ students being no exception. Continued follow-up and research will be necessary to explore the long-term effects, and these changes in the education system have had on the well-being and academic abilities of American children.[53]

What Is the Intervention?

As part of our clinical assessment of youth, we explore sexual orientation and sexual behavior history in our clinical spaces. If done in a safe and nonjudgmental manner,

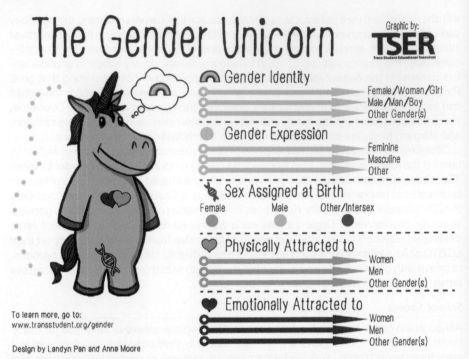

Fig. 1. The Gender Unicorn presents a framework and shared langue to explore youth's gender and sexuality.

youth often reveal gaps in knowledge or questions about sexuality and sexual health. Much sex education happening within family units or within the context of health class at school is delivered from a heteronormative and cisgender orientation. LGBTQ youth may find themselves completely absent from the conversation, further intensifying internalized homophobia or transphobia. We can help explore these concerns and provide informed sex and health education for LGBTQ youth to safely explore intimacy and sexuality. We may also encourage schools to adopt more inclusive sex education curricula in their health classes.

Child and adolescent psychiatrists can play an important role in advocating for all students and leveraging a relationship with school to help assess and treat patients. Teachers and mentors can be enlisted to complete screening tools to aid providers in diagnosis and treatment monitoring. Child and adolescent psychiatrists must advocate for their patients in the political arena, fighting to ensure they are treated with respect and able to access a free and fair education regardless of how sexual orientation or gender identity. Physicians can also be involved in meetings involving supportive services such as a 504 Plan or Individualized Education Plan.[54–56]

Community Sphere

LGBTQ youth may experience unique challenges in the community sphere when compared with their cisgender and heterosexual peers. Up to one-third of LGBTQ youth report subsequent verbal, psychological, and even physical abuse on disclosing their identity to family, and many are forced out or choose to leave their homes for their own well-being. LGBTQ youth are disproportionately represented in populations of homeless youth; despite making up less than 10% of the population, up to 40% of homeless youth identify as LGBTQ.[57]

At the same time, LGBTQ youth are disproportionately represented in the foster care system. For those in foster care, pressure to conform to traditionally masculine or feminine roles to find placement can be demoralizing. A significant percentage of these children have reported harassment or discrimination due to their sexual orientation or gender identities in foster homes or group facilities.[58]

Without support from their families or guardians, LGBTQ youth without stable housing may resort to various means to put a roof over their heads and food on their tables. For a sample of transgender women living in Los Angeles, for example, a study found that about half had used sex work to pay rent. This inevitably puts these young people at a higher chance of engaging in riskier behavior such as substance use and unprotected sex, both of which can increase the likelihood of sexually transmitted infections. Data have shown the prevalence of the human immunodeficiency virus (HIV) in adult transgender female sex workers to be just over 25%.[59,60]

Such survival behaviors often result in LGBTQ youth engaging with America's law enforcement and legal systems as well. Incarceration rates for LGBTQ youth may be three times higher than the general population. Despite being somewhere between 5% and 8% of the total population of American youth, LGBTQ youth comprise about 15% of the population in juvenile detention centers. Finally, one in six transgender individuals and almost 50% of Black transgender individuals report having being incarcerated at some point in their life.[61]

What Is the Intervention?

Child and adolescent psychiatrists can play a vital role in helping LGBTQ youth navigate their community sphere. Providers should assess for housing and food instability given the high risk for homelessness. Other social determinants of health such as access to healthy foods and educational, employment, and health care resources should also be explored. At-risk youth can be counseled on substance use and sexual activity. Clinicians can coordinate with pediatricians to ensure proper health care follow-up for basic medical cares and evidence-based testing for high-risk behaviors. Finally, physicians can provide information and resources for community support centers able to help patients struggling to find safe housing or job opportunities.[55]

Clinical Sphere

LGBTQ individuals have experienced extensive stigmatization from psychiatry over its recent past, necessitating careful advocacy within the clinical sphere. It was not until the 1970s that homosexuality was removed from the paraphilias section of the Diagnostic and Statistical Manual of Mental Disorders (DSM), a diagnosis that reflected discriminatory societal views rather than the presence of psychological distress.[62] Just a few years later, the diagnosis of gender identity disorder (GID) first appeared in the DSM-IV, again seeming to pathologize what we now consider to be "normal and expectable dimensions of human development."[63] GID was replaced by the new diagnosis of gender dysphoria in DSM-5, reflecting a shift whereby the psychological distress, not the gender identity itself, is the "clinical problem."[10]

Stigma and discrimination continue in modern day health care. In a survey of over 5000 LGBTQ adults, 30% of LGB respondents and 51% of transgender and gender nonconforming adults believed that had been treated differently by a health care professional due to their sexual orientation and/or gender identity.[64]

It is unsurprising then, considering psychiatry's past and present, there remains some level of distrust of the medical establishment by LGBTQ individuals. LGBTQ youth may avoid seeking care when medically necessary or may not disclose their sexual orientation and/or gender identity, thereby obfuscating the clinician's history and clinical reasoning. Transgender and gender nonconforming youth have the added hurdle of required mental health assessments to proceed with gender-affirming medical care which can create systemic inequity with challenges around access.[65]

What Is the Intervention?

It is the child and adolescent psychiatrist's role, within their clinical care sphere, to build bridges and deliver affirming care on an individual and system-level scope. As labels and attitudes and guidelines around the care of LGBTQ youth are constantly changing, the clinician must adopt a sense of cultural humility and continually strive to learn more and do better. Within one's office, one can ask open-ended and gender-neutral questions when taking a sexual history and affirming a transgender patient's name (instead of their name assigned at birth or "dead name"). Clinicians should acknowledge and apologize for using a patient's name assigned at birth or their incorrect pronouns. The clinician may need to have a more nuanced conversation with the child about which name and pronouns they would prefer in different settings, such as with a parent in the room or in the medical record. Respect for confidentiality is paramount in clinical care and documentation, especially in an era where parents may have access to a child's medical record.

Clinicians can also advocate on behalf of their LGBTQ patients at the systems level. Workshops such as safe space can be useful for all patient-facing staff to promote a safe and welcoming clinical setting. Waiting rooms and offices can include signage indicating inclusivity of all sexual orientations and gender identities. Serving transgender and gender nonconforming youth admitted to inpatient psychiatry may create unique dilemmas. Clinicians should seek to affirm a child's gender by allowing them to room with a peer of their identified gender, for example, while balancing the implications that may arise around confidentiality and disclosures to their families or other patients. Anecdotally, there have been some LGBTQ-specific inpatient psychiatry units created to help mitigate these clinical care quandaries while fostering connectedness in an affirming and supportive environment.

SUMMARY

Working with LGBTQ youth can present a uniquely challenging opportunity for clinicians. In many ways, youth are exploring gender and sexuality in ways that are completely new and foreign to the current generation of providers, pioneering new phraseology and expression. The care of LGBTQ youth is an ever-changing landscape that requires humility and openness to life-long learning. Yet, perhaps nowhere is there a greater need for competent providers given the paucity of LGBTQ youth-friendly services, especially in more rural settings.[65]

At the same time, working with LGBTQ youth can be exquisitely rewarding and impactful. Mental health providers have the opportunity to approach treatment holistically, think outside the box, and tailor their interventions to the highest yield spheres of influence. Providers are called not only to use the range of their clinical acumen on the individual level but also to consider a youth's strengths and challenges in their home, school, and community. When LGBTQ youth are supported at every sphere, we give them the best chance to survive and thrive into adulthood.

CLINICS CARE POINTS

- Gender and sexuality are integral parts of identity and development for all youth but may be especially salient for gender and/or sexual minority youth.

- Gender-affirming care, including medical and non-medical interventions, are safe and effective for transgender and gender non-binary youth.
- Mental health clinicians working with LGBTQ youth must assess and intervene on the individual, family, school, community, and clinical spheres to optimize patient care and wellbeing.

DISCLOSURE

The authors have no conflicts of interests or disclosures to declare.

REFERENCES

1. Conron K. LGBT Youth Populations in the United States. Williams Institute. Available at: https://williamsinstitute.law.ucla.edu/wp-content/uploads/LGBT-Youth-US-Pop-Sep-2020.pdf. Accessed July 1, 2022.
2. Griffiths DA. Shifting syndromes: sex chromosome variations and intersex classifications. Soc Stud Sci 2018;48(1):125–48.
3. Karkanaki A, Praras N, Katsikis I, Kita M, Panidis D. Is the Y chromosome all that is required for sex determination? Hippokratia 2007;11(3):120–3.
4. DeLamater J, Friedrich WN. Human sexual development. J Sex Res 2002; 39(1):10–4.
5. Bao A-M, Swaab DF. Sexual differentiation of the human brain: relation to gender identity, sexual orientation and neuropsychiatric disorders. Front Neuroendocrinol 2011;32(2):214–26. https://doi.org/10.1016/j.yfrne.2011.02.007.
6. Blakemore JEO, Berenbaum SA, Liben LS. Gender development, xi. Psychology Press; 2009. p. 519.
7. Answers to your questions for a better understanding of sexual orientation and homosexuality. American Psychological Association. Available at: https://www.apa.org/topics/lgbtq/orientation. Accessed July 1, 2022.
8. Savin-Williams RC, Diamond LM. Sexual identity trajectories among sexual-minority youths: gender comparisons. Arch Sex Behav 2000;29(6):607–27.
9. Steensma TD, Kreukels BP, de Vries AL, Cohen-Kettenis PT. Gender identity development in adolescence. Horm Behav 2013;64(2):288–97.
10. American Psychiatric Association. Diagnostic and Statistical Manual of Mental Disorders. 5th edition. Washington, DC: American Psychiatric Association; 2013
11. Malpas J. Between pink and blue: a multi-dimensional family approach to gender nonconforming children and their families. Fam Process 2011;50(4):453–70.
12. Wallien MS, Cohen-Kettenis PT. Psychosexual outcome of gender-dysphoric children. J Am Acad Child Adolesc Psychiatry 2008;47(12):1413–23.
13. Littman L. Parent reports of adolescents and young adults perceived to show signs of a rapid onset of gender dysphoria (vol 13, e0202330, 2018). PLoS One 2019;14(3). https://doi.org/10.1371/journal.pone.0214157.
14. Bauer GR, Lawson ML, Metzger DL, Team TYCR. Do clinical data from transgender adolescents support the phenomenon of "rapid onset gender dysphoria"? J Pediatr 2022;243:224.
15. Standards of Care for the Health of Transsexual, Transgender, and Gender Nonconforming People. The World Professional Association for Transgender Health. https://www.wpath.org/media/cms/Documents/SOC%20v7/SOC%20V7_English.pdf. Published 2012. Accessed July 6, 2022.

16. Rew L, Young CC, Monge M, Bogucka R. Review: puberty blockers for transgender and gender diverse youth-a critical review of the literature. Child Adol Ment Health 2021;26(1):3–14.

17. Kimberly LL, Folkers KM, Friesen P, et al. Ethical issues in gender-affirming care for youth. Pediatrics 2018;142(6). https://doi.org/10.1542/peds.2018-1537.

18. Conversion Therapy. American Academy of Child and Adolescent Psychiatry. https://www.aacap.org/aacap/Policy_Statements/2018/Conversion_Therapy. aspx. Published 2018. Accessed July 6, 2022.

19. DeCamp M, DeSalvo K, Dzeng E. Ethics and spheres of influence in addressing social determinants of health. J Gen Intern Med 2020;35(9):2743–5.

20. Karches K, DeCamp M, George M, et al. Spheres of influence and strategic advocacy for equity in medicine. J Gen Intern Med 2021;36(11):3537–40.

21. Stone DM, Luo FJ, Ouyang LJ, Lippy C, Hertz MF, Crosby AE. Sexual orientation and suicide ideation, plans, attempts, and medically serious attempts: evidence from local youth risk behavior surveys, 2001-2009. Am J Public Health 2014; 104(2):262–71.

22. Kuper LE, Mathews S, Lau M. Baseline mental health and psychosocial functioning of transgender adolescents seeking gender-affirming hormone therapy. J Dev Behav Pediatr 2019;40(8):589–96.

23. Moyer DN, Connelly KJ, Holley AL. Using the PHQ-9 and GAD-7 to screen for acute distress in transgender youth: findings from a pediatric endocrinology clinic. J Pediatr Endocrinol Metab 2019;32(1):71–4.

24. Herman J, Brown T, Haas A. Suicide thoughts and attempts among transgender adults. Williams Institute. Available at: https://williamsinstitute.law.ucla.edu/ publications/suicidality-transgender-adults/. Published April 9, 2020. Accessed July 1, 2022.

25. Green AE, Price MN, Dorison SH. Cumulative minority stress and suicide risk among LGBTQ youth. Am J Community Psychol 2022;69(1–2):157–68.

26. Meyer IH. Prejudice, social stress, and mental health in lesbian, gay, and bisexual populations: conceptual issues and research evidence. Psychol Bull 2003; 129(5):674–97.

27. Hendricks RJT ML. A conceptual framework for clinical work with transgender and gender nonconforming clients: an adaptation of the Minority Stress Model. Prof Psychol Res Pract 2012;43(5):460–7.

28. Johns MM, Poteat VP, Horn SS, Kosciw J. Strengthening our schools to promote resilience and health among LGBTQ youth: emerging evidence and research priorities from the State of LGBTQ Youth Health and Wellbeing Symposium. LGBT Health 2019;6(4):146–55.

29. Pachankis JE. Uncovering clinical principles and techniques to address minority stress, mental health, and related health risks among gay and bisexual men. Clin Psychol Sci Pr 2014;21(4):313–30.

30. Janssen A, Leibowitz S. Affirmative mental health care for transgender and gender diverse youth : a clinical guide. 1st ed. Imprint: Springer: Springer International Publishing; 2018. p. 1, online resource (XVIII, 214 pages 4 illustrations in color.

31. Tordoff DM, Wanta JW, Collin A, Stepney C, Inwards-Breland DJ, Ahrens K. Mental health outcomes in transgender and nonbinary youths receiving gender-affirming care. JAMA Netw Open 2022;5(2). https://doi.org/10.1001/ jamanetworkopen.2022.0978. ARTN e220978.

32. Olson KR, Durwood L, DeMeules M, McLaughlin KA. Mental health of trans-gender children who are supported in their identities. Pediatrics 2016;137(3). https://doi.org/10.1542/peds.2015-3223. ARTN e20153223.
33. Turban JL, King D, Carswell JM, Keuroghlian AS. Pubertal suppression for trans-gender youth and risk of suicidal ideation. Pediatrics 2020;145(2). https://doi.org/10.1542/peds.2019-1725. ARTN e20191725.
34. Barbee H, Deal C, Gonzales G. Anti-transgender legislation-a public health concern for transgender youth. JAMA Pediatr 2022;176(2):125–6.
35. Van der Miesen AIR, Hurley H, De Vries ALC. Gender dysphoria and autism spec-trum disorder: a narrative review. Int Rev Psychiatry 2016;28(1):70–80.
36. Russell ST, Fish JN. Mental health in lesbian, gay, bisexual, and transgender (LGBT) youth. Annu Rev Clin Psycho 2016;12:465–87.
37. Rosario M, Schrimshaw EW, Hunter J. Disclosure of sexual orientation and sub-sequent substance use and abuse among lesbian, gay, and bisexual youths: crit-ical role of disclosure reactions. Psychol Addict Behav 2009;23(1):175–84.
38. D'augelli AR. Mental health problems among lesbian, gay, and bisexual youths ages 14 to 21. Clin Child Psychol Psychiatry 2002;7(3):433–56.
39. Klein A, Golub SA. Family rejection as a predictor of suicide attempts and sub-stance misuse among transgender and gender nonconforming adults. LGBT Health 2016;3(3):193–9.
40. Ryan C, Russell ST, Huebner D, Diaz R, Sanchez J. Family acceptance in adoles-cence and the health of LGBT young adults. J Child Adolesc Psychiatr Nurs 2010; 23(4):205–13.
41. Trans Student Educational Resources, 2015. "The Gender Unicorn." Available at: http://www.transstudent.org/gender.
42. National Research Council (US) Panel to Review the Status of Basic Research on School-Age Children, Collins WA, eds. Development During Middle Childhood: The Years From Six to Twelve. Washington (DC): National Academies Press (US); 1984.
43. Murdock TB, Bolch MB. Risk and protective factors for poor school adjustment in lesbian, gay, and bisexual (LGB) high school youth: variable and person-centered analyses. Psychol Schools 2005;42(2):159–72.
44. Kosciw JG, Clark CM, Truong NL, et al. The 2019 National School Climate Survey: The Experiences of Lesbian, Gay, Bisexual, Transgender, and Queer Youth in Our Nation's Schools. A Report from GLSEN. 2020.
45. Russell ST, Seif H, Truong NL. School outcomes of sexual minority youth in the United States: evidence from a national study. J Adolescence (London, England) 2001;24(1):111–27.
46. Marx RA, Kettrey HH. Gay-straight alliances are associated with lower levels of school-based victimization of LGBTQ+ youth: a systematic review and meta-analysis. J Youth Adolesc 2016;45(7):1269–82.
47. Ioverno S, Russell ST. Homophobic bullying in positive and negative school cli-mates: the moderating role of gender sexuality alliances. J Youth Adolesc 2020;50(2):353–66.
48. Veale JF, Peter T, Travers R, Saewyc EM. Enacted stigma, mental health, and pro-tective factors among transgender youth in Canada. Transgender Health 2017; 3(1):27–216. https://doi.org/10.1089/trgh.2017.0031.
49. McPhee C, Jackson M, Bielick S, et al. National Household Education Surveys Program of 2016: Data File User's Manual (NCES 2018-100). National Center for Education Statistics, Institute of Education Sciences, US Department of Edu-cation, Washington, DC. 2018.

50. Riley G. A qualitative exploration of the experiences of individuals who have iden-tified as LGBTQ and who have homeschooled or unschooled. Other Educ 2018; 7:3–17.
51. Murphy J. Riding history: the organizational development of homeschooling in the US. Am Educ Hist J 2013;40(1/2):335.
52. Nearly 93% of Households With School-Age Children Report Some Form of Dis-tance Learning During COVID-19 (2020).
53. Salerno JP, Williams ND, Gattamorta KA. LGBTQ populations: psychologically vulnerable communities in the COVID-19 pandemic. Psychol Trauma 2020; 12(S1):S239–42.
54. Protecting Students with Disabilities. Office for Civil Rights. Avaialble at: https:// www2.ed.gov/about/offices/list/ocr/504faq.html#introduction. Published January 10, 2020. Accessed July 6, 2022.
55. Janssen A, Coyne C, Poquiz J, et al. Gender and Sexual Diversity in Childhood and Adolescence. In: Dulcan's Textbook of Child and Adolescent Psychiatry. Washington, DC: American Psychiatric Association Publishing; 2022:565–580.
56. Adelson SL. Practice parameter on gay, lesbian, or bisexual sexual orientation, gender nonconformity, and gender discordance in children and adolescents. J Am Acad Child Adolesc Psychiatry 2012;51(9):957–74.
57. Lolai D. You're going to Be straight or you're not going to live Here: child support for LGBT homeless youth. Tul JL Sex 2015;24:35.
58. Ashley B. The Challenge of LGBT Youth in Foster Care. The Forum: A Tennessee Student Legal Journal. 2014;1(1).
59. Garofalo R, Deleon J, Osmer E, Doll M, Harper GW. Overlooked, misunderstood and at-risk: exploring the lives and HIV risk of ethnic minority male-to-female transgender youth. J Adolesc Health 2006;38(3):230–6. https://doi.org/10.1016/ j.jadohealth.2005.03.023.
60. Wilson EC, Garofalo R, Harris RD, et al. Transgender female youth and sex work: HIV risk and a comparison of life factors related to engagement in sex work. AIDS Behav 2009;13(5):902–13.
61. Robinson BA. The lavender scare in homonormative times: policing, hyper-incarceration, and LGBTQ youth homelessness. Gend Soc 2020;34(2):210–32.
62. Kamens SR. On the proposed sexual and gender identity diagnoses for DSM-5: history and controversies. Humanistic Psychol 2011;39(1):37–59.
63. AACAP Statement Responding to Efforts to ban Evidence-Based Care for Trans-gender and Gender Diverse Youth. American Academy of Child and Adolescent Psychiatry. Available at: https://www.aacap.org/AACAP/Latest_News/AACAP_ Statement_Responding_to_Efforts-to_ban_Evidence-Based_Care_for_ Transgender_and_Gender_Diverse.aspx. Published November 8, 2019. Ac-cessed July 6, 2022.
64. When Health Care Isn't Caring: LGBT People and People Living with HIV Speak Out. Lambda Legal. Available at: https://www.lambdalegal.org/sites/default/files/ publications/downloads/whcic-insert_lgbt-people-and-people-living-with-hiv-speak-out.pdf. Published 2010. Accessed July 7, 2022.
65. Hadland SE, Yehia BR, Makadon HJ. Caring for lesbian, gay, bisexual, trans-gender, and questioning youth in inclusive and affirmative environments. Pediatr Clin North Am 2016;63(6):955.

Immigrant/Acculturation Experience

Tanuja Gandhi, MD[a], Aditi Hajirnis, MD[a], Otema A. Adade, MD, MA[b],
Rameshwari V. Tumuluru, MD[c],*

KEYWORDS

- Acculturation • Immigrants • Acculturative stress • Culture

KEY POINTS

- Acculturation is a process of cultural contact and exchange through which a person or group acquires certain values and practices of another culture that is not originally their own while still retaining their distinct cultural characteristics.
- Immigrant children and families are subjected to unique challenges and stress during the process of migration and acculturation that can result in both positive and negative outcomes.
- Understanding the impact of acculturation, addressing the stigma associated with access to mental health services, and using a cultural lens while delivering care are crucial components to improving behavioral health outcomes of diverse immigrant groups.

INTRODUCTION

The United States is a nation of immigrants with an estimated 44.5 million immigrants, accounting for 14% of the population in the year 2020. With increasing globalization, technological advances, and climate change resulting in international migration between countries, and a rapid influx of immigrants into the United States,[1,2] there is increasing diversity in the population. The process of migrating from one's native country and adapting to the host country can have a long-standing impact on first-generation immigrants and their subsequent generations.[3–5] Acculturation is the balance between adopting the attitudes and behaviors of the dominant culture while retaining the traditions, values, and beliefs of one's own culture.[6] It has also been described as "the process of cultural change and adaptation that occurs when individuals from diverse cultures come in contact with each other"[2] or when individuals living

[a] Department of Psychiatry and Human Behavior, Warren Alpert Medical School of Brown University, 1011 Veterans Memorial Parkway, Riverside, RI 02915, USA; [b] Lotus: The Center for Behavioral Health and Wellness, 401 15th Street South East, Unit 100-C, Washington, DC 20003, USA; [c] University of Pittsburgh School of Medicine, 3811 O'Hara Street, Pittsburgh, PA 15213, USA
* Corresponding author.
E-mail address: tumulururv@upmc.edu

in multicultural societies encounter each other.[1] This process of acculturation can have a significant impact on the mental health and well-being of immigrant populations. Acculturation has thus become an important area of interest and research.

The goal of this article is to provide a brief overview of the process of acculturation, its impact on the mental health of immigrant families, and highlight how child and adolescent psychiatrists can better address the unique mental health needs of immigrant populations.

BACKGROUND/HISTORY OF IMMIGRATION

Immigration to the United States has occurred over several decades in four major waves. **Table 1** reflects the corresponding periods, countries of origin, and key factors influencing migration.

Over 86 million individuals legally immigrated to the United States between 1783 and 2019.[9] The United States has experienced waves of both forced and voluntary immigration onto its soil. Although the 2020 census bureau report indicates that the population in the United States has become increasingly multiracial and multicultural (**Table 2**), the immigration system remains fragmented with an uneven application of immigration policies[9,10] leading to hardship among immigrant populations. Thus, it is important to note that immigrant health outcomes are affected by geopolitical determinants related to governments, geographies, policies, the interests of countries, and the relationships between them.

Acculturation

The classic definition of acculturation comes from cultural anthropology wherein Redfield et al[11] state that "Acculturation comprehends those phenomena which result when groups of individuals having different cultures come into continuous first-hand contact, with subsequent changes in the original cultural patterns of either or both groups." However, Berry[12] describes acculturation as a "dual process of cultural and psychological change that takes place as a result of contact between two or more cultural groups and their individual members."

At the core,[12–15] acculturation is a process of adaptation wherein all acculturating populations are faced with two main issues: (1) a relative preference for maintaining one's heritage culture and identity and (2) a relative preference for identification with the adopted culture. The interplay between these two issues can lead to acculturation through four possible strategies, including integration, assimilation, separation, and marginalization.[12,13,15] Following intercultural contact, all cultural groups change and can adopt different strategies of acculturation. However, not all individuals or groups acculturate in the same way or at the same rate, and these strategies themselves are dynamic and susceptible to change with situational and other factors. In general, integration has been found to be the most beneficial strategy for mental health[12,16–18] with better adaptation[19] than marginalization which is considered least beneficial. Assimilation and separation strategies are correlated with intermediate levels of stress and adaptation[12] (**Table 3**).

The process of acculturation is influenced by multiple factors of both the immigrant community and the receiving culture, including the circumstances around immigration.[20] Migration trajectories before, during, and after relocation can determine the level of adversity faced by immigrant populations. Premigration trajectories can disrupt one's social networks, education in children, and employment in adults, and separate individuals from extended family and communities. During migration, immigrants can face uncertainty, exposure to deprivation, violence, and poor living

Table 1
Waves of immigration

1st Wave (1607–1820)	2nd Wave (1820–1890)	3rd Wave (1890–1930)	4th Wave (1930–present)
Northern Europe Western Europe Africa	Ireland Germany	Southern Europe Eastern Europe	Latin America Asia Africa
Influenced by better economic opportunities, political freedom, religious freedom, freedom from slavery, and the Transatlantic slave trade	Driven by improvements in transportation, European strife, and the "American Dream"	Secondary to expansive industrialization and urbanization	High incidence of highly skilled immigrants
	Experienced widespread hostility and organized opposition	First restrictive immigration law passed by the State Congress in 1917 Immigration law of 1924—reduced annual quota for immigrants based on country of origin	Immigration and Nationality Act of 1965—established preferential system for immigrants from eastern hemisphere No pathway for lower skilled workers. 28 million undocumented immigrants from 1965 to 1986 Diversity Visa Program of the Immigration Act of 1990—favored European, mainly Irish immigrants

Source: "Immigration and Relocation in U.S. History." Library of Congress, https://www.loc.gov/classroom-materials/immigration/.[7]

conditions that can result in hopelessness, a lack of agency over one's future, and contribute to depression and anxiety. Though initially, hopeful immigrants face continued challenges post-migration stressors, including discrimination, poverty, racism, and adjustment to a new culture can result in ongoing stress. Language and monetary barriers, along with lack of access to culturally affirming care increase the stress along with the inherent stigma of seeking behavioral health care. Further, premigration issues, violence, deprivation, and pre-existing mental health issues can predispose an immigrant child to behavioral health issues. Precipitating factors, such as experiences of bullying, intrafamilial violence, and linguistic factors, can perpetuate behavioral health issues, whereas support within communities, religious beliefs, and inner resilience can serve as protective factors.[21]

In summary, the process of acculturation is multifaceted, complicated, and has an impact on mental health outcomes thus highlighting the need for continued education and research to "reconceptualize acculturation" in the current times.[20,22]

Table 2 US population by race and ethnicity	
White Alone	76.3%
Black or African American alone	13.4%
American Indian and Alaskan Native alone	1.3%
Asian alone	5.9%
Native Hawaiian and other Pacific Islander alone	0.20%
Two or more races	2.8%
Hispanic or Latino	18.5%
White alone, not Hispanic or Latino	60.1%

Source: US Census 2020 Report; https://www.census.gov/newsroom/press-releases/2021.[8]

Acculturative Stress and Mental Health

Literature indicates that acculturation has an impact on both physical and mental health. The process of acculturation can itself be a challenging experience. Berry describes the stress reaction in response to the unique stressors that immigrants experience during the process of acculturation as acculturative stress.

A variety of individual and group characteristics can influence this experience of acculturative stress. Individual characteristics, including age, gender, race, ethnicity, and social support can influence the experience and perception of the acculturation and immigrant experience both before and during the process of acculturation. Other factors that can influence acculturative stress include the circumstances of migration,[24,25] level of education,[17] language proficiency,[17,24] financial difficulties,[17] experiences of discrimination,[26] and familial factors, such as family cohesion.[24,27]

Being treated like a minority or foreigner for the first time, fear of deportation, detainment, or family separation, navigating social support networks, and learning a new language can also contribute to acculturative stress.[28] For example, studies have

Table 3 Glossary of terms	
Acculturation	The process of cultural and psychological change resulting from contact between cultural groups and their members
Acculturative stress	A negative psychological or emotional reaction to the experience of acculturation
Assimilation	A process of acculturation in which individuals do not wish to maintain their heritage culture and seek to participate in the larger society by adopting the cultural values, behaviors, and beliefs of the predominant culture.
Cultural identity	How an individual thinks about himself/herself in relation to their two cultural groups
Immigrant	An individual born outside of the host country or born in the host country and raised by foreign born parents
Integration	An acculturation method in which an individual seeks to maintain his/her heritage culture and participate in the larger society.
Marginalization	An acculturation style in which an individual does not seek to maintain his/her heritage culture or participate in the larger society.
Separation	An acculturation approach in which an individual seeks to maintain his/her heritage culture and avoid participation in the larger society.

Adapted from: Berry J. 2004; Schwartz S. et al 2006

found forced separation to have a negative impact on family functioning and developmental outcomes.[28] Other studies found evidence of the negative impact of acculturative stress on the mental health of immigrant youth.[23,28,29] Sirin et al[29] conducted a longitudinal study on first- and second-generation urban immigrant adolescents, and found that exposure to greater levels of acculturative stress was related to more anxiety, depression, and somatic symptoms. Intergenerational conflict can serve as another layer to acculturative stress, as the next generation adopts more attributes of the dominant culture. Experiences of discrimination and anti-immigrant attitudes can also have negative effects on immigrant youth during adolescence, a developmental phase when they are exploring their identity. Internalized negative views about their group can lead to conflict between the immigrant adolescents and their parents and impact their self-image.[28]

In contrast, family cohesion and social support can serve as protective efforts and help buffer the impact of acculturative stress[27,30] When both the youth and their parents strike a balance between maintaining old and adopting new practices, they benefit from the protective effect of familial and community support.[28,31] Thus, the experience of acculturative stress can be variable across immigrant generations and communities.

It would seem that the stressors of immigration, limited access to resources, and the challenges faced with acculturation would impact and lead to relatively poor health, education, and development outcomes in recent immigrants. However, the literature indicates a paradoxical phenomenon, commonly described as the immigrant paradox wherein recent immigrants can have better health- and education-related outcomes compared to more established or nonimmigrants. For instance, Marks et al[32] describe that "children and adolescents who recently immigrated to the United States have better developmental outcomes when compared to children who have been living in the United States longer or who were born in the United States to immigrant parents." In contrast, Hofferth et al[5] describe how recent immigrant children have higher educational achievement in comparison to children of native-born US parents.

It is important to note that although interesting, the paradox may not be a consistent or uniform experience across generations and cultural groups. Although it highlights the strengths and resilience of immigrant families, it also highlights the risks and challenges associated with acculturation and adaptation to a new culture and community.[4,5] Notably, Breslau et al[4] found that the level of risk for a psychiatric disorder can change within a generation of immigration. Nevertheless, it is essential to describe the immigrant paradox as understanding this effect is vital to appreciating the nuances of cultural, parental, and familial factors that influence acculturation and the associated stress.

Discussion

As described earlier, the influence and interplay between several factors contribute to the stress of acculturation. To better understand the mental health needs of immigrant populations, it is essential for clinicians to have a broader understanding of the often-complex experience of migration and immigration and an appreciation of the process of acculturation and adaptation.

Using clinical vignettes, we discuss and emphasize different clinical and ethical questions that can arise when working with immigrant families. We highlight clinical pearls that can be helpful for clinicians in the context of cross-cultural encounters.

Case Vignette 1

Jane is a 15-year-old child of Bhutanese origin who came to the United States as a refugee with her family. She was born in a settlement camp in Nepal. She is the oldest of three children and is a good student in a local high school. She was seen following a suicide attempt and for treatment of worsening depression. Her pertinent history included bullying at school and peers making fun of her lunches because they smelled funny. She reported being sexually assaulted by a family member and that the family allowed the perpetrator to live in the community and did not alert the authorities.

During the interview, Jane shared that she is the caregiver for her family, who needs her help to translate and help make phone calls because they are not fluent in English. Overall, she shared that she and her family are accepted in the community but the kids in school can be mean. During the COVID-19 pandemic, Jane shared feeling afraid that her family would get hurt because of their Asian appearance and often wished that she could change her appearance. These struggles resulted in her presentation for treatment. The family needed much support as seeking behavioral health care was not as prevalent.

Exploring the child and family's experience with racism and discrimination and the fear of retaliation are important issues to explore. This is not uncommon where children are often parentified and the family depends on them to navigate the system. The ongoing xenophobia in the host culture can be devastating as the family may have faced similar discrimination before immigration.

The effect of migration and its effect on children can be divided into premigration, migration, and post-migration. Prior to the migration, Jane was born in a settlement camp, and it is unclear what the living conditions and the family status were but in talking to the parents it appears that they faced economic hardships and there was a lack of educational support for the children, they lived in harsh settlement camps where they faced an uncertain future and deprivation. After Jane moved, she faced all of the stresses related to adaptation, including access to education, bullying acculturation stress related to religious vies, ethnic food, intergenerational conflict, exclusion, and discrimination.[21]

The use of broaching, a technique used to better understand the impact of cultural, racial, and ethnic nuances that may influence the child and family's presentation for treatment, is important. This technique will also help us to better understand the family's and child's experiences within and outside their community of origin.[33]

Clinical pearls

- When assessing the immigrant child, supportive listening without reacting is important. The fear of judgment and shame may prevent the child from sharing his/her trauma. A common issue in some immigrant cultures where the loss of "face" is particularly important.
- Supporting the family is an implicit message given to immigrant culture. Exploring the child's experiences at school is important as the child has to navigate the continued immersion of the culture of their cultural heritage while navigating the cultural nuances of the dominant host culture.
- Exploring the child and family's experience with racism and discrimination is important. Fear of retaliation may be an additional issue to explore.
- The role of the child psychiatrist would be to utilize the tenets of cultural formulation interview and cultural humility to better understand the child, the family, the community, and the cultural underpinnings to formulate a cogent plan.

Case Vignette 2

Jill is an 11-year-old girl who recently immigrated to the United States. She lives with her mother who primarily speaks Spanish, but Jill is bilingual and speaks both English and Spanish. She presents with anxiety, depression, and passive thoughts of suicide and reports a history of self-harm behaviors in the context of bullying. She feels like she doesn't fit in at school or anywhere and misses her extended family that lives in her country of origin. Jill feels that her mother doesn't understand her experience and the stress associated with having to adjust to a new school and culture.

Jill is presenting with symptoms of anxiety and depression with thoughts of self-harm in the context of the stress of "fitting in" and figuring out where she belongs. Children who are recent immigrants, especially in their preadolescent or adolescent years can struggle with reconciling their cultural and individual identity, with the stress of immigration adding to the stress of this stage of development. Children can often be torn between the desire to fit in, the need or pressure to fit in, and the inherent struggle with fitting into a new cultural, social, and emotional landscape.

Family sessions were conducted with the assistance of an interpreter. Jill's mother actively participated in treatment but doesn't know about the severity of her daughter's symptoms. She shares her worries about Jill being labeled as mentally ill if she is hospitalized or started on medications. The mother believes that the spirits of her ancestors are upset, and she needs to consult her community's spiritual leader for guidance.

In many cultures, there is a significant stigma toward mental health with different beliefs about the practice of Western medicine and psychiatry. The terminology, understanding, stigma, and cultural concepts around mental health can vary across cultures[34,35] and even within families from the same culture. As described earlier, cultural, religious, and linguistic factors can also play a role in the expectations of and experience in treatment. Immigrant families may thus struggle with understanding, accepting, and participating in treatment. In addition, understanding the impact of culture on the patient's illness narrative is also critical in treatment. For instance, in their article on the health care needs of African immigrants, Omenka et al[35] describe culture, religion, and spirituality as important factors influencing the health care experience and mistrust in the health care system, and the lack of affordable, culturally competent care as barriers to accessing care.

In treatment, Jill discloses traumatic experiences that occurred during the process of migration and potential abuse by a relative who lives in the country of origin with whom she no longer has any contact. She also reports a history of physical discipline in childhood by her father and sometimes by her mother who would spank her. She is also hesitant to share the history of abuse by the relative with her mother.

In the context of cross-cultural interactions, it is vital for clinicians to have an open and honest conversation with patients about the different aspects of confidentiality and its limitations. Utilizing transparency in discussions, clinicians may present situations in which confidentiality might need to be broken to protect the patient and to follow state-specific legal responsibilities, including child abuse reporting, and discuss what this would mean for the patient.[25] Exploring the cultural understanding, expectations, or worries about the concept of confidentiality and potential conflicts of interest need to be discussed and addressed to maintain and foster trust in the treatment relationship between the clinician and immigrant family. This is just as important when the clinician and immigrant families share similar or same cultural or ethnic backgrounds.

Jill is eager to try an antidepressant but worries that her mother might not agree with her. Her mother is relatively open to the idea of medications but also worries that medications might impair Jill in her daily life.

The process of informed consent is fundamental to a patient's right to make voluntary decisions and is based on the ethical principles of autonomy and respect for the patient. It also includes the right to refuse treatment. When working with immigrant populations, the process of informed consent can be influenced by many factors, including the patient's level of literacy, language proficiency, knowledge, understanding, and perception of the health care system. Patients may have worries about the process of consent itself, what it entails, their right to refuse treatment, and the process of signing relevant documents. Families may hesitate to share their concerns, worry about the clinician's perceptions of their families' cultural or religious views, and have concerns about the impact or consequences of refusing treatment. It is also important to note that in many cultures treatment decisions are made in consultation with and participation of other family members whose beliefs and perceptions can also influence treatment.[34]

Clinical pearls

- An open, empathetic, and reflective stance can create a safe space for conversations about difficult and conflicting emotions.
- Clinicians should be careful when applying cultural concepts to immigrant families based on the culture of origin, as these can vary across families of the same culture.
- An honest conversation about the tenets of patient confidentiality, including its limitations is crucial to building and maintaining trust in the therapeutic alliance.
- When using interpreter services to obtain informed consent, it is important to have a clear discussion about the different aspects of the treatment, including the right to refuse treatment.

Case Vignette 3

Chioma, a Nigerian American second-year psychiatry resident, was assigned to work with Esther, a 19-year-old Ghanaian born, Liberian with a history of depression, who was admitted for a sixth suicide attempt. Esther was born in Ghana and the daughter of a Liberian asylum seeker who immigrated to the United States following the political unrest in Liberia. She was identified as Ghanaian, whereas her 37-year-old mother was identified as a Liberian. The inpatient team thought that the second-year Nigerian American resident would be a good fit for the patient because they came from "similar cultures." However, Chioma was born in the United States, had never visited Nigeria, and was unfamiliar with the civil war in Liberia. When Chioma approached Esther, the patient instantly felt apprehensive and distrustful of her doctor. Chioma was surprised by how quickly Esther shut down. The treatment team found it difficult to understand why Esther did not gravitate toward Chioma.

Esther and Chioma are both from West Africa, but they were from diverse cultures and had very different immigrant experiences. Chioma was a first-generation immigrant and raised by her parents in an affluent neighborhood. Esther had humble but stable beginnings in Ghana and then moved to a low-income city in the United States. Their backgrounds and upbringings were dissimilar. The resident and the treatment team were faced with a unique opportunity to learn about a new culture. They must not only ask open ended questions but approach Esther with a stance of cultural humility.

Esther had suffered from depression throughout her adolescence and was estranged from her mother, with whom she reunited at the age of 13. The patient was raised from birth by her maternal aunt in Ghana, whereas her mother lived in the United States. Esther had two younger brothers who were born in the United States and lived with their mother throughout their lives.

Within the same family, siblings may be born in different geographic locations. Immigrant children may be raised by different family members and reunite with their parents later in life, thereby affecting the parent–child relationship. Use the experiences shared to draw a family genogram, which includes information reflective of the immigrant experience, such as the location of birth, length of stay in different locations, special circumstances, and additional details about family relationships and emotional relationships.

When Esther arrived in the United States, her mother was not welcoming or loving toward her because she was the product of rape. The patient's mother often told Esther she reminded her of the Liberian rebel fighter who kidnapped and sexually assaulted her. Esther and her mother had a very distant relationship and during arguments, her mother would tell her she wished that she was never born.

Traumatic experiences have a profound impact on the immigrant experience and family dynamics. Ask open-ended questions and seek to understand a patient's narrative of why they immigrated to the host country. Also, be aware that individuals within the same family may have vastly different narratives.

Esther's mother was not supportive or sympathetic when she endured bullying in high school because of her foreign name, accent, and the way she dressed when she first arrived in the United States. Esther did not feel like she fit in anywhere and was shunned by her fellow black peers. She missed her life in Ghana and often asked her mother to send her back to her maternal aunt. Esther became severely depressed and had multiple suicide attempts. However, her mother did not believe in psychotropic medications and utilized a religious healer instead of mental health providers. Esther did not start an antidepressant until she was 18 years and found it hard to find providers because she had Medicaid.

As clinicians, it is important to be aware that immigrants, both young and old, may have experienced a better quality of life in their country of origin because the transition to the host country often presents economic and social hardships. Immigrant youth may express fond memories of their country of origin compared to their current circumstances. Parents' standpoint of seeking new opportunities and a "better life," may feel invalidating and be challenged by the youth's desires to return to their country of origin. Clinicians should also be aware that self-advocacy can place immigrant youth at odds with their parent's beliefs. This is because cultural beliefs impact one's receptiveness toward seeking mental health care over community elders or religious leaders.

Clinical pearls

- Coming from the same geographic region, neighboring countries or the same country does not mean cultural homogeneity. When learning about a new culture the individual should be approached with a stance of curiosity and cultural humility.
- Genograms serve as an important part of the assessment phase of treatment. A genogram can help organize the information obtained about an individual's immigrant experience.
- It is important to understand the inter- and intragenerational trauma associated with genocide and civil war, and how they impact attachment and familial cohesiveness.

- Immigrants and their children may have different opinions about their experiences in the host country. Family interventions should account for these nuances and an array of perspectives.
- Reaching the age of consent presents an important milestone for an immigrant youth whose parents are not in support of seeking mental health care.

SUMMARY

In this nation of immigrants, the acculturative process has impacted the lives of those seeking a new life. Geopolitical factors have influenced the different waves of immigrant populations and changed the landscape of this nation's racial and ethnic makeup.

Upon immigrating, children ad families are left to navigate a new world without the social networks of their country of origin while adopting aspects of the new culture. Berry's study referred to the unique stressors that immigrants experience during the acculturation process as acculturative stress.[23] Family cohesion and social support can buffer the profound effect of leaving one's country of origin.[31] However, the stress which accompanies the process of acculturation may negatively impact the mental health of immigrant populations.

In their review, Balidemaj et al[36] concluded that "acculturation, ethnic identity and mental health are related to one another, affecting both individuals and communities." Their review also reported higher psychological well-being is associated with a higher level of acculturation and ethnic identity.

The acculturative experience is as variable as the immigrant communities. Both individual and community experiences need to be taken into account when evaluating immigrant children and families. There cannot be a one size fits all evaluation and categorization of experiences. Child and adolescent psychiatrists must therefore have an awareness and understanding of the unique issues immigrants face. Clinicians should bear in mind the cultural, religious, and linguistic factors which may influence treatment. Awareness of one's own biases, preconceived notions, and assumptions helps to foster openness to learning about a new culture and understanding how an individual's culture impacts their illness narrative. It is important to be mindful and use principles of cultural humility and broaching as a clinical tool to engage diverse populations in patient-focused communication with continuous self-evaluation by the provider.[33]

Clinicians may also serve as advocates. Providers not only assess, treat, and engage patients but also can serve as advocates to support immigrant families while they navigate larger systems, such as school and other community resources, such as fair housing, religious support, food stamps, and culturally affirming behavioral health and medical care. Educating teachers, employers, behavioral health, and medical providers with culturally affirming care is necessary to support the immigrant family. Furthermore, training community members to be peer support may help engage immigrant families and assist them in seeking much-needed medical and mental health treatment. These efforts will help support immigrant families' ability to integrate into the host communities and acculturate without censure.

In summary, the process of acculturation is a dynamic, bidirectional, and everevolving process. Working with immigrant children and families requires providers to be flexible in their methodology and thinking and not apply a "one size fits all approach."

This article serves as an overview on how to approach matters of forging a therapeutic alliance, supportive listening without reacting, informed consent, and confidentiality, with cultural humility and nonjudgmental curiosity. We also discuss the use of broaching to better understand a child and family. The clinical pearls can be applied to different clinical scenarios and a variety of cross-cultural encounters.

CLINICS CARE POINTS

Clinical Care Points: Recommendations for Clinicians
- Awareness of the impact of culture on the patient's illness narrative and acknowledging the stress experienced with acculturation are essential to the process of treatment.
- Understanding the stigma attached to receiving mental health treatment and empathetic listening can be more effective than imposing treatment.
- Educating providers in schools and integrating community organizations, religious groups, and peer support is important.
- It is crucial to have an honest conversation about the limits of patient confidentiality and the impact on patients when confidentiality needs to be breached.
- It is essential for clinicians to empathize and acknowledge the trauma experienced with migratory experiences while supporting the patient's dignity.
- Clinicians need to be aware of political rhetoric, which may be causing concern in the culturally diverse immigrant communities.
- Training all providers in providing culturally affirming care is of vital importance.
- Diversity among providers is essential while caring for diverse patients. It is also important to recognize that providers and patients may not be culturally homogeneous despite similarities in geographic origins and native cultural practices.
- Patients originating from the same geographic areas of origin and shared cultural identity may have different levels of acculturation and variability in clinical presentations.

DISCLOSURE

The authors have nothing to disclose.

REFERENCES

1. Berry JW. Acculturation. In: Spielberger C, editor. Encyclopedia of applied psychology. Elsevier Inc.; 2004. p. 27–34.
2. Gibson MA. Immigrant adaptation and patterns of acculturation. Human Develop 2001;44(1):19–23.
3. Harker K. Immigrant generation, assimilation, and adolescent psychological well-being. Soc Forces 2001;79(3):969–1004.
4. Breslau J, Aguilar-Gaxiola S, Borges G, et al. Risk for psychiatric disorder among immigrants and their US-born descendants: evidence from the national comorbidity survey-replication. J Nerv Ment Dis 2007;195(3):189.
5. Hofferth SL, Moon UJ. How do they do it? The immigrant paradox in the transition to adulthood. Soc Sci Res 2016;57:177–94.
6. Delgado-Romero EA, Mollen D, Ridley CR. Counseling of racial and ethnic minorities. Encyclopedia Appl Psychol 2004;3:211 5.
7. Immigration and relocation in U.S. History. Library of congress. Available at: https://www.loc.govclassroom-materials/immigration/. Accessed Feburary 22, 2022.
8. US census 2020 report. Available at: https://www.census.gov/library/stories/2021/08/improved-race-ethnicity-measures-reveal-united-states-population-much-more-multiracial.html. Accessed Feburary 22, 2022.

9. Institute Cato, M Baxter A, Nowrasteh A. A Brief History of U.S. Immigration Policy from the Colonial Period to the Present Day (August 3, 2021). Cato Institute, Policy Analysis, No. 919.

10. Samari G, Nagle A, Coleman-Minahan K. Measuring structural xenophobia: US State immigration policy climates over ten years. SSM-Population Health 2021; 16:100938.

11. Redfield R, Linton R, Herskovits MJ. Memorandum for the study of acculturation. Am Anthropol 1936;38(1):149–52. https://doi.org/10.1525/aa.1936.38.1.02a00330.

12. Berry JW. Acculturation: living successfully in two cultures. Int J Intercultural Relations 2005;29(6):697–712.

13. Berry JW. Immigration, acculturation, and adaptation. Appl Psychol 1997; 46(1):5–34.

14. Berry JW. Globalisation and acculturation. Int J Intercultural Relations 2008;32(4): 328–36.

15. Handelsman MM, Gottlieb MC, Knapp S. Training ethical psychologists: an acculturation model. Prof Psychol Res Pr 2005;36(1):59.

16. Yoon E, Chang CT, Kim S, et al. A meta-analysis of acculturation/enculturation and mental health. J Couns Psychol 2013;60(1):15.

17. Choy B, Arunachalam K, Gupta S, et al. Systematic Review: acculturation strategies and their impact on the mental health of migrant populations. Public Health Pract 2021;2:100069.

18. Behrens K, del Pozo MA, Großhennig A, et al. How much orientation towards the host culture is healthy? Acculturation style as risk enhancement for depressive symptoms in immigrants. Int J Soc Psychiatry 2015;61(5):498–505.

19. Sam DL, Berry JW. Acculturation: when individuals and groups of different cultural backgrounds meet. Perspect Psychol Sci 2010;5(4):472–81.

20. Schwartz S, Montgomery M, Briones E. The role of identity in acculturation among immigrant people: theoretical propositions, empirical questions, and applied recommendations. Human Develop 2006;49:1–30.

21. Kirmayer LJ, Narasiah L, Munoz M, et al. Common mental health problems in immigrants and refugees: general approach in primary care. CMAJ 2011;183(12): E959–67.

22. Salant T, Lauderdale DS. Measuring culture: a critical review of acculturation and health in Asian immigrant populations. Soc Sci Med 2003;57(1):71–90.

23. Berry JW, Phinney JS, Sam DL, et al. Immigrant youth: acculturation, identity, and adaptation. Appl Psychol 2006;55(3):303–32.

24. Lueck K, Wilson M. Acculturative stress in Asian immigrants: the impact of social and linguistic factors. Int J Intercultural Relations 2010;34(1):47–57.

25. Lewis FJ, Paik SE, Tseng CF. Deconstructing the legal process for the immigrant population in the United States: ethical implications for mental health professionals. Contemp Fam Ther 2017;39(3):141–9.

26. Joseph TD. "My life was filled with constant anxiety": anti-immigrant discrimination, undocumented status, and their mental health implications for Brazilian immigrants. Race Social Probl 2011;3(3):170–81.

27. Vidal de Haymes M, Martone J, Muñoz L, et al. Family cohesion and social support: protective factors for acculturation stress among low-acculturated Mexican migrants. J Poverty 2011;15(4):403–26.

28. Sirin SR, Sin EJ, Clingain C, et al. The antiimmigrant sentiment and its impact on immigrant families. In: Halford WK, van de Vijver F, editors. Cross-cultural family

research and practice. Elsevier Academic Press; 2020. p. 415–36. https://doi.org/10.1016/B978-0-12-815493-9.00014-4.

29. Sirin SR, Ryce P, Gupta T, et al. The role of acculturative stress on mental health symptoms for immigrant adolescents: a longitudinal investigation. Develop Psychol 2013;49(4):736.
30. Sirin SR, Sin E, Clingain C, et al. Acculturative stress and mental health: implications for immigrant-origin youth. Pediatr Clin North Am 2019;66(3):641–53.
31. Borrego J Jr, Ortiz-González E, Gissandaner TD. Ethnic and Cultural Considerations. In: Pediatric Anxiety Disorders. Academic Press; 2020. p. 461–97. https://doi.org/10.1016/B978-0-12-813004-9.00021-9.
32. Marks AK, Ejesi K, García Coll C. Understanding the US immigrant paradox in childhood and adolescence. Child Develop Perspect 2014;8(2):59–64.
33. Day-Vines N, Cluxton-Keller F, Agorsor C, et al. Strategies for broaching the subjects of race, ethnicity, and culture. J Couns Dev 2021;99:348–57.
34. Yeung A, Kam R. Ethical and cultural considerations in delivering psychiatric diagnosis: reconciling the gap using MDD diagnosis delivery in less-acculturated Chinese patients. Transcultural Psychiatry 2008;45(4):531–52.
35. Omenka OI, Watson DP, Hendrie HC. Understanding the healthcare experiences and needs of African immigrants in the United States: a scoping review. BMC Public Health 2020;20(1):1–13.
36. Balidemaj A, Small M. The effects of ethnic identity and acculturation in mental health of immigrants: A literature review. Int J Soc Psychiatry 2019;65(7-8):643–55. https://doi.org/10.1177/0020764019867994. PMID: 31478453.

Clinical Considerations for Immigrant, Refugee, and Asylee Youth Populations

Vincenzo Di Nicola, MPhil, MD, PhD[a,b,c,d,*], Marissa Leslie, MD[e,*],
Camila Haynes, MD[f], Kanya Nesbeth, MD[f]

KEYWORDS

• Immigrant • Refugee • Asylum • Child • Adolescent • Youth

KEY POINTS

• Immigration policies that have positive effects on child mental health and promote healthy child development prioritize family preservation and child development, improve care and appropriate custody of children and ensure access to social safety nets for immigrant children and families.

• The COVID-19 pandemic had disproportionately greater effects on immigrant, refugee, and asylee populations.

• Overall, youth of immigrant backgrounds are better adjusted in countries with better immigrant integration and multicultural policies.

INTRODUCTION

Throughout global history, migration has persisted. According to the United Nations, youth ages 19 or under comprise 14% of the world's migrant population and half of the world's refugees (. In the first half of 2021, there were *26.6 million* refugees in the world—the highest ever seen; 50.9 million internally displaced people; and. 4.4 million asylum-seekers.[1] Over the years, there have been increasing numbers of refugees and asylum seekers trying to escape unfavorable conditions in their homelands. In response, many countries—including the US—developed extreme policies to deter mass numbers of refugees seeking entry into the country.

Funded by: CANADALETR.
[a] Canadian Association of Social Psychiatry (CASP); [b] World Association of Social Psychiatry (WASP); [c] Department. of Psychiatry & Addictions, University of Montreal; [d] Department of Psychiatry & Behavioral Sciences, The George Washington University; [e] Georgetown University School of Medicine; [f] Howard University Hospital
* Corresponding authors.
E-mail addresses: vincenzodinicola@gmail.com (V.D.N.); mleslie@ahm.com (M.L.)

Child Adolesc Psychiatric Clin N Am 31 (2022) 679–692
https://doi.org/10.1016/j.chc.2022.06.010
1056-4993/22/© 2022 Elsevier Inc. All rights reserved.

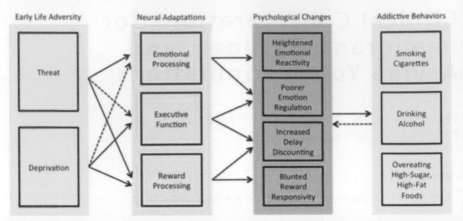

Fig. 1. The effect of 2 dimensions of early life adversity (ELA)–threat and deprivation–on brain development. Neural adaptions to ELA affect emotion, reward, and cognitive networks. These neural adaptions affect 4 psychological processes that have downstream consequences for health-risk behaviors. Smoking cigarettes, drinking alcohol, and overeating highly palatable foods further heighten emotional regulation, increase delay discounting, and blunt reward responsivity, leading to a positive feedback loop for addictive behaviors. Duffy, K.A., McLaughlin, K.A. and Green, P.A. (2018), Early life adversity and health-risk behaviors: proposed psychological and neural mechanisms. Ann. N.Y. Acad. Sci., 1428: 151–169. https://doi.org/10.1111/nyas.13928.

UNACCOMPANIED MINORS AND FAMILY SEPARATION

One such strategy of deterring immigration in the United States was "forced separation" of children and adolescents from their parents, despite the credible warning of the inevitable "traumatic psychological injury."[2,3] This was conducted without a systematic plan for reunification in place.[2] Quite often "reunification has failed for migrant children in custody as relatives or kinship members may be undocumented or parents may be deported."[4] Many if not most arrivals to the border already experienced significant trauma only for the children and adolescents to be met with the trauma of being separated from their parents. Such an experience would be considered an Adverse Childhood Event (**Fig. 1**).[5,6] "ACEs are linked with the disruption of neurodevelopment and with negative effects on social, emotional, and cognitive functioning.[7,8] ACEs have also been associated with negative intergenerational effects.[9]" Repeated adverse events put them at risk for developing toxic stress as well as overtime developing poor coping strategies and resorting to substance use, violence and likely developing mental illness[10,75]

Children can navigate "great hardship in the presence of parents with whom they feel protected and cared for." The act of separating the 2 compromises the child's ability to self-regulate and develop resilience.[6,11] It was theorized that the separation "exacerbated pre-existing trauma from events and incidents in their home country." Hampton and colleagues demonstrated that even after reunification, "most met diagnostic criteria for post-traumatic stress disorder (PTSD), major depressive disorder (MDD), or generalized anxiety disorder (GAD)."[2]

For both parents and children, psychiatric symptoms were present at the time of the family separation as well as the time of the examination postreunification. Chief concerns included feelings of confusion, general upset to severely depressed mood, constant worry/preoccupations, frequent crying, difficulty sleeping, difficulty eating (loss of appetite), recurring nightmares, and overwhelming anxiety. The asylum-seekers also reported physiologic manifestations of anxiety and panic (racing heart, shortness of breath, and headaches) as well as experiencing "pure agony," emotional and mental despair, hopelessness, and being "incredibly despondent.[2]"

"The children exhibited reactions that included regression in age-appropriate behaviors, such as crying, not eating, having nightmares and other sleeping difficulties, excessive parental attachment, clinging to caregivers, urinary incontinence, and recurring feelings of fear following reunification with their parents."[2]

Though less common, some asylum-seeking children have also been known to develop pervasive refusal syndrome (PRS). PRS is a "severe life-threatening condition that affects young asylum seekers" typically with comorbid depression, anxiety, or PTSD. Depressive Devitalization (DD) forms within the spectrum of this condition but is a more passive form of refusal. PRS typically requires hospitalization and even nasogastric feedings as part of management. "A premorbid high-achieving, perfectionist, conscientious personality seems to play an important role in the etiology of PRS generally, as can a psychiatric history of parents or child."[12]

Family is the cornerstone "for emotional and social support for resettled refugee youth." The structure allows them to develop resilience and adapt in the face of the adversity associated with "war and displacement." In the absence of the "secure attachments" formed with parents, these minors can find it difficult to develop a sense of identity. For refugee minors who remained unaccompanied, it makes sense that they would make efforts to develop a sense of a support system or simulated family dynamics, with "employees, foster parents, significant others" social workers and so forth as they moved toward integration.[13]

PSYCHIATRIC SEQUALAE OF FAMILY SEPARATION AND THERAPEUTIC OPTIONS

Asylum-seeking youth typically experience numerous external, internal, and community-based losses starting from the premigration period.[14,15] Even after reunification, they might experience "the psychological absence of parents who are very overwhelmed themselves by the magnitude of their losses." Additionally, the stresses that a parent may have due to resettling, such as concern about finances, can impact the mental health of the minor.[14]

There is an "increasing interest in systemic approaches to refugee care, moving beyond the individual level and emphasizing dynamics within family and community contexts." This is largely based on the understanding that "cultural idioms of distress" common to a culture or family can be an important manifestation of mental health symptoms[14] and might even inform management strategies.

"Migrant adolescents are at a higher risk than their native-born counterparts of psychiatric disorders, and their care is a public health issue." Not only do they often require treatment of longer periods of time, but their condition is often resistant to the "First Line Therapists (FLT)." As a result, alternative therapeutic techniques must be considered. One such alternative is "transcultural psychotherapy" (developed in France). "The clinical approach relies on elements from systemic and psychoanalytic family therapy, narrative therapy, and cultural mediation. The patient, accompanied by his or her family, is received by a group of therapists (psychiatrists, psychologists, and nurses) of diverse cultural origins, trained in transcultural psychotherapy; the group also includes trainees." This technique provides a better foundation for a therapeutic alliance to develop. Other countries such as the US are encouraging strategies such as teaching providers' cultural competency, "ethnic matching" of therapist and patient as well as supervision and developed models relying on interpreters and cultural mediators.[16]

EFFECTS OF THE COVID-19 PANDEMIC

Coronavirus disease 2019 (COVID-19) has profoundly affected life all over the world. Factors such as isolation, contact restrictions, and economic shutdown imposed a "complete change in the psychosocial environment of affected countries." The situation has affected children, adolescents, and their families in distinct ways.[2,76]The life course of children and adolescents who are refugees, asylum, and unaccompanied minors were fraught with adverse childhood experiences (ACEs) prepandemic, ultimately making them more susceptible to the effects of the pandemic than children without said experiences. Most significantly, ACEs are associated with a higher risk for developing mental health problems.[13] Maltreatment has been associated with consequent heightened neural response to signals of threat[17] which leads to an increase in emotional reactivity and a decrease in emotional regulation.[18] This suggests that children and adolescents who experienced adversity before the pandemic are at higher risk to develop anxiety and adopt dysfunctional strategies to cope with the COVID-19-associated challenges such as developing addictive behaviors.[13,18]

"Pandemics such as COVID-19 have population-level mental health effects, with vulnerable groups such as migrants" (Qiu and colleagues, 2020)[19] "having a greater mental health risk" (Morganstein, Fullerton, Ursano, Donato, & Holloway, 2017).[20] "Social distancing measures and the closing of schools and places of work also meant increased boredom and isolation as well as reduced daily structure, negatively affecting overall functioning of children and youth."[21] At the same time, some clinicians noted that "having experienced violence and war before migration, families showed resilience while adapting to the current crisis."[21] Reasons for this could be varied. Further insight into the level of trauma-informed work and coping tools already provided to these specific children and families would be useful in understanding the contributing factors to their ability to cope with the stress induced by the pandemic.

Encounters at the border, including those with unaccompanied minors, plummeted in early 2020 amid the beginnings of the COVID-19 pandemic but have since risen steadily, reaching an all-time high—with nearly 150,000 unaccompanied minors at or near the US–Mexico border in 2021. About 76% of unaccompanied children in federal care are 15 years of age or older, though authorities have detained infants and toddlers.[22] Immigration detention facilities are congregate settings whereby the infection rate and death toll from COVID-19 are disproportionately high.[23] The number of people per month who tested positive for SARS-CoV-2 in ICE detention between April and August 2020 was between 5.7 to 21.8 times higher than the case rate of the US general population during that same time.[24] Eighty percent of refugees in ICE detention centers reported never being able to maintain a six-foot distance from others in their eating area. 96% reported that they were less than six feet from their neighbor while sleeping. Eighty-two percent of people reported not having access to hand sanitizer anywhere in the detention facility. Interviewees reported long wait times to see a medical professional, with an average wait time of 100 hours.[25] Further, studies have shown that "airway infections are a leading cause for acute morbidity in underage refugees." They are often subjected to refugee camps and communal living spaces before arriving in their destination country which makes them more susceptible to communicable diseases such as COVID-19.[26]

Exacerbating this, refugees often come across language barriers in the country of destination and because of this they often do not get the latest information regarding COVID-19-preventive measures and guidelines.[27,28] This, as well as administrative, financial, and legal barriers, cumulatively prevent refugees from accessing health care services and thus, they remain excluded from COVID-19 testing and treatment.[29–31] This may be more exaggerated for unaccompanied refugees who have limited adult guidance and supervision with regards to hand hygiene, social distancing and mask wearing. This population has always struggled with access to care due to barriers such as lack of transportation, "navigating complex medical and insurance systems, overcoming language and cultural barriers, institutional mistrust, and the residual impacts of trauma."[32] However, the disruptions and duration of the pandemic presented new barriers and enhanced some that already existed. These barriers are primarily rooted in a lack of resources available to marginalized and underserved populations. While the use of technology such as computers and access to the internet became the norm for many, access to these "could not be presumed when working with this population."[33] Even when technology and internet were present to facilitate tele-medicine, these children and adolescents still faced these barriers as a result of their family and home structures such as lack of privacy, sharing rooms with other members of the household, inadequate or insufficient interpretation services and "reduced proficiency in technology."[33,34] Many parents were laid off which led to food and housing insecurity, and increased difficulty in accessing health insurance. Because of undocumented status, many families were unable to receive government relief packages.[21,35] Schools implemented remote education which simply was not feasible for many who had technological barriers.[21]

COVID-19 also created barriers to access to legal support for refugees. Widespread border closures prevented refugees from their right to seek asylum. Movement restrictions coupled with legal status concerns can limit access to health care services and hamper the delivery of medical supplies and doctors.[36] The closure of courts and the reduced activities of authorities caused even slower asylum processes and the postponement of legal decisions concerning refugee status associated with a general reduction of administrative services.[28] Also, some search and rescue operations were put on hold due to logistical difficulties in the context of lockdowns and travel bans.[31]

In addition to restrictions on daily activities requiring families to stay at home together, many refugee parents have also suddenly been required to fulfill the full-time role of childcare and educator for children as school and day-care were no longer open.[37] Alternatively, many refugee parents work in jobs that are deemed to be "essential service" jobs in the context of COVID-19, which often leaves children unsupervised. Consistent with family stress models of children's mental health difficulties, this stress increases susceptibility to relational conflict and in extreme cases, family violence.[38,39] Compounding this is the reality that many refugees (parents and children) have limited access to the police, legal and social services and safe shelters owing to the lack of registration and a prevalent fear of authorities.[31]

In 1959, the UN declared that all children have a right to protection, education, health care, shelter, and good nutrition.[40] While we know the refugees, asylum, and unaccompanied minors are often not protected in these regards, the pandemic has further challenged these basic rights. The "pandemic highlights entrenched inequalities in health, education, and economic opportunity and the effects of racism and xenophobia through COVID-19's disproportionate harm to minorities and vulnerable populations."[21]

IDENTITY FORMATION AND YOUTH IMMIGRANT POPULATIONS

The development of one's personal identity is a complex process. Education and interpersonal relationships are important pillars and have implications for adolescent adjustment and psychological well-being.[41] There are 2 processes involved in establishing personal identity: exploration, which refers to the active questioning and weighing of alternative roles, beliefs, values, and life plans, before deciding which to adopt and pursue; and commitment making, which involves personal investment in particular alternatives, and the adoption of a course of action that will lead to the implementation of these choices.[42] For refugees and immigrants, their development of identity is further complicated by their immigrant status. Ethnic Identity refers to the sense of membership one has with regard to his/her cultural background, ethnic heritage, or racial phenotype while national identity refers to the sense of belonging to the nation.[43] In a longitudinal study in Greece, which investigated immigrant adolescents in middle school, it was found that exploration and commitment to ethnic, national and personal identities all occurred simultaneously. Ethnic and national identities were linked negatively over time and were disconnected from the youths' formation of personal identity which authors attributed to the assimilatory society which discouraged the achieving of dual identities.

Four acculturation strategies are defined: assimilation, separation, integration, and marginalization. Assimilation is the adopting the receiving culture and discarding the heritage culture; separation, the rejecting of the receiving culture and retaining the heritage culture; integration, the adopting the receiving culture and retaining the heritage culture; and marginalization, rejecting both the heritage and receiving cultures.[44] The "need" for ethnic identity within a given immigrant group may be directly related to that group's extent of perceived cultural difference from the dominant host-national group.[45] Perceived rejection from the host-national group may cause immigrants to detach from the national identity and from the labels that the ethnic group imposes on them. Some ethnic groups may even make their own labels to distinguish themselves from other members of the nation and to express pride in that distinction. Examples include Chicano (Mexican Americans) and Boricua (Puerto Ricans residing on the United States mainland).[46]

Native residents, as well as second-generation immigrants with only one foreign-born parent, are more likely to be in favor of assimilation compared with first-generation immigrants and second-generation immigrants with 2 foreign-born parents. First- and second-generation immigrants (with both parents born abroad) are more supportive of multiculturalism than natives are. The preference for multiculturalism among residents with an immigration background is in keeping with the theoretic argument that this model creates less acculturation stress. In one longitudinal study in Luxembourg, support for assimilation among the native population increased significantly within a 10-year period. As realistic group conflict theory implies, this increase in preference for assimilation can be attributed to the increased diversity of the society during this period. Interestingly, nonnatives also displayed a very similar growth in support of assimilation. Authors proposed that these results might be explained by the fact that the heterogeneity of these multilingual and multinational societies forces all residents to find common ground on which they can live together, resulting in increased support for assimilation and decreased support for multiculturalism, even among residents with a migratory background.[47]

School and home are very important aspects of adolescents' lives and the shaping of their identities through interactions. Adolescents' acculturation orientations are influenced by the perceived acculturation orientations endorsed by their migrant parents and the perceived acculturation preferences of their nonmigrant classmates. Parents' influences are significantly stronger than classmates' influences with regard to adolescents' adoption of the destination culture. This suggests that parents are perceived as the primary socialization context, particularly as it pertains to the adaptation of destination culture.[48] This does not minimize the role school plays in acculturation and identity formation. In fact, positive teacher–student relationships are linked to higher self-esteem[49] as well as a more positive attitude toward the majority group.[43] Ethnic identity may also be a protective factor by buffering the negative effect of perceived teacher discrimination on children's academic attitudes and school belonging.[50] Higher mainstream language fluency indirectly encourages adopting parts of the destination culture as it has been linked to better grades, lower school absenteeism, and less disruptive behavior in class[51] as well as to greater support from classmates. Cross-ethnic friendships are also linked to positive outcomes such as greater well-being, greater conflict-solving ability, higher self-esteem, and better social adjustment.[52]

The general society can also shape immigrant adolescents' ethnic and national identities as well. Assimilationist societies force immigrants to choose between their ethnic and cultural identities thus generating conflict between both while multicultural societies which are more receptive give immigrant youth the space and option to nurture, explore and keep both which leads to less conflict between the 2.[53] Large, united immigrant groups may be viewed as most threatening to host nationals and natives' views are most negative during times of mass immigration.[54] When the majority group believes that the minority group is threatening their economic, cultural, and future societal position, they become less open to diversity and prefer assimilative strategies. Even in a country with objectively low levels of realistic and symbolic threat and a generally positive attitude toward the foreign community, threat perceptions seem to be closely linked to native residents' acculturation preferences. Stronger perceptions of threat are related to more support for assimilation among all residents and to less support for multiculturalism among native residents and culturally close immigrants. More contact with natives is associated with more support for assimilation among culturally close immigrants and with more threat perceptions among culturally distant immigrants, which is indirectly associated with more support for assimilation.[55] A higher level of education was associated with more positive attitudes toward unaccompanied refugee minors (URM).[56]

Politics also influence identity of the URM population. Defensive measures such as travel bans and deportation of illegal immigrants may be the result of increased perceived threat and this in turn also stifle the immigrants' identity. As ethnic and national identity influence personal identity, hostility toward these groups may also impact personal identity. Some states have banned ethnic-centered classes as a way to prevent the ethnic community from developing. Defensive policies hinder immigrant bicultural development.[57] Right-wing political attitudes led to a lower acceptance of URM, showing that a more conservative political attitude led to lower levels of acceptance regarding the intake of more refugees than a more liberal attitude.[58]

The different types of acculturation have also been connected with mental illness. Stronger ethnic identity is linked to fewer depressive symptoms and internalizing and externalizing behaviors, greater self-esteem, well-being, life satisfaction, school engagement, academic achievement, and better physical health.[59] Those who endorsed a marginalized acculturation style showed the strongest association between severity of acculturative hassles and PTSD. Older age was found to attenuate the relationship between trauma and symptoms of depression. The marginalized and separated groups reported higher depression symptom levels than the assimilated and integrated groups, suggesting that having an acculturative style that excludes participation in the host culture or both the host culture and ethnic culture has a potential negative effect of not feeling a sense of identification, and it may create additional challenges.[60] Studies have highlighted that first-generation immigrants show poorer psychological adaptation (lower life satisfaction, self-esteem, and greater psychological problems) compared with the second generation.[61]

Overall, youth of immigrant backgrounds are better adjusted in countries with better immigrant integration and multicultural policies.[62] Initial high levels of ethnic identity may help the refugee youth to establish supportive relationships with other members of their ethnic group, which in turn may provide more psychological safety. The maintenance and further development of one's ethnic identity provide a certain amount of continuity in their self-perception and identity.[63] Studies suggest that 4 or 5 years after arrival, refugees "return to normal life" wherein they adapt to aspects of majority culture while their attachment to the country and culture of origin are less complicated.[63]

POLITICS AND EFFECTS ON YOUTH MENTAL HEALTH

As policies relating to asylum and immigration differ across the world, several key concerns have been raised about the management of unaccompanied children or the effects of family separation on child development and well-being.[64] Whereas immigration policies affect the mental health of children fleeing persecution, many policies are not developed with the consideration of a child's mental health or well-being.[64]

Asylum procedures are often guided by concerns about enforcement instead of protection. Tasked with a law-enforcement mandate, US Customs and Border Patrol (CBP) facilities have been described as "inhumane" with references to lack of bedding and bathing facilities, inadequate access to food and water, open toilets, confiscation of belongings, and lack of access to essential medical care, sexual violence by staff against children custody, inappropriate use of solitary confinement, and lack of timely medical treatment contributing to the death of at least 9 children under immigration custody since 2018.[65]

Political, ethical, and logistical challenges are created because of this debate between enforcement versus protection.[66] Deterring migrants from crossing borders were implicit in US immigration policy from 2016 to 2020.[66] The increased focus on enforcement had social, emotional, and developmental repercussions for the children involved in migration to the US–Mexico border.

In the US when children come to the border, they are placed in CBP. Under the trafficking victims protection reauthorization act, unaccompanied children must be transferred within 72 hours from CBP custody to the Office of Refugee Resettlement which manages 170 shelters, group homes, foster care and therapeutic facilities across the country. The increase of children and families in immigration detention was amplified by the "zero tolerance" policy in April 2018, which criminalized crossing the border to seek asylum.[67]

In contrast, Canada's immigration policies embrace different priorities. Immigration is a part of the economic growth strategy of Canada.[68] Therefore, immigration policies allow for a temporary pathway to permanent residency.[68] Immigration is easier for applicants seeking Canadian residence status who work in "essential" jobs. These jobs include cashiers, janitors, and butchers. In addition, graduate students and health care workers can seek a temporary pathway to permanent Canadian residency.[68] Before the COVID-19 pandemic, Canadian immigration previously prioritized English-speaking skilled workers.[68] Since the 2019 COVID-19 pandemic, the criteria for pathways to Canadian residency have broadened.[68]

Steele and colleagues (2002) looked at health and social policy changes in Ontario, Canada, and the effect on recent immigrants and refugees in inner-city Toronto. They postulated that socio-economic factors are likely more important as determinants of health for immigrants versus nonimmigrants and that, therefore, during times of policy change affecting the socio-economic environment, immigrants are more vulnerable.

Women seemed to bear disproportionately higher burden as primary caregivers whose financial independence is affected by cuts to welfare, home care support, and community services.[69]

When thinking about immigrant children today, we are likely to picture clusters of youth crowded into unsanitary detention centers, scared and crying behind wired fences[70] The zero-tolerance policy enacted in April 2018 in the United States put a spotlight on the more than 5400 children separated from their parents at the US–Mexico border, along with thousands more kept in detention with their families.[70] But, the category of immigrant children is significantly larger than those caught in the turbulence at the US southern border. Immigrant children, defined comprehensively as all children of all immigrants living anywhere within the United States, represent 19.6 million children, nearly 1/4 of all children in the United States.[71,72] This is a heterogeneous group that includes refugees, asylum-seekers, recipients of the deferred action for childhood arrival policy or of special temporary status, and unaccompanied minors.[70] The group also includes first-generation Americans- US citizens by birth, any children born to immigrant parents or those living in households in which at least one parent is an immigrant.[70]

The topic of immigration and child mental health shines a light on what some call "political determinants of health."[70] This is the idea that nearly all of the social determinants of health are affected by political decisions.[70] Policy making can also positively impact children. For example, social safety net programs such as the Children's Health Insurance Program (US), the Canada Child Benefit are products of political wrangling that led to policies of value for children's health.[70]

Policies such as child and family separation, however, have been associated with negative mental health effects such as trauma exacerbation, fear, anxiety, and depression. If conditions in detention facilities for youth in detention are substandard, the consequence can even be death.[70]

Immigration policies that have positive effects on child mental health and promote healthy child development have 4 characteristics.[73,74] Bassett and Yoshikawa, 2020 recommend[73]:

1. Prioritize Family Preservation
2. The policies prioritize child development by enlisting trained and licensed child welfare professionals with expertise in children's psychological, emotional and physical needs and ensuring hygienic, child-friendly spaces for screening and processing children's cases.
3. Improve care and appropriate custody of children.
4. Ensure access to social safety nets for immigrant children and families.

Children are innocent bystanders in the varying political conflicts and tensions in the global immigration debate. In the Universal Declaration of Human Rights, the United Nations has proclaimed that childhood is entitled to special care and assistance. As clinicians and child advocates, we are uniquely positioned to offer scientific and clinical input into policy for the ultimate benefit of immigrant, refugee children, children of recent immigrants, and children seeking asylum.

CLINICS CARE POINTS

- It is important to evaluate ACE risk factors in migrant youth.
- Consider alternative therapeutic techniques in migrant youth demonstrating resistance to psychotherapy.

- Assessing the stressors parents or caregivers of migrant youth are encountering can contribute to more effective treatment of the child.
- If working in an immigration assessment setting, advocate for hygienic and child-friendly spaces during screening and processing.

DISCLOSURE

Authors have nothing to disclose.

REFERENCES

1. USA for UNHCR. Refugee statistics. Available at: https://www.unrefugees.org/refugee-facts/statistics/. Accessed March 20, 2022.
2. Hampton K, Raker E, Habbach H, Camaj Deda L, Heisler M, Mishori R. The psychological effects of forced family separation on asylum-seeking children and parents at the US-Mexico border: a qualitative analysis of Medico-legal documents. PLOS ONE 2021;16(11). https://doi.org/10.1371/journal.pone.0259576.
3. Barajas J. Trump administration was warned of 'traumatic psychological injury' from family separations, official says. PBS. 2018. Available at: https://www.pbs.org/newshour/politics/trump-administration-was-warned-of-traumatic-psychological-injury-from-family-separations-official-says. Accessed March 6, 2022.
4. Monico C, Mendez-Sandoval J. Group and child–family migration from Central America to the United States: forced child–family separation, reunification, and Pseudo adoption in the Era of Globalization. Genealogy 2019;3(4):68.
5. Oral R, Ramirez M, Coohey C, et al. Adverse childhood experiences and trauma informed care: the future of health care. Pediatr Res 2016;79(1–2):227–33. https://doi.org/10.1038/pr.2015.197.
6. Teicher MH. Childhood trauma and the enduring consequences of forcibly separating children from parents at the United States border. BMC Med 2018;16(1). https://doi.org/10.1186/s12916-018-1147-y.
7. Felitti VJ, Anda RF, Nordenberg D, Williamson DF, Spitz AM, Edwards V, et al. Relationship of childhood abuse and household dysfunction to many of the leading causes of death in adults: the adverse childhood experiences (ACE) study. Am J Prev Med 2019. https://doi.org/10.1016/j.amepre.2019.04.001. PMID: 31104722.
8. Oh DL, Jerman P, Marques SS, Koita K, Ipsen A, Purewal S, et al. Systematic review of pediatric health outcomes associated with adverse childhood experiences (aces). https://doi.org/10.1016/j.amepre. 2018.11.030 PMID: 30905481
9. Lê-Scherban F, Wang X, Boyle-Steed KH, Pachter LM. Intergenerational associations of parent adverse childhood experiences and child health outcomes. Pediatrics 2018;(6):141. https://doi.org/10.1542/peds.2017-4274. PMID: 29784755.
10. Wood LCN. Impact of punitive immigration policies, parent-child separation and child detention on the mental health and development of children. BMJ Paediatr Open 2018;2(1):e000338.
11. MacKenzie MJ, Bosk E, Zeanah CH. Separating families at the border - consequences for Children's health and well-being. N Engl J Med 2017;376(24): 2314–5. https://doi.org/10.1056/NEJMp1703375.
12. Ngo T, Hodes M. Pervasive refusal syndrome in asylum-seeking children: review of the current evidence. Clin Child Psychol Psychiatry 2020;25(1):227–41. https://doi.org/10.1177/1359104519846580.

13. Fegert JM, Vitiello B, Plener PL, Clemens V. Challenges and burden of the coronavirus 2019 (COVID-19) pandemic for Child and adolescent mental health: a narrative review to highlight clinical and research needs in the acute phase and the long return to normality. Child Adolesc Psychiatry Ment Health 2020; 14(1). https://doi.org/10.1186/s13034-020-00329-3.

14. Rabiau MA. Culture, migration, and Identity Formation in adolescent refugees: a family perspective. J Fam Social Work 2018;22(1):83–100. https://doi.org/10. 1080/10522158.2019.1546950.14.

15. Andersson ES, Skar AMS, Jensen TK. Unaccompanied refugee minors and resettlement: Turning points towards integration. Eur J Social Psychol 2021;1–30. https://doi.org/10.1002/ejsp.2761.

16. Grau L, Carretier E, Moro MR, et al. A qualitative exploration of what works for migrant adolescents in transcultural psychotherapy: perceptions of adolescents, their parents, and their therapists. BMC Psychiatry 2020;20(1):564.

17. Hein TC, Monk CS. Research Review: neural response to threat in children, adolescents, and adults after child maltreatment - a quantitative meta-analysis. J Child Psychol Psychiatry 2017;58(3):222–30. https://doi.org/10.1111/jcpp. 12651.

18. Duffy KA, McLaughlin KA, Green PA. Early life adversity and health-risk behaviors: proposed psychological and neural mechanisms. Ann N Y Acad Sci 2018; 1428(1):151–69. https://doi.org/10.1111/nyas.13928.

19. Qiu J, Shen B, Zhao M, Wang Z, Xie B, Xu Y. A nationwide survey of psychological distress among Chinese people in the COVID-19 epidemic: implications and policy recommendations [published correction appears in Gen Psychiatry. Gen Psychiatry 2020;33(2):e100213.

20. Morganstein JC, Fullerton CS, Ursano RJ, Donato D, Holloway HC. Pandemics: health care Emergencies. In: Ursano RJ, Fullerton CS, Weisaeth L, Raphael B, editors. Textbook of Disaster Psychiatry. 2nd ed. Cambridge: Cambridge University Press; 2017. p. 270 84. https://doi.org/10.1017/9781316481424.019.

21. Endale T, Jean N St, Birman D. Covid-19 and refugee and immigrant youth: a community-based mental health perspective. Psychol Trauma 2020;12(S1). https://doi.org/10.1037/tra0000875.

22. Cheatham A, Roy D. U.S. detention of child migrants. Council on Foreign Relations. 2021. Available at: https://www.cfr.org/backgrounder/us-detention-child-migrants#chapter-title-0-2. Accessed March 10, 2022.

23. Press A. US extends heightened border enforcement during coronavirus. VOA. 2020. Available at: https://www.voanews.com/a/usa_immigration_us-extends-heightened-border-enforcement-during-coronavirus/6189600.html. Accessed March 10, 2022.

24. Carmody| S. ACLU files class action lawsuit to press for release of ice detainees. Michigan Radio. 2020. Available at: https://www.michiganradio.org/law/2020-04-27/aclu-files-class-action-lawsuit-to-press-for-release-of-ice-detainees. Accessed March 10, 2022.

25. Praying for hand soap and masks. Physicians for Human Rights. 2021. Available at: https://phr.org/our-work/resources/praying-for-hand-soap-and-masks/. Accessed March 10, 2022.

26. Müller F, Hummers E, Hillermann N, et al. Factors influencing the frequency of airway infections in underage refugees: a Retrospective, cross Sectional study. Int J Environ Res Public Health 2020;17(18):6823.

27. Høvring R. 10 things you should know about coronavirus and refugees. NRC. Available at: https://www.nrc.no/news/2020/march/10-things-you-should-know-about-coronavirus-and-refugees/. Accessed March 10, 2022.

28. Kluge HH, Jakab Z, Bartovic J, D'Anna V, Severoni S. Refugee and migrant health in the COVID-19 response. Lancet 2020;395(10232):1237–9.

29. Alemi Q, Stempel C, Siddiq H, Kim E. Refugees and COVID-19: achieving a comprehensive public health response. WHO 2020. Available at: https://www.who.int/bulletin/volumes/98/8/20-271080.pdf. Accessed March 10, 2022.

30. Vonen HD, Olsen ML, Eriksen SS, Jervelund SS, Eikemo TA. Refugee camps and COVID-19: can we prevent a humanitarian crisis? Scand J Public Health 2021; 49(1):27–8. https://doi.org/10.1177/1403494820934952.

31. Bohnet H, Rüegger S. Refugees and Covid-19: beyond health risks to insecurity. Swiss Polit Sci Rev 2021;27(2):353–68. https://doi.org/10.1111/spsr.12466.

32. Hunter K, Knettel B, Reisinger D, et al. Examining Health Care Access for refugee children and families in the North Carolina triangle area. North Carolina Med J 2020;81(6):348–54. https://doi.org/10.18043/ncm.81.6.348.

33. Birkenstock L, Chen T, Chintala A, et al. Pivoting a community-based participatory research project for mental health and immigrant youth in Philadelphia during COVID-19. Health Promotion Pract 2021;23(1):32–4. https://doi.org/10.1177/15248399211033311.

34. Brickhill-Atkinson M, Hauck FR. Impact of covid-19 on resettled refugees. Prim Care Clin Off Pract 2021;48(1):57–66. https://doi.org/10.1016/j.pop.2020.10.001.

35. Page KR, Venkataramani M, Beyrer C, Polk S. Undocumented U.S. immigrants and covid-19. New Engl J Med 2020;(21):382. https://doi.org/10.1056/nejmp2005953.

36. Lau LS, Samari G, Moresky RT, et al. Covid-19 in humanitarian settings and lessons learned from past epidemics. Nat Med 2020;26(5):647–8. https://doi.org/10.1038/s41591-020-0851-2.

37. Heymann DL, Shindo N. WHO scientific and Technical Advisory group for infectious Hazards. COVID-19: what is next for public health? Lancet 2020; 395(10224):542–5. https://doi.org/10.1016/S0140-6736(20)30374-3.

38. Thompson LA, Rasmussen SA. What does the coronavirus disease 2019 (COVID-19) mean for families? JAMA Pediatr 2020;174(6):628. https://doi.org/10.1001/jamapediatrics.2020.0828.

39. Browne DT, Smith JA, Jde Basabose. Refugee children and families during the COVID-19 crisis: a resilience framework for mental health. J Refugee Stud 2021;34(1):1138–49. https://doi.org/10.1093/jrs/feaa113.

40. Convention on the rights of the child - unicef.org. Available at: https://www.unicef.org/turkmenistan/sites/unicef.org.turkmenistan/files/2019-09/GC-21-EN.pdf. Accessed March 11, 2022.

41. Dimitrova R, Buzea C, Taušová J, Uka F, Zakaj S, Crocetti E. Relationships between identity domains and life satisfaction in minority and majority youth in Albania, Bulgaria, Czech Republic, Kosovo, and Romania. Eur J Developmental Psychol 2018;15(1):61–82. https://doi.org/10.1080/17405629.2017.1336997.

42. Kroger J, Marcia JE. The identity statuses: origins, meanings, and interpretations. Handbook Identity Theor Res 2011;31–53. https://doi.org/10.1007/978-1-4419-7988-9_2.

43. Umaña-Taylor AJ, Kornienko O, McDermott ER, Motti-Stefanidi F. National identity development and friendship Network dynamics among immigrant and non-immigrant youth. J Youth Adolescence 2020;49(3):706–23. https://doi.org/10.1007/s10964-019-01181-1.

44. Berry JW, Padilla AM. Acculturation: theory, models and some new findings. Acculturation as varieties of adaption 1980;9:25.

45. Rudmin FW. Critical history of the acculturation psychology of assimilation, separation, integration, and marginalization. Rev Gen Psychol 2003;7(1):3–37. https://doi.org/10.1037/1089-2680.7.1.3.

46. Schwartz SJ, Meca A, Ángel Cano M, Lorenzo-Blanco EI, Unger JB. Identity development in immigrant youth. Eur Psychol 2018;23(4):336–49. https://doi.org/10.1027/1016-9040/a000335.

47. Callens M-S, Valentová M, Meuleman B. Do attitudes towards the integration of immigrants change over time? A comparative study of Natives, second-generation immigrants and foreign-born residents in Luxembourg. J Int Migration Integration 2013;15(1):135–57. https://doi.org/10.1007/s12134-013-0272-x.

48. Karataş S, Crocetti E, Schwartz SJ, Rubini M. Understanding adolescents' acculturation processes: new insights from the intergroup perspective. New Dir Child Adolesc Development 2020;2020(172):53–71. https://doi.org/10.1002/cad.20365.

49. Agirdag O, Van Houtte M, Van Avermaet P. Ethnic school segregation and self-esteem. Urban Education 2012;47(6):1135–59. https://doi.org/10.1177/0042085912452154.

50. Brown CS, Chu H. Discrimination, ethnic identity, and academic outcomes of Mexican immigrant children: the importance of school context. Child Development 2012;83(5):1477–85. https://doi.org/10.1111/j.1467-8624.2012.01786.x.

51. Motti-Stefanidi F, Masten AS. School success and school engagement of immigrant children and adolescents. Eur Psychol 2013;18(2):126–35. https://doi.org/10.1027/1016-9040/a000139.

52. Jugert P, Feddes AR. Children's and adolescents' cross-ethnic friendships., . The Wiley Handbook of Group Processes in Children and Adolescents. Hoboken: Wiley; 2017. p. 373–92.

53. Ward C, Geeraert N. Advancing acculturation theory and research: the acculturation process in its ecological context. Curr Opin Psychol 2016;8:98–104. https://doi.org/10.1016/j.copsyc.2015.09.021.

54. Coenders M, Lubbers M, Scheepers P, Verkuyten M. More than two decades of changing ethnic attitudes in The Netherlands. J Social Issues 2008;64(2):269–85. https://doi.org/10.1111/j.1540-4560.2008.00561.x.

55. Callens M-S, Meuleman B, Marie V. Contact, perceived threat, and attitudes toward assimilation and multiculturalism: evidence from a majority and minority perspective in Luxembourg. J Cross-Cultural Psychol 2019;50(2):285–310. https://doi.org/10.1177/0022022118817656.

56. Plener PL, Groschwitz RC, Brähler E, Sukale T, Fegert JM. Unaccompanied refugee minors in Germany: attitudes of the general population towards a vulnerable group. Eur Child Adolesc Psychiatry 2017;26(6):733–42. https://doi.org/10.1007/s00787-017-0943-9.

57. Thijs J, Verkuyten M. Ethnic attitudes of minority students and their contact with majority group teachers. J Appl Developmental Psychol 2012;33(5):260–8. https://doi.org/10.1016/j.appdev.2012.05.004.

58. Bullard SM. Attitudes toward refugees entering the United States of America. The Aquila Digital community. 2015. Available at: https://aquila.usm.edu/honors_theses/323/. Accessed March 8, 2022.

59. Rivas-Drake D, Syed M, Umaña-Taylor A, et al. Feeling good, happy, and proud: a meta-analysis of positive ethnic-racial affect and adjustment. Child Development 2014;85(1):77–102. https://doi.org/10.1111/cdev.12175.

60. Lincoln AK, Lazarevic V, White MT, Ellis BH. The impact of acculturation style and acculturative hassles on the mental health of Somali Adolescent Refugees. J Immigrant Minor Health 2015;18(4):771–8. https://doi.org/10.1007/s10903-015-0232-y.

61. Schachner MK, Juang L, Moffitt U, van de Vijver FJ. Schools as acculturative and Developmental Contexts for Youth of immigrant and refugee background. Eur Psychol 2018;23(1):44–56. https://doi.org/10.1027/1016-9040/a000312.

62. Dimitrova R, Chasiotis A, van de Vijver F. Adjustment outcomes of immigrant children and youth in Europe. Eur Psychol 2016;21(2):150–62. https://doi.org/10.1027/1016-9040/a000246.

63. Keles S, Friborg O, Idsøe T, Sirin S, Oppedal B. Resilience and acculturation among unaccompanied refugee minors. Int J Behav Development 2018;42(1):52–63. https://doi.org/10.1177/0165025416658136.

64. Hasson R, Crea T, McRoyT, Le A. Patchwork of Promises: a Critical analysis o f immigration policies for unaccompanied undocumented children in the United States. Child Fam Soc Work 2019;24:275–92.

65. U.S. Commission on Civil Rights. Trauma at the Border: The Human Cost of Inhumane Immigration Policies Briefing Report. United States Commission on Civil Rights. 2019.

66. Song S. Mental health of unaccompanied. Children: effects of U.S. Immigration policies. *BJPsych* Open 2021;7(6):e200.

67. U.S Department of Justice (DOJ) Attorney general Announces zero-tolerance policy for criminal illegal entry. DOJ 2018. Available at: https://www.justice.gov/opa/pr/attorney-general-announces-zero-tolerance-policy-criminal-illegal-entry [Google Scholar].

68. Coletta A. Canada wants immigrants but the pandemic is in the way. So it's looking to keep people already there. Wash Post 2021.

69. Steele LS, Lemieux-Charles L, Clark JP, Glazier R. The impact of policy changes on the health of recent immigrants and refugees in the inner city. Can J Public Health 2002;93(2):118–22.

70. Mishori R. Children's health. Am Fam Physician 2020;101(4):202–4.

71. Child Trends. Immigrant children. 2018. Available at: https://www.childtrends.org/indicators/immigrant-children. Accessed March 14,2022.

72. Zong J, Batalova J, Burrows M. Frequently requested statistics on immigrants and immigration in the United States. 2019. Available at: https://www.migrationpolicy.org/article/frequently-requested-statistics-immigrants-and-immigration-united-states. Accessed March 14,2022.

73. Bassett L, Yoshikawa H. Our immigration policy has done Terrible Damage to Kids. *Scientific Am* Opin 2020.

74. United Nations General Assembly. Convention on the Rights of the Child. United Nations, 1989.Google Scholar.

75. Di Nicola V. Family, psychosocial, and cultural determinants of health. In: Sorel E, editor. *21st Century Global Mental Health*. Burlington, MA: Jones & Bartlett Learning; 2012. p. 119–50.

76. Di Nicola V, Daly N. Growing up in a pandemic: Biomedical and psychosocial impacts of the COVID-19 crisis on children and families. World Soc Psychiatry 2020;2(2):148—151. https://doi.org/10.4103/WSP.WSP_52_20.

The Color of Child Protection in America
Antiracism and Abolition in Child Mental Health

Rupinder K. Legha, MD[a],*, Kimberly Gordon-Achebe, MD[b]

KEYWORDS

- Antiracism • Racism • White supremacy • Child mental health • History of medicine

KEY POINTS

- Antiracist approaches to child mental health require confronting the color of child protection.
- Existing medical educational frameworks for understanding racism erase the enduring histories of white supremacist violence shaping public education, child welfare, juvenile justice, and mental health systems.
- Bold and radical frameworks, such as abolition, decolonization, and critical race theory, provide the necessary lexicon for confronting the color of child protection while protecting minoritized children against these systems of harm.
- This article delineates a daily antiracist practice whereby child mental health providers connect minoritized children and families' stories to racist inequities; then challenge these inequities along with the historical arcs driving them; protect minoritized children and families against the systems of care designed to harm them; and work toward the longer-term goal of abolishing these systems altogether.
- Child mental health providers' fundamental oath to first do no harm requires protecting children of the global majority from the systems of harm designed to protect white children.

Authorship Note: Dr R.K. Legha (she/her) led the conception and design of this article, its initial drafting and its critical revision. Dr K. Gordon-Achebe (she/her) participated in the conception and design of this article and its initial drafting, and reviewed the critical revisions. Inquiries about this article, including presentations or educational content pertaining to it, should be directed toward Dr R.K. Legha.

[a] 4859 West Slauson Avenue, #693, Los Angeles, CA 90056, USA; [b] Department of Psychiatry, Division of Child and Adolescent Psychiatry, University of Maryland School of Medicine, 701 West Pratt Street, 4th Floor, Baltimore, MD 21201, USA
* Corresponding author.
E-mail address: antiracistmd@gmail.com

Child Adolesc Psychiatric Clin N Am 31 (2022) 693–718
https://doi.org/10.1016/j.chc.2022.05.004
1056-4993/22/© 2022 Elsevier Inc. All rights reserved.

Abbreviations	
ADHD	attention deficit hyperactivity disorder
ODD	oppositional defiant disorder
IEP	individualized educational plan
CPR	cardiopulmonary resuscitation
PTSD	posttraumatic stress disorder
SAT	standardized achievement test
IQ	intelligence quotient
CNN	cable news network
NAACP	National Association for the Advancement of Colored People
ACLU	American Civil Liberties Union
MD	Medical Doctor
LGBTQIA	lesbian, gay, bisexual, transgender, queer, (questioning), intersex, asexual, and (agender)

INTRODUCTION
Answer the Call to Action by Saying Their Names

How does a child mental health profession originating in a white supremacist country traverse its racist past to promote meaningful antiracist action now to protect children of the global majority in the future?

Begin by saying their names (**Table 1**). Their lives and deaths embody the color of child protection[a] in the United States, where public education, child welfare, juvenile justice, and mental health systems harm—and even kill—children of the global majority[b] (**Fig. 1**).[1,2] These same systems protect white children, serving as vehicles for the white supremacy nurturing their development.[3] These violences reverberate across communities and generations, breaking hearts, shortening telomeres, denying human rights, and flooding bloodstreams with cortisol.[4]

Continue by rejecting existing medical education frameworks through which racism is framed and whiteness is deliberately obscured.[5] The social determinants of health, cultural competency, and implicit bias make no mention of the policing, family separation, and apartheid social institutions assaulting minoritized children's mental health. They ensure the racist status quo because—by design—they obscure the traumas and violences of the racist problem.[3]

Embrace a new direction inspired by better questions. Bold and radical frameworks such as abolition, decolonization, and critical race theory inoculate against whitewashing the histories giving rise to systems of "care" designed to harm the people of the global majority (**Box 1**).[3] They offer blueprints for reimagining them as instruments of healing nurturing all children's mental health, body, and soul.[3] They inspire the reflective questions opening many of this article's sections.[6]

Answer the call to action. Kalief Browder. Michael Brown. Ma'Khia Bryant. Latasha Harlins. Kendrick Johnson. Emmet Till. Trayvon Martin. Diane Ramirez. Nigel Shelby. Thousands of indigenous children disappeared during the boarding school era. We say your names to honor to issue a mandate. We are seeding the antiracist practices

---

[a] The term "color of child protection" is borrowed from legal scholar Dorothy Roberts, specifically her book entitled *Shattered Bonds: The Color of Child Welfare*.

[b] There are numerous ways to refer to children who are not white. Some examples include "minoritized," "Black, Indigenous, People of Color," and "nonwhite." Although we use these terms interchangeably, we primarily use the term children of the global majority—a term borrowed from Campbell-Stephens—to affirm nonwhite people's inherent power as the majority of the world's population.

Table 1 **Deaths in the name of "protection": children of the global majority murdered by systems of education, justice, and welfare**	
Children	**Voices of the Children, their Families, and Communities**
Kalief Browder (1993–2015)	"Haunted by the mental and physical torture he was subjected to [at] Rikers….Kalief took his own life in 2015 at our home shortly after he was released….The stress of fighting for justice and the pain over her son's death literally broke my mother's heart, resulting in her premature death at age 63 from complications of a heart attack."—Deion Browder (sister)[81]
Michael Brown (1996–2014)	"Burn this b***h down!"—Louis Head's outrage after the jury failed the indict the police officer who murdered his son. He (not the police officer) was investigated for inciting a riot[82]
Ma'Khia Bryant (2004–2021)	"When I watched Ma'Khia Bryant's TikTok videos I saw my middle niece in her. I saw [her] joy, creativity, potential, and humanity. No child's life should be judged and dissected based on one day and one event. Some of the hot takes about [her] have been truly awful."—Michael Hollingsworth (community member)[83]
Latasha Harlins (1976–1991)	"The most important thing to me is that my family is always protected by a shield so that they won't be harmed by dangerous, ruthless, uncaring people"—Poem by Latasha about her plans to become a lawyer[84]
Kendrick Johnson (1995–2013)	"Kendrick went to school with a bookbag and came home in a body bag"—Sign of community member protesting for justice on behalf of Kendrick Johnson and his family after his death was ruled an accident not a homicide[85]
Emmett Till (1941–1955)	"Let the people see what they did to my boy."—Mamie Till-Mobley (mother) on why she chose an open-casket funeral for her son's brutalized body[86]
Trayvon Martin (1995–2012)	"The children of other mothers dying, those are triggers…. I can't equate it to anything but PTSD. We are never ever going to recover from this….We live it every day. We carry the pain every single day.—Sybrina Fulton (mother)[87]
Diane Ramirez (2002–2019)	"She was supposed to be protected and she wasn't protected,"—Albert Ramirez (father) after Diane died while in the care of a foster parent[88]
Nigel Shelby (2004–2019)	"I don't want him to be remembered as a kid who was bullied for being gay and who took his own life. He was so much more than that. He was sunshine. . . . [H]e had so much more love to give."—Camika Shelby (mother)[89]
Indigenous children who died in government boarding schools	"When I look at these suicide figures…. I see [a] manifestation of deep historical trauma. . . . This isn't some kind of isolated history chapter — that it happened and now it's better. It's not better. We're all still paying for it. But you can see that the pattern over time is disappearing Native people; they're disappearing our nations."—Jackie Thompson Rand (community member)[90]

Review the names and voices of these children, families, and communities. Look up their and their families' stories if they are unfamiliar. Commit to a daily practice of learning the story of one child, family, and community each day. These stories humanize the systems of harm failing to protect while fueling a lifelong antiracism in child mental health journey that does.

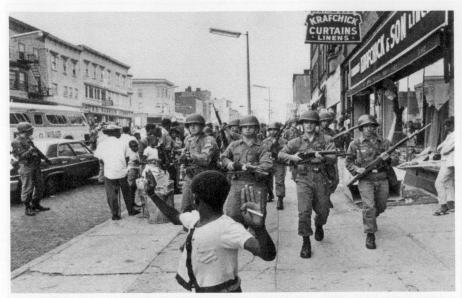

Fig. 1. Charles, DH. National Guard members clearing Springfield Ave. in Newark on July 14, 1967. In several days of rioting amid racial tensions, at least 20 people were killed and 700 injured. The New York Times. https://www.nytimes.com/slideshow/2017/12/25/us/the-photographs-of-don-hogan-charles.html. Published December 25, 2017. Accessed March 17, 2022. Don Hogan Charles/The New York Times/Redux.

that would have made it our responsibility to save your lives by first imploring our colleagues to mourn your deaths.

Reconfigure the colorblind oath to first do no harm and pledge an antiracist one stating the color of child protection.[7] Embrace the antiracist practice described here: connecting minoritized children and families' stories to racist inequities; then challenging these inequities along with the historical arcs driving them; protecting children and families against the systems of care designed to harm them; and working toward the longer-term goal of abolishing these systems altogether.[3,6,8,9] We focus on 3 systems of harm[c]—child welfare, public education, and juvenile justice—and how they intersect with the child mental health system's deep-seeded racism and whiteness, covered in our previous study.[3] We close by illuminating how abolition and Black, Indigenous, People of Color (BIPOC) love and resistance provide gateways to antiracist awakening in child mental health.

Authors' Positionality and Disclosures

How do you enter this antiracist child mental health endeavor, and how does the delusion of whiteness cloud your ability to dismantle the systems of harm benefiting you and your families?

---

[c] Child protection generally refers to the safeguarding of children from violence, exploitation, abuse, and neglect. This article takes a more expansive view of child protection by emphasizing child welfare, public education, and juvenile justice. We use the term child welfare—referring to systems involved with child abuse and neglect—interchangeably with child protective services and the child welfare system. The term "systems of harm" is meant to indicate how racist and damaging these instruments of child protection are to minoritized children.

Box 1
Major conceptual frameworks

Abolition[9,91]
- *Abolition* seeks to undo the way of thinking and doing things that sees prison and punishment as solutions for all kinds of social, economic, political, behavioral, and interpersonal problems. It calls for defunding the police, removing police from schools, repealing laws that criminalize survival, and providing safe housing for everyone. An act of radical imagination, it demands reorganizing and reimagining and rejects reform.
- *Abolition medicine* involves constructing new systems of community-based care that challenge the medical-industrial complex rooted in slavery, to build a new, healthier, more just society committed to healing. It reimagines the work of medicine as an antiracist practice; calls for the abolition of race-based diagnostic tools and treatment guidelines that reinforce biological race; and demands longitudinal antiracist training in medical education, desegregating the profession, and reparations for communities devastated by medical experimentation.

Critical Race Theory[92]
- A theoretic framework providing a critical analysis of race and racism to illuminate and combat root causes of structural racism and highlighting the relationship between race, racism, and power.
- Key concepts include: (1) *Ordinariness* (racism and white supremacy in postcivil rights society are integral and normal rather than aberrational); (2) *Centering in the margins* (shifting discourses' starting point from the majority group's perspective—eg, whiteness—to that of marginalized groups); (3) *Social construction of race* (race was fabricated based on historical, contextual, and political considerations); (4) *Intersectionality* (the multidimensionality of oppressions—race, gender identity, class, national origin, sexual orientation—resulting in disempowerment); (5) *Activism* (commitment to social justice, scholars assume an active role in "eliminating racial oppression as a broad goal of ending all forms of oppression"); (6) *Race consciousness* (explicit acknowledgment of the workings of race and racism in social contexts or in one's personal life); and (7) *Critical consciousness* (digging beneath the surface to develop deeper understandings of concepts, relationships, and personal biases).

Decolonization[93]
- Decolonizing mental health care seeks healing through culturally affirming practices and decenters mental health care away from the dominant white, heteronormative, patriarchal, gender-binary narrative.
- It dismantles harmful mental health practices that derive from and reinforce systemic privilege and whiteness. It recognizes the heavily Euro-centric approach to mental health as colonizing and that existing mental health practices do not adequately account for colonization, global issues, and cultural variables. It advances a movement to seek justice and liberation through education, collective care, and activism. It centers the needs of Black, Indigenous, People of Color and the LGBTQIA2S + community, honors the full neurodiversity spectrum, and advocates for mental health care accessibility for people with disabilities.

Disclosing our self-interest and proximity to the historically triumphant communities we serve provides an accountability crucial for antioppression work. We represent diverse backgrounds and experiences. The survival strategies our ancestors encoded in our DNA guide some of us to assimilate to whiteness so we can one day annihilate it. We outwardly endorse the colorblind frameworks that never would have saved Daniel Prude or Dr Susan Moore's lives while internally lamenting the ways in which they delete us.[10,11] Others have fled the oppressive confines of academia and the inpatient setting, vowing never again to inject or restrain a Black child victimized by our colleagues' white rage.[12] No matter which strategy we choose, antiracism is always a trauma and a triumph. The more courageous the endeavor, the more retaliatory the whitelash. Our lives, livelihoods, and bodies are always on the line; however, the echoes of their names (see **Table 1**) remind us we have no choice. We dare anyone to police, punish, or subjugate our efforts. We name this likelihood to shield ourselves from the anticipated assault.[13]

We ask that you model the same critical and reflective lens requisite for antiracist action and adopt the same urgency.[5,14] As beneficiaries of racism's productivity,[d] you can elect to silence the call to action, refusing to dismantle the systems of oppression feeding your community while ravaging ours.[15] High-risk for abusing your power to exploit children of the global majority, you owe their parents the full informed consent stating the dangers of receiving your care.[16] Your professionalism and codified standards of practice do not hold you to it. Our tone, gravitas, and imperative statements do. Likely offensive to your whiteness, they answer to the families whose children were stolen from them (see **Table 1**)—not the ivory towers that protect you and would have us forget their names. We refuse the taxation of defining basic terms crucial to the antiracist lexicon and offering hope rather than despair.[17,18] Look up the unfamiliar while processing your antiracist awakening. Being "objective" or "apolitical" is no longer an excuse.[19] The time for the child mental health professions to get off the racist sidelines to honor an antiracist practice is long overdue.[6] In a white supremacist society, refusing to antiracist constitutes clinical negligence and malpractice devastating our most vulnerable youth.[5] Commence the lifelong journey of antiracism from within.[20]

THE COLOR OF CHILD PROTECTION: UNITING HISTORIES OF HARM AND DEMONIZING IDEOLOGIES

In your clinical care today, which historical arcs of oppression neglected and traumatized BIPOC children while overserving and coddling white children's development? Can you see yourself and your own family's origin story in the eyes of the children and families you took an oath to first do no harm? Which racist stereotypes and tropes denigrating BIPOC and glorifying white people influenced your and your colleagues' clinical decision-making?

Uniting Histories

Historical patterns pervading systems of harm inform subsequent explorations of their inequities while identifying touchpoints for enacting antiracism to protect children of the global majority.[8,21] Exposing their racist, white supremacist roots validates our closing calls to abolish, rather than reform, them.[9] Unpacking their justifying ideologies positions child mental health providers to challenge their related stereotypes as part of a clinical activism guarding minoritized children and families against degrading and dehumanizing "care."[8,21] Just as they live in our social institutions' DNA, they are expressed in our clinical decision-making.[5] The following themes emerge: family separation, punishing and policing, white innocence and BIPOC blame, harm in the name of help, and white normativity and BIPOC deviancy.[3]

American family separation originated in slavery and the indigenous genocide. The domestic slave trade's Second Middle Passage (1790–1861) tore millions of Black families apart to support the country's booming cotton industry and westward expansion, compounding the intergenerational traumas wrought during the Transatlantic Slave Trade (**Fig. 2**).[22] Between 1860 and 1978, the Bureau of Indian Affairs operated more than 300 boarding schools, where thousands of indigenous children kidnapped from their parents were beaten, sexually abused, and killed by white teachers and

---

[d] Racism's "productivity" is wording borrowed from sociologist Dr Ruha Benjamin and described in greater detail in her book *The New Jim Code*.

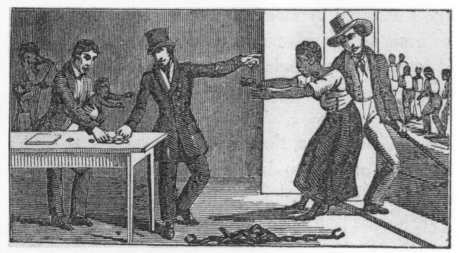

Fig. 2. *Black Mother being separated from her baby.* Schomburg Center for Research in Black Culture, Manuscripts, Archives and Rare Books Division, The New York Public Library. https://digitalcollections.nypl.org/items/510d47dd-e86f-a3d9-e040-e00a18064a99. Published 1862. Accessed March 17, 2022.

missionaries. "Kill the Indian, Save the Man" white assimilationist genocidal policies also displaced thousands of indigenous children in white foster homes to annihilate their cultural practices and languages.[23] White supremacist state violence severed Black and indigenous parents' legal, moral, and biological rights and then poured acid into their wounds by punishing them for obeying their parental instinct to fight back or resist.[22,23] Ta-Nehisi Coates describes, "Here we find the roots of American wealth and democracy – in the for-profit destruction of the most important asset available to any people, the family. The destruction was not incidental to America's rise; it facilitated that rise."[24]

Family separation continues today with disturbingly violent force and comparable fiscal incentive, profiting billions for the foster industrial and prison industrial complexes through BIPOC suffering.[7,25,26] Mass incarceration, family regulation,[e] and immigrant detention and deportation (**Fig. 3**) compound the intergenerational traumas wrought by slavery, colonization, and their aftermaths.[22,27] The toxic stress, ruptured attachments, battered neurologic development, and deep psychological wounds are criminal.[27] The concurrent assault on culture, language, and the spiritual practices is genocidal.[28] Removing BIPOC children from their homes through juvenile justice and child protective services (CPS) must be understood in this broader historical context as a perpetual mechanism of white supremacist state violence.[25] Child mental health providers' good intentions cannot disentangle their interventions from this interference; they obscure it.[5,8] BIPOC harm in the name of child protection must not only be weighed; it should be assumed. Medicating children and imposing behavioral

---

[e] Legal scholar Dorothy Roberts contends that, similar to the criminal "justice" system, the "child welfare" system is misnamed and could be more accurately referred to as the "family regulation system" to reflect how they punish and regulate black and other marginalized people. This term also speaks to the big business incentives—rather than social protection imperative—surrounding the foster industrial complex and its surveillance of people of color.

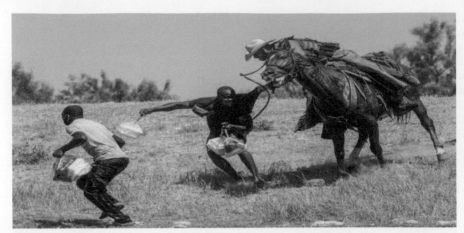

Fig. 3. Sullivan, E, Kanno-Youngs, Z. Images of Border Patrol's Treatment of Haitian Migrant-sPrompt Outrage. New York Times. https://www.nytimes.com/video/us/100000007986229/haitians-texas-border.html. Published Sept. 21, 2021. Updated Oct. 19, 2021. Accessed March 17, 2022.

strategies on their parents as their families are ravaged is how we clinically pour acid into the wounds of people devastated by these legacies. They should not be separated at all.[3]

Organized child protection's origin story and mission must also be understood within this context. New Yorker Henry Bergh founded the nation's first child protection society in 1874 after police refused to intervene on behalf of a 9-year-old white child abused by her parents. By 1922, 300 privatized child protection societies existed nationwide. As the founder of the American Society for the Prevention of Cruelty to Animals, Bergh extended his activism to protect animals from abuse but not to the thousands of black children lynched, murdered, and terrorized during the Jim Crow era.[29] The nation's emerging orphanage system also shunned black children, segregating them into a few destitute facilities during the first part of the twentieth century. Not until the 1960s did private orphanages—by then residential treatment centers for emotionally disturbed children—welcome black children equally. Even still, they were less likely than white children to be placed in private facilities where they might receive psychiatric help and more likely to be placed in correctional settings.[30] Innocent white children deserve sanctuary. Deviant black ones need confinement.[5]

Indicting and traumatizing nonwhite children, while protecting and sanctifying the healthy development of white ones, is an age-old pattern of American child protection—and child psychiatry.[3] In the 1900s, the nascent profession's child guidance clinics, intertwined with the burgeoning juvenile court system, targeted poor, immigrant families based on racist, classist beliefs that they were unable to raise their children "correctly" for modern society. It construed delinquent children as having a "psychic constitutional deficiency" in need of remedy, establishing an early, enduring pattern of condemning minoritized children for their behaviors instead of the social structures assailing them.[31] This white, middle-class nuclear family ideal exalted white children as normal, while condemning BIPOC children as pathologic.[3] The implications were violent. Black youth were coerced into juvenile court caseloads for behaviors that would have been sanctioned if they were white.[32,33] They were also thrown into adult prisons with one 1890 census revealing that nearly 20% of Black prisoners were youth (https://www.youtube.com/shorts/mNsxdCV-zAw).[32] Thousands, including black women and girls, were sentenced to slave labor and sexually assaulted through the convict leasing and chain gang systems that often kidnapped them based on fabricated charges.[34,35] Slavery had not been abolished. It had simply evolved, and the "justice" system became the next vehicle for legitimizing its white supremacist violence.[26]

As child welfare transitioned from the private to the public sector, its apartheid nature persisted, segregating white children into resourced care, while imprisoning BIPOC ones in correctional facilities. Sending black children without homes to adult prisons or reform schools continued through the mid-twentieth century and endures in their overrepresentation in juvenile detention facilities today.[32] These carceral practices extend to school and community settings where BIPOC children are terrorized for their hair, clothing, and behavior; traumatized by police and coercive school surveillance (https://www.youtube.com/shorts/mNsxdCV-zAw); and subjected to excessive suspensions and expulsions, devastating their developmental trajectories.[36,37] Meanwhile their white peers are funneled into advanced placement (AP) classes and referred for mental health care if they struggle.[38,39] There is no educational "achievement gap," only a ruinous education debt seeded centuries ago when enslaved black children were denied any formal education and tortured for trying to access it.[40] This racialized bifurcation of protection and punishment, of nurturing and abuse, laid the foundation for child welfare, public education, and juvenile justice's apartheid nature, reflected in their enduring white–black racist inequities today.

Demonizing Ideologies

A spawn of the white supremacist parental state, child protection's primary goal has always been to normalize whiteness and its violences while demonizing people of the global majority standing in the way of its colonizing agenda.[41] Racist ideologies and tropes justify cruelty and violence.[42] Black children have been portrayed as criminals, aggressors, and superpredators, even as crimes against humanity prey on them (see **Figs. 1** and **2**). They have been dehumanized from children into adults even as the adults responsible for them have violated them.[42]

Fabricated during slavery to justify black children's exploitation, adultification persists in white adults' hypersexualizing black girls and believing they experience less pain and suffering compared with their white peers. It erases black children's innocence, framing their "transgressions" as conniving and deserving of rebuke.[43] "Tangle of pathology" stems from the 1965 Moynihan Report condemning the black family as a flawed institution of absent, weak fathers and domineering matriarchs who emasculated sons and defeminized daughters.[44] Moynihan's conclusions emerged from white normative conceptions of ideal families requiring breadwinning fathers, stay-at-home mothers, and parent–children familial units isolated from larger communites.[42] They degraded the kinship network BIPOC communities have cultivated for centuries as a key survival strategy against white supremacist state violence and structural racism.[45]

Incriminating and indicting BIPOC humanity fuels zero-tolerance, tough-on-crime, and other racist policies.[42] Configuring poverty as individual failure or laziness, rather than the legacy of slavery and colonization, naturalizes denying social protections and educational and treatment opportunities.[3] Racist tropes—whether the licentious Jezebel, the absent black father, the foreign immigrant, or the savage native—point the finger of blame at individuals' "choices," not the external causes requiring social change.[42] They undergird white savior behavioral health agendas focused on protecting children of the global majority from their parents' alleged ineptitude instead of structural assault making it impossible for them to parent.[46] They constitute a violence, demonizing BIPOC to subhuman status (see **Fig. 3**) while cementing the structures causing them harm (see **Fig. 1**). They poison clinical decision-making, dictating which children get restrained, secluded, and labeled as oppositional and difficult while their parents are reported and which children are showered with compassion and empathy, their anxiety and sadness validated while their parents are lauded.[3,8]

ANTIRACISM IN CHILD MENTAL HEALTH: CONFRONTING THE SYSTEMS OF HARM

These historical arcs manifest in the key racist inequities pervading these systems of harm and the various forms of racism that collide when they intersect with the child mental health system. Delineating racism's presence—the policing, punishing, measuring, blaming, criminalizing, pathologizing, regulating, and separating of minoritized children and families—positions providers to engage in clinical activism that protects children against it. Brief vignettes realistically portray this racism, whereas clinical strategies outline immediate measures to thwart it (**Table 2**).

Child Welfare: Family Regulation and Family Separation

Case A: 12-year-old black child needs a life-saving cardiac procedure. The all-white pediatrics team documents: "Parents are noncompliant, refusing care, despite imminent risk of death, raising concerns for medical neglect." Wishing to report the parents to CPS, they contact the child psychiatry service for support.

Case B: A severely depressed, nonbinary, neurodivergent 13-year-old black child presents for a child psychiatry intake with both parents. They report that their house is "too loud" and that they fight with her 16-year-old sister often. Their mother, severely depressed since her brother was killed while imprisoned 1 year ago, is unable to work; and their maternal aunt, who recently moved in after being evicted, is not taking her bipolar medication. The mother clarifies that the older sister threw a magazine, not a book, and that she spoke to her about not doing it again.

Case C: A white orthopedic surgery intern covering the emergency room evaluates an 8-year-old black child who broke his arm while skating. The child reports living "nowhere." His mother clarifies that she was recently laid off and evicted, so she and her 3 children have been living with family members. The intern tells the white child psychiatry fellow: "My attending said this seems fishy. Single mom, homeless, kid with a broken arm.... We should contact child psych and call CPS just to be safe."

Most child welfare cases—up to 75%—pertain to neglect stemming from poverty, rather than abuse or exploitation.[7] Poverty is highly racialized, reflecting the damning impact of redlining, gerrymandering, and discrimination: for every dollar of wealth non-Hispanic white child households have, black ones have just one cent.[47] Poverty creates environments of desperation whereby nonwhite parents must fight for their children's basic needs—pertaining to housing, education, and (mental) healthcare—in a white supremacist war zone where their every move is scrutinized. With no choice but to depend on social services—such as food stamps, subsidized housing, or public health insurance—the state surveillance of their parenting increases and the war zone becomes more perilous.[48]

Remarkably, more than one-third of children are investigated by CPS before their 18th birthdays. Although only a quarter of white children are investigated, more than half of black and indigenous children are. Very few cases are substantiated.[48,49] Black children are more likely than white children to be investigated, placed in foster care, and permanently separated from their biological parents.[48,49] The results are

Table 2
Antiracist clinical strategies: scripts, documentation, and clinical activism

	Psychoeducation and Evaluation: Examples of Antiracist Scripts for Children (C) and Parents (P)	Documentation: Antiracist Narrative Inspiration	Clinical Activism
Child welfare: family regulation and family separation	• Health-care providers are required to report suspected child abuse and neglect. This process is racist. More than half of black and indigenous children are reported before age 18. Doctors have prowhite biases and may be more likely to test you for drugs or call child protective services (CPS) thinking they are keeping your child safe from you." (P) • Being reported to CPS is scary. Most cases are for neglect, not abuse. Very few reported cases are investigated or substantiated. An even smaller percentage of kids are removed from their homes. This risk is higher for Black youth." (P) • My number one goal is to keep you and your child safe. If I ever have to report, I will tell you directly. My oath to not harm you is antiracist. I vow to never police you. My responsibility is to consider the high likelihood of your child being reported. I	• Do not guess a child's race based on phenotype or prior notes. Ask the child's family which racial demographic (if any) they want documented in the chart • Document the various forms of racism (related to housing, education, health care) the child and family have been subjected to and triumphed over • Do a genogram to identify all members of the family (biological and otherwise) involved. Reach out to them and document how these extensive kinship networks nurture and protect the child • Recognize that when families are threatened with CPS involvement for "refusing" to follow medical advice, this is racial coercion. Document all the efforts that went into—or failed to go into—explaining treatment options and recommend caring for parents, not policing and threatening them	• Never order urine drug screens for BIPOC without a thorough informed consent, warning them of their greater risk of being criminalized for substance use, first. Always document the consent (or refusal to consent) • Document the child and parents' consent (or refusal) for using racial identifiers in the chart • When reporting to CPS, consider saying "I do not know" for racial demographics because of the racist algorithms used to determine which families are investigated • Interrogate the positionality of the other providers involved in care. Be attuned to how their whiteness may lead them to police these families or elicit a trauma response from them • Educate colleagues about the racist inequities and harms involved with CPS involvement

(continued on next page)

Table 2
(continued)

	Psychoeducation and Evaluation: Examples of Antiracist Scripts for Children (C) and Parents (P)	Documentation: Antiracist Narrative Inspiration	Clinical Activism
	will document carefully, anticipating this likelihood." (P)	• Document how Black, Indigenous, People of Color (BIPOC) parents are "involved," "agreeable," and "collaborative" to rewrite "tangle of pathology" stereotypes	
Public education: segregation, testing, punishment, and assimilation into whiteness	• Schools perpetuate racism through discipline, testing, classroom (mis)placement, and (mis)allocating financial and teaching resources. Asking specific questions about teachers and students' racial demographics and racist practices sounds unusual but this information matters for your child's development and wellbeing." (P) • White teachers perpetrate anger and adultification biases that rob Black and Brown children of their innocence while setting them up to be punished, suspended, and expelled. They also have lower expectations for black children,	• Write school letters of support for (all) minoritized children, especially those who are labeled "behavioral problems." They demonstrate parents' advocacy and show the school another set of (MD) eyes is monitoring the racism • Make school letters holistic and antiracist. Highlight children's multiple talents and their families' strong advocacy. Provide clear antiracist recommendations about not policing and over punishing children and link this to literature demonstrating how toxic this and other kinds of racism are to children's health • Articulate adultification and racialized anger biases' harms.	• Never diagnose a minoritized child with oppositional defiant disorder; instead excavate the oppression the child is opposing • Never diagnose a minoritized child with conduct disorder, which amounts to a clinical racist trope • Never dissect what is wrong with the child; look for what was done to the child • Ask every parent of minoritized children about their school/district's racial demographics (children and staff alike) using the narrative scripts provided • Recognize that children of the global majority are policed, traumatized, assailed, and punished by the adults charged with protecting them at school.

	which impacts placement in special education classes." (P) • You are so talented. I am surprised to hear that school has been hard. Do your teachers care for you or punish you? Are they white or Black? Do other kids put you down because of the color of your skin?" (C) • I ask all kids certain questions to take care of them. I want to avoid making you feel judged or like a 'bad kid' because you are perfect. Do you feel comfortable telling me whether you vape (drink alcohol, smoke cannabis, and so forth)?" (C)	Provide specific recommendations regarding how to care for and nurture the children. Render the invisibility of whiteness visible to show schools their racism and its health effects are being scrutinized clinically • Help parents draft letters requesting 504 or IEP evaluation—especially parents who do not speak English • Document school-based racism in the chart to prevent misdiagnosing children with behavioral problems and to implicate providers in protecting children from school settings, not implicating them as the source of pathologic condition	Name this trauma as the pathology, not the child's symptoms signaling it
Juvenile injustice: criminalization and traumatization	• The juvenile justice system is racist. This racism manifests at every stage of involvement—from what is considered delinquent behavior, who gets stopped by the police and how often, who is diverted and who is detained; adjudication, disposition, and placement in residential facilities, too." (P/C) • Juvenile facilities have historically been spaces of abuse and mistreatment for BIPOC	• Avoid language that criminalizes BIPOC children: "aggressive," "assaultive," "delinquent," "illicit drug use," "convicted," "repeat offender." • For one-liners, never refer to children as "male" or "female," which adultifies them. Use gender inclusive language that makes it clear that (BIPOC) children are young and innocent (eg, "child" or "youth")	• Connect families to the NAACP or ACLU for legal support to ensure children are not pressured to plead guilty to felony and other life-changing charges. Sometimes, they can contact district attorneys to support charges being dropped • Recognize that juvenile injustice, part of the prison industrial complex, is a big business that evolved from slavery and is designed to assail

(continued on next page)

Table 2
(continued)

	Psychoeducation and Evaluation: Examples of Antiracist Scripts for Children (C) and Parents (P)	Documentation: Antiracist Narrative Inspiration	Clinical Activism
	children. They also promote family separation, which is damaging to children's health." (P) • Do you feel like your attorney is trying to get you out of here as quickly as possible so you can go home? Or do you feel pressured to plead guilty or to plead guilty to more serious charges? Is your lawyer involving your parents and family in these important decisions?" (C) • I am so sorry you have to be in this facility locked in a cage. No child deserves this. I want to make sure you are safe while you are here. Do you feel abused, mistreated, neglected, or unfairly targeted?"	• Do not refer to detention facilities as "camp" or other terms that make it sound like a fun, recreational alternative to children's structurally violated and overpoliced neighborhoods • When documenting or writing reports for justice-involved children, avoid (residential) placements fueling family separation. Cite literature to back up recommendations to redirect children toward community-based interventions and psychiatric services that support the trauma, grief and liberation of BIPOC • Write forensic reports that avoid diagnostic and behavioral condemnation and instead expose the racism and white supremacy (related to policing in the community, at school, placement in lower-level classes, over suspension and expulsion) that have assailed youth, causing sustained chronic trauma, and toxic health effects	black and brown children by design. Instead of asking kids to develop coping skills while caged, insist that why should not be caged in the first place. Connect their oppression to historical patterns so they are clear they did nothing wrong • Connect kids and families to abolition-oriented community organizations (eg, Youth Justice Coalition) that validate the violence and oppression they are experiencing • Recognize the color of child protection is white. Providers uphold whiteness by allocating more time and resources to over advantaged white families

devastating. Mothers who lose custody of their children are more likely to attempt and complete suicide; die from avoidable and unavoidable causes; and endure poor mental health outcomes.[50-52] Children displaced into foster care and facilities are at high-risk for abuse and more likely to experience physical and mental illness.[53-55] Complicit with the family regulation system, doctors—whose prowhite implicit bias and related harms are well-established—overreport minoritized children and overdrug screen their mothers during pregnancy.[56,57]

Because more than half of black and indigenous children are reported to CPS before age 18, providers must anticipate this likelihood. Nonwhite families deserve psychoeducation detailing their unique risks of being reported to CPS for normal family dynamics distorted by white supremacy. Sibling discord misperceived by a neurodivergent black child (Case B, see **Table 2**), miscommunicated to a well-intentioned white school counselor can be racistly misreported to CPS— "just to be safe." Colleagues deluded by white saviorist desires to rescue BIPOC children from their "tangle of pathology" families by reporting them, need antiracist remediation, not white complicity allowing them to sleep at night. Instead of colluding with colleagues by calling CPS to create "safety," child psychiatry fellows can shield families from their colleagues' racism. Document strengths and clarify that poverty—which is crippling, not "fishy"—does not equal neglect (Case C). Instead of promoting pediatrics services' indictment of black parents terrified of all-white teams holding their children's lives in their hands, child psychiatry services can uphold the most basic standard of care. Document the racialized traumas behind parents' hesitation and discourage policing their emotions to implicate pediatric service in a more humane—and more effective—consent for care (Case A). Explore providers' and one's own positionality (see "Authors' Positionality and Disclosures" section) to cultivate the critical and race consciousness necessary for unveiling whiteness' influence on clinical decision-making.[58] The typical one-liner stating the patient's racial demographics and reasons for presentation is supplanted by an antiracist one noting the providers' identity and exposing their complicity with systems of oppression and risk of perpetrating harm.

All-white clinical teams bear particular responsibility for the noxious harms they perpetrate when reporting nonwhite families.[59,60] Reporting as an option of convenience or instrument of racial coercion when parents do not "obey" is an act of medical brutality that should constitute malpractice (Case A).[12] Health-care providers operating in a white supremacist society, however, are unlikely to face repercussions, likely assuming that reporting is protecting children from harm. Because of family separation's toxic health effects, every clinical decision—documentation, psychoeducation, and urine drug screens alike—is inextricably linked to CPS's overintrusive reach into minoritized children's lives, mandating a clinical activism actively safeguarding families against it (see **Table 2**).

Public Education: Segregation, Testing, Punishment, and Assimilation into Whiteness

Case A: X, a 17-year-old child arrives at the emergency department (ED), due to suicidal ideation, in 4-point restraints, thrashing, yelling, and surrounded by police. The legal hold reads, "The police were called after X got into an altercation with a teacher and ran into the street. She refused to get on the gurney, and required restraints to transport her to the emergency room." ED staff order X to cooperate, proceed to interrogate their drug use, and threaten to administer intramuscular (IM) medication, due to their perceived risk of danger to others. A previous ED visit documents the following: "17-year-old African-American female with oppositional defiant disorder brought in by police in restraints after parents stated the child made suicidal comments. Child was aggressive and uncooperative and given IM Thorazine."

Case B: A 10-year-old child announcing "I'm Black and proud!" presents to a county mental health clinic with his grandmother because "school says he has ADHD and ODD." He is in the principal's office everyday for "disrupting class and clowning around." The child psychiatrist reviews the child's IEP, initiated during fourth grade and reporting "in utero drug exposure from addict mother"—which his grandmother adamantly denies. When asked what happened in the fourth grade to warrant the IEP, the child says his father died. His grandmother tearfully clarifies that the child witnessed his father die 1 year ago from a heart attack as he tried to perform CPR while calling 911. There is no mention of this trauma or PTSD in the IEP.

Despite decades of integration efforts since Brown v. Board (1954), most American schoolchildren still attend racially concentrated school districts that are either predominantly nonwhite or white.[61] The latter receive 23 billion dollars more in funding, despite enrolling the same number of students, due to community wealth stolen through land theft and redlined loans and walled off from the children of the global majority by gerrymandering.[62] Standardized testing and disciplinary practices (see **Fig. 4**) compound this segregation of resources and opportunities.[38,63,64] Various aptitude tests, achievement assessments, and college entrance exams—including the SAT and IQ testing—originated in eugenics and were designed to favor white, upper-income individuals. Better proxies for race and privilege, not aptitude or potential, they stifle academic advancement, bar scholarship opportunities, and prevent high school graduation for BIPOC children, resulting in their higher rates of unemployment and imprisonment.[65–67]

White teachers, comprising 80% of the public school workforce, abuse and neglect nonwhite students, damaging their developmental trajectories without consequence. Their lower expectations for black students than white students exacerbate the former's overrepresentation in special education classes.[68] Their "racialized anger bias," derived from tropes about black criminality, imagines anger among black children where none exists.[69,70] This virulent antiblackness terrorizes these children, who are suspended and expelled with gusto. Along with LatinX students, they are hurled down the school-to-prison pipeline. Their white schoolteachers are never censured for failing their jobs entirely by extinguishing educational opportunities while ruining life chances.[37,43,71] Meanwhile, white peers engaging in the same behaviors are either ignored or referred for mental health treatment.[39]

The schoolhouse offers children of the global majority no sanctuary, inflaming neurons burned by the traumas of being policed in their communities while inspiring fear and alienation (see **Fig. 4**).[60,72] The white assimilative ghost of the American Indian Boarding School era haunts the next generation of BIPOC children through whitewashed curricular content romanticizing the white supremacist nation-building project while gaslighting away its devastation of their communities.[73] English-only and school dress code policies and unlawful policing of black children's hairstyles scream the same white civilizing agenda.[36,74] Black students are more likely to be suspended for discretionary (ie, unnecessary) reasons such as dress code or long hair violations—neither of which is predictive of student misconduct—and to endure punishment for behaviors normalized, sanctioned, and ignored among white students (see **Fig. 4**).[36] It is no wonder that when teachers, resource officers, and the police come for them, they flee (Case A). The message is clear: you do not belong. This is how American public education sustains the legacies of colonization and slavery and their bloody massacres, pogroms, forced relocations, and racial terrorism. Through a racial apartheid whereby white children are overadvantaged financially, behaviorally, and intellectually to cement their supremacy by denying their nonwhite peers the same life opportunities.[75]

The standard of care for minoritized children mandates comprehensive mental health assessments rooting out the racism assailing them through erasures of their traumas (Case B), diagnostic condemnation of their behaviors (Case A and B), criminalization and punishment of their suffering (Case A and B), and police involvement (Case A) and racist tropes brutalizing their humanity (eg, addict mother, Case B). Providers owe children explicit reformulations that they are perfect and there is nothing wrong with them, only something wrong with what is being done to them (see **Table 2**). Questions about their behaviors and health history—especially pertaining to substance use and sexual health, which are highly racialized and degrading— must promise to not interrogate and adultify them, rather understand them while opening a pathway to healing (see **Table 2**). Mental health providers must never replicate educational violence—such as calling police and punishing distress stemming from white supremacy—through unnecessary clinical roughness such as seclusion and restraint or misgendering, misracializing, and misdiagnosing children (Case A). Instead of extending the carceral reach, amputate it. Instead of conspiring with the systems of harm, shield children and offer them a soothing balm.

Juvenile Injustice: Criminalization and Traumatization

Case A: 16-year-old child (he/him) has a promising music career inspired by his remarkable desire to support his younger siblings and mother, who has terminal lung cancer. She has relied on public assistance—despite having a college degree—due to severe PTSD related to witnessing her brother being shot by police during a "routine" traffic stop (the child witnessed it, too) and her newborn child being killed during childbirth when she went into premature labor the following day.

Unable to save money while keeping his siblings clothed and fed, the child steals musical equipment from a van one night to expand his career prospects. Due to multiple prior traumas involving police (police stops, uncle's murder, George Floyd's lynching), he runs away terrified when the police approach him and draw guns. The 4 officers—all white men—physically take him down to the ground and label him "combative." When they find $200 he earned from a music gig, they accuse him of selling drugs. First-time offenses, the 2 felony charges for robbery and reckless evading, are reduced to probation, court-ordered anger management and drug treatment, and going home with an ankle monitor.

No longer allowed to play musical gigs, he becomes severely depressed and his grades plunge. Without funds from his job, his mother struggles to care for his younger siblings, 2 of whom are placed in foster care for neglect. He skips court-ordered "treatment" which, led by all-white staff, feels alienating, the transportation too expensive to afford. He is kicked out of his honors classes, and teachers send him to detention regularly, lamenting "you used to be a good kid." Denied any compassion and mental health treatment from the adults surrounding him, he smokes cannabis to cope and is "caught" during a routine urine drug screen. Rather than being diverted to intensive mental health care, he is detained for several months with no end date. His mother—heartbroken by her family's separation—dies during this time. On the night before her funeral, he is placed in solitary confinement for getting into a physical fight with a peer who called his mother a "dead b**ch." He is then disallowed from attending the funeral. Despondent and hopeless, orphaned and alone, he commits suicide the following day by hanging himself. His younger siblings are devastated by this additional horrifying loss.

Case B: Police stop a 16-year-old child driving into oncoming traffic on a 2-way street while intoxicated. When offered a breathalyzer, he declines, saying "talk to my parents' attorney." As officers prepare to detain him, he cries out that he is suicidal and is placed on a legal hold and taken to a local emergency room unrestrained. His parents, notified by the police, meet him at the emergency room and thank the officers—who do not press charges—for keeping their child "safe." "He seems like a good kid. Make sure to keep him out of trouble," they say. Finding him acute low risk for suicide, the child psychiatry fellow discharges him home. She advises follow-up with the outpatient child psychiatrist who has been treating him for ADHD, for which he has a 504 plan. Before discharging, his mother states, "He has a big test tomorrow but it's been such a hard night. Junior year is a big year, and if he fails, it could really mess with his college prospects. Do you mind writing him a doctor's note so he can miss class tomorrow?" The fellow happily obliges.

The juvenile justice system's stated goal is to help young people avoid future delinquency and mature into law-abiding adults. Its apparent role is to devastate BIPOC children's developmental trajectories while punishing the adaptive strategies they invoke to survive the white supremacist attack on their well-being. Despite constituting one-third of the US adolescent population, youth of color represent two-thirds of those incarcerated. Racism assails them during every stage of the juvenile justice process, including which behavior is considered delinquent; who gets stopped by the police; whether or not they are referred to juvenile justice system; whether they are admitted to it or diverted from it; and later stages including adjudication, disposition, and aftercare.[76] Although youth incarceration has recently been cut in half, black and American Indian youth are still overwhelmingly more likely to be held in custody than their white peers: 5 times as likely for the former, 3 times as likely as the latter; 42% more likely for Latinx youth.[77]

Get-tough approaches to juvenile justice—which play on racist tropes such as black criminality and juvenile "superpredator"—fail to change behavior and damage children's health irreparably, amplifying the racist assaults from school and the child welfare system. Compared with white peers, black children experiencing police contact before the eighth grade have 11 times the odds of being arrested when they are aged 20 years.[78] Psychological distress, not prior "delinquent" behavior, partially mediates these results. A recent systematic review examining 40 years of research found that police stops, even those providing assistance, result in poor mental health, substance use, and impaired safety for black children, especially boys.[60] In addition to being criminogenic, policing and incarceration traumatize children, leading to premature death including by suicide.[59] The juvenile justice system does not make people safe. It is—in scholar-activist Mariame Kaba's words—a "death-making institution."[79]

Protecting children from the global majority against juvenile injustice involves fighting back at racism at every stage of the process (see **Table 2**). "It is not what is wrong with you, it is what was done to you" as a guiding mantra positions providers to actively reject adultifying and criminalizing youth while galvanizing them to take action. The risk–benefit analysis for injustice-involved minoritized children weighs the likelihood of death and integrates all forms of racism jeopardizing entire families across generations (Case A). Connect families to civil rights attorneys who may be more likely than overburdened district attorneys to fight for diversion and not pressure terrified children with underdeveloped frontal lobes into accepting felony charges (see **Table 2**). Say Khalif Browder's name to remind yourself of the unnamed suicides of the most promising BIPOC youth falsely accused of crimes they never committed, their dreams and souls extinguished as a result.[80] Never forget the color of child protection is also white. It is manifested in which kids get 504 plans for ADHD so they can receive

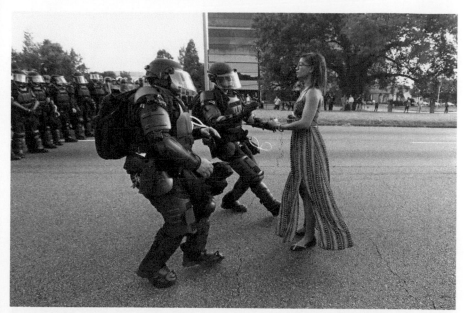

Fig. 4. Cole, T. The Superhero Photographs of the Black Lives Matter Movement. New York Times. https://www.nytimes.com/2016/07/31/magazine/the-superhero-photographs-of-the-black-lives-matter-movement.html. Published July 26, 2016. Accessed March 17, 2022. Jonathan Bachman / Reuters Pictures.

extra time on their SATs as white supremacy catapults them to the top of the racist hierarchy—despite their dangerousness and ineptitude (Case B). The extra time, care, and protection child psychiatrists grant the most privileged families (Case B) stem from the same concern, connection, and commitment they deny the country's most desperate children of—including by never seeing in the first place (Case A). The results can be deadly.

Conclusion: Black, Indigenous, People of Color Love and Resistance

"Tenderness is what love feels like in private. Justice is what love looks like in public."

—*Dr Cornel West*

We close by saying their names again (see **Table 1**). Their lives and deaths provide *the* inspiration for a child mental health profession originating in a white supremacist country to traverse its racist past, promote meaningful antiracist action now, and protect children of the global majority in the future.[3] Abolition (see **Box 1**) reimagines the work of health care as an antiracist practice, one dichotomizing all actions and decisions as either racist or antiracist, and issuing an ultimatum in which child mental health providers are either part of the problem or part of the solution.[3,8,9,21] It ensures probing historical confrontation, rather than a superficial celebration of diversity and differences, and instills fierce scrutiny seeking to remake a child mental health profession steeped in whiteness—not reform it.[3] The antiracist practice prescribed here offers immediate strategies for engaging this remaking. However, by highlighting child welfare, public education, and juvenile injustice's deep-seeded racism and

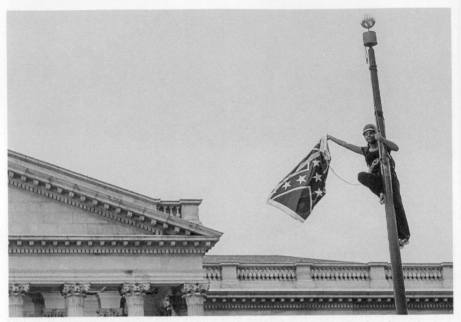

Fig. 5. Ms. Newsome scaled a flagpole to remove the Confederate battle flag from the State Capitol in Columbia, S.C., in 2015. Adam Anderson Photo/Reuters.

whiteness—which intersect with child mental health's—we make it clear that immediate antiracist action cannot supplant the necessary tearing down of systems of harm. BIPOC love and resistance inspires the antiracist reimagining while pointing to the people who should lead the charge.

Because for as long as racism and white supremacy have assailed people of the global majority, their love and resistance have assured their survival and triumph. Mothers have hurled their bodies across their children being stripped away from them at the auction block (see **Fig. 1**). Women have scaled capitol buildings and faced down armed police to say no more state violence (**Figs. 4** and **5**). Fanny Lou Hamer and Ida B. Wells and the Black Panthers have exposed the lynching, forced sterilization, and racist experiments experimentation terrorizing their communities while ensuring safe, supportive health care where otherwise none would be found. This BIPOC love and resistance reminds us that no amount of diversity and inclusion, implicit bias training, or cultural sensitivity will ever help us work our way out of systems designed to destroy us. BIPOC love and resistance supplant the policing, punishing, measuring, blaming, criminalizing, pathologizing, regulating, and separating of children and families of the global majority—reminding our profession to begin by getting out of the way.

CLINICS CARE POINTS

- Child mental health providers lay the foundation cementing antiracist practices by saying the names of children of the global majority killed by systems of harm (child welfare, public education, juvenile injustice) and connecting their lives and stories to the children they see (or do not see) each day.

- Antiracist child mental health care requires child mental health providers to first inform children and families of the global majority of the various racist risks they face when entering these systems of harm voluntarily or involuntarily.

- It proceeds by challenging enduring histories of policing, punishing, measuring, blaming, criminalizing, pathologizing, regulating, and separating children and families of the global majority by first acknowledging these risks intrinsic to these systems of harm.

- Colorblind approaches to mental health care, such as cultural competency, implicit bias, and the social determinants of health fail to protect children of the global majority from systems of harm because they erase the ongoing white supremacist violence assailing them.

- Bolder and more radical frameworks such as abolition, critical race theory, and decolonization position clinicians to engage in clinical activism whereby they avoid punitive, coercive, carceral practices; recognize and explain racism and white supremacy's pervasiveness and harm; and promote intergenerational healing rather than tolerating intergenerational harm within systems of harm.

DISCLOSURE

The authors have no conflicts of interest to disclose.

REFERENCES

1. Harris M, Benton H. Implicit bias in the child welfare, education and mental health systems. National Center for Youth Law 2021.
2. Campbell-Stephens RM. Educational leadership and the global majority: decolonising narratives. New York, NY: Springer Nature; 2021.
3. Legha RK, Clayton A, Yuen L, et al. Nurturing all the children's mental health body and soul: confronting American child psychiatry's racist past to reimagine its antiracist future. Child Adolesc Psychiatr Clin N Am 2022;31(2):277–94.
4. Goosby BJ, Heidbrink C. The transgenerational consequences of discrimination on African-American health outcomes. Sociol Compass 2013;7(8):630–43.
5. Legha RK. Teaching antiracism to the next generation of doctors. Sci Am 2020.
6. Asmerom B, Legha RK, Mabeza RM, et al. An abolitionist approach to antiracist medical education. AMA J Ethics 2022;24(3):194–200.
7. Roberts D. Shattered bonds: the color of child welfare. Child Youth Serv Rev 2002;24(11):877–80.
8. Legha RK, Miranda J. An anti-racist approach to achieving mental health equity in clinical care. Psychiatr Clin North Am 2020;43(3):451–69.
9. Iwai Y, Khan ZH, DasGupta S. Abolition medicine. Lancet 2020;396(10245):158–9.
10. Dahlberg B. Rochester hospital released Daniel Prude hours before fatal encounter with police. NPR. 2020. Available at: https://www.npr.org/sections/health-shots/2020/09/29/917317141/rochester-hospital-released-daniel-prude-hours-before-fatal-encounter-with-polic. Accessed December 10, 2021.
11. Maybank A, Jones CP, Blackstock U, et al. Say her name: Dr susan Moore. Washington post. 2020. Available at: https://www.washingtonpost.com/opinions/2020/12/26/say-her-name-dr-susan-moore/. Accessed March 17, 2022.
12. Legha RK. Medical brutality, social media, and collective activism. Kevin MD. Available at: https://www.kevinmd.com/post-author/rupinder-k-legha. Accessed June 24, 2022.

13. Blackstock U. Why Black doctors like me are leaving faculty positions in academic medical centers. Stat 2020;16.
14. Legha RK, Richards M, Kataoka SH. Foundations in racism: a novel and contemporary curriculum for child and adolescent psychiatry fellows. Acad Psychiatry 2021;45(1):61–6.
15. Gravlee C. How whiteness works: JAMA and the refusals of White supremacy. Somatosphere 2021.
16. Sabin JA, Greenwald AG. The influence of implicit bias on treatment recommendations for 4 common pediatric conditions: pain, urinary tract infection, attention deficit hyperactivity disorder, and asthma. Am J Public Health 2012;102(5):988–95.
17. Cyrus KD. Medical education and the minority tax. JAMA 2017;317(18):1833–4.
18. Mensah MO. Majority taxes - toward antiracist allyship in medicine. N Engl J Med 2020;383(4):e23.
19. Devakumar D, Selvarajah S, Shannon G, et al. Racism, the public health crisis we can no longer ignore. Lancet 2020;395(10242):e112–3.
20. Singh AA. The racial healing handbook: practical activities to help you challenge privilege, confront systemic racism, and engage in collective healing. Oakland, CA: New Harbinger Publications; 2019.
21. Legha RK, Williams DR, Snowden L, et al. Getting our knees off Black people's necks: an anti-racist approach to medical care. 2021.
22. Brown D. Barbaric': America's cruel history of separating children from their parents. Washington Post. 2018. Available at: https://www.washingtonpost.com/news/retropolis/wp/2018/05/31/barbaric-americas-cruel-history-of-separating-children-from-their-parents/. Accessed October 3, 2021.
23. Haaland DA. Memorandum from the secretary of the interior : federal Indian boarding school initiative. Washington, D.C: U.S. Department of the Interior; 2021.
24. Coates T-N. The case for reparations. In: Sid H, editor. The best American magazine writing 2015. New York, NY: Columbia University Press; 2015. p. 1–50.
25. Roberts D. Abolishing policing also means abolishing family regulation. The Imprint. 2020. Available at: https://imprintnews.org/child-welfare-2/abolishing-policing-also-means-abolishing-family-regulation/44480. Accessed October 3, 2021.
26. Alexander M. The new Jim Crow: Mass incarceration in the age of Colorblindness. New York, NY: The New Press; 2020.
27. Miranda J, Legha R. The consequences of family separation at the Border and beyond. J Am Acad Child Adolesc Psychiatry 2019;58(1):139–40.
28. Nations U. United Nations Office On Genocide Prevention And The Responsibility To Protect. Published online 2015.
29. Myers JEB. A Short history of child protection in America. Fam L Q 2008;42(3):449–63.
30. Morton MJ. Institutionalizing Inequalities: black children and child welfare in cleveland, 1859-1998. J Social Hist 2000;34:141–62.
31. Jones KW. Taming the troublesome child: American families, child guidance, and the Limits of psychiatric Authority. Cambridge, MA: Harvard University Press; 1999.
32. Bell JR. Repairing the Breach: a Brief history of youth of color in the justice system. Oakland, CA: W. Haywood Burns Institute of Youth Justice Fairness & Equity; 2016.

33. Chavez-Garcia M. States of delinquency. Oakland, CA: University of California Press; 2012.

34. LeFlouria TL. Chained in silence: black women and convict labor in the new South. Chapel Hill, NC: UNC Press Books; 2015.

35. Keeler CO. The crime of crimes: or, the convict system Unmasked. Washington, D.C.: D. C. Pentecostal era Company; 1907.

36. Henderson H, Wyatt Bourgeois J. Penalizing Black hair in the name of academic success is undeniably racist, unfounded, and against the law. Published online 2021.

37. BLACK GIRLS MATTER: PUSHED OUT, OVERPOLICED AND UNDERPROTECTED. Human Rights Documents Online. Published online 2018.

38. Ford JE, Triplett N. E(race)ing Inequities | Students of color take fewer honors courses than white peers, new report finds. Published online August 21, 2019.

39. Ramey DM. The social structure of criminalized and medicalized school discipline. Sociol Educ 2015;88(3):181–201.

40. Ladson-Billings G. From the achievement gap to the education debt: understanding achievement in U.S. Schools. Educ Res 2006;35(7):3–12.

41. Johnson-Farias R. Uniquely common: the cruel heritage of separating families of color in the United States. Harv L Pol'y Rev 2019;14:531.

42. Kendi IX. Stamped from the Beginning: The Definitive History of Racist Ideas in America. Hachette (United Kingdom):Bold Type Books (Queens, New York); 2016.

43. Epstein R, Blake J, Gonzalez T. Girlhood interrupted: the erasure of black girls' childhood. Washington, D.C.: Georgetown Law Center on Poverty and Inequality; 2017.

44. Moynihan DP, Rainwater L, Yancey WL. The Moynihan report and the politics of controversy. Cambridge, MA: Massachusetts Institute; 1967. Published online.

45. White C. Federally mandated destruction of the black family: the adoption and safe families act. Nw JL Soc Pol'y 2006;1:303.

46. Raz M. What's wrong with the poor?: psychiatry, race, and the war on poverty. Chapel Hill, NC: UNC Press Books; 2013.

47. Percheski C, Gibson-Davis C. A Penny on the dollar: racial Inequalities in wealth among households with children. Socius 2020;6. 2378023120916616.

48. Putnam-Hornstein E, Ahn E, Prindle J, et al. Cumulative rates of child protection involvement and terminations of parental rights in a California Birth cohort, 1999–2017. Am J Public Health 2021;111(6):1157–63.

49. Kim H, Wildeman C, Jonson-Reid M, et al. Lifetime Prevalence of investigating child maltreatment among US children. Am J Public Health 2017;107(2):274–80.

50. Wall-Wieler E, Roos LL, Bolton J, et al. Maternal mental health after custody loss and death of a child: a retrospective cohort Study using linkable Administrative Data. Can J Psychiatry 2018;63(5):322–8.

51. Wall-Wieler E, Roos LL, Nickel NC, et al. Mortality among mothers whose children were taken into care by child protection services: a discordant sibling analysis. Am J Epidemiol 2018;187(6):1182–8.

52. Wall-Wieler E, Roos LL, Brownell M, et al. Suicide attempts and completions among mothers whose children were taken into care by child protection services: a cohort Study using linkable Administrative Data. Can J Psychiatry 2018;63(3):170–7.

53. Benedict MI, Zuravin S, Somerfield M, et al. The reported health and functioning of children maltreated while in family foster care. Child Abuse Negl 1996;20(7):561–71.

54. Benedict MI, Zuravin S, Brandt D, et al. Types and frequency of child maltreatment by family foster care providers in an urban population. Child Abuse Negl 1994;18(7):577–85.
55. Turney K, Wildeman C. Mental and physical health of children in foster care. Pediatrics 2016;138(5).
56. Cort NA, Cerulli C, He H. Investigating health disparities and disproportionality in child maltreatment reporting: 2002-2006. J Public Health Manag Pract 2010; 16(4):329–36.
57. Kunins HV, Bellin E, Chazotte C, et al. The effect of race on provider decisions to test for illicit drug use in the peripartum setting. J Womens Health 2007;16(2):245–55.
58. Hardeman RR, Karbeah J 'mag, Kozhimannil KB. Applying a critical race lens to relationship-centered care in pregnancy and childbirth: an antidote to structural racism. Birth 2020;47(1):3–7.
59. Dudley RG. Childhood trauma and its effects: Implications for police. Published online 2015.
60. Jindal M, Mistry KB, Trent M, et al. Police exposures and the health and well-being of Black youth in the US: a systematic review. JAMA Pediatr 2022; 176(1):78–88.
61. Chang A. School segregation didn't go away. It just evolved. Vox. 2017. Available at: https://www.vox.com/policy-and-politics/2017/7/27/16004084/school-segregation-evolution. Accessed June 24, 2022.
62. EdBuild. Available at: https://edbuild.org/. Accessed June 24, 2022.
63. Ford JE, Triplett N, Story RT. E (race) ing Inequities| How access to Advanced Placement courses breaks down by race. Published online August 12, 2019.
64. Artiles AJ, Trent SC. Overrepresentation of minority students in special education: a continuing debate. J Spec Educ 1994;27(4):410–37.
65. Apology to people of color for APA's role in promoting, perpetuating, and failing to challenge racism, racial discrimination, and human hierarchy in U.S. PsycEXTRA Dataset. Published online 2021.
66. Pope-Davis D, Moore JL III, Ford D. Time will tell: three black scholars Ponder APA's Apology for silence and complicity in Perpetuating racism. Diversity issues in higher education. 2021. Available at: https://www.diverseeducation.com/opinion/article/15286201/time-will-tell-three-black-scholars-ponder-apas-apology-for-silence-and-complicity-in-perpetuating-racism. Accessed December 20, 2021.
67. FairTest. Racial justice and standardized educational testing. Available at: https://fairtest.org/racial-justice-and-standardized-educational-testin. Accessed June 24, 2022.
68. Gershenson S, Papageorge N. THE POWER of TEACHER EXPECTATIONS: how racial bias hinders student attainment. Education Next 2018;18(1):64–71.
69. Halberstadt AG, Castro VL, Chu Q, et al. Preservice teachers' racialized emotion recognition, anger bias, and hostility attributions. Contemp Educ Psychol 2018; 54:125–38.
70. Halberstadt AG, Cooke AN, Garner PW, Hughes SA, Oertwig D, Neupert SD. Racialized emotion recognition accuracy and anger bias of children's faces. Emotion. Published online July 2, 2020.
71. Riddle T, Sinclair S. Racial disparities in school-based disciplinary actions are associated with county-level rates of racial bias. Proc Natl Acad Sci U S A 2019;116(17):8255–60.
72. Del Toro J, Lloyd T, Buchanan KS, et al. The criminogenic and psychological effects of police stops on adolescent black and Latino boys. Proc Natl Acad Sci U S A 2019;116(17):8261–8.

73. White supremacy in education. Teaching Tolerance. Published online Spring 2021.
74. Motha S. Race, Empire, and English language teaching: Creating responsible and Ethical anti-racist practice. New York, NY: Teachers College Press; 2014.
75. McArdle N, Acevedo-Garcia D. Consequences of segregation for children's opportunity and wellbeing. Cambridge, MA: Harvard University; 2017.
76. The Annie E. Casey Foundation. Youth incarceration rates in the United States. The Annie E. Casey Foundation. 2021.
77. Rovner J. Racial Disparities in youth incarceration persist. Washington, D.C.: The Sentencing Project; 2021.
78. McGlynn-Wright A, Crutchfield RD, Skinner ML, et al. The usual, racialized, suspects: the consequence of police contacts with black and white youth on adult arrest. Soc Probl 2020;69(2):299–315.
79. Taylor KY. The emerging movement for police and prison abolition. New York, NY: The New Yorker; 2021. Available at: https://www.newyorker.com/news/our-columnists/the-emerging-movement-for-police-and-prison-abolition.
80. Gonnerman J. Kalief Browder, 1993–2015. New York, NC: New Yorker; 2015.
81. Browder D. My mom died trying to preserve the legacy of her son. Keeping kids out of solitary will preserve hers. USA Today. 2019. Available at: https://www.usatoday.com/story/opinion/policing/spotlight/2019/04/23/kalief-browder-suicide-solitary-confinement-venida-browder-policing-the-usa/3540366002/. Accessed March 17, 2022.
82. McMurtry-Chubb TA. Burn this Bitch down: mike Brown, emmett till, and the gendered Politics of black parenthood. Nev LJ 2016;17:619.
83. @mike4brooklyn. When I watched Ma'Khia Bryant's TikTok videos I saw my middle niece in her. I saw Ma'Khia's joy, creativity, potential, and humanity. 2021. Available at: https://twitter.com/mike4brooklyn/status/1385807583399849990. Accessed March 17, 2022.
84. Javier C. Say Latasha harlins' name. Splinter. 2017. https://splinternews.com/say-latasha-harlins-name-1794671969.
85. Skinner P. Photo of Kendrick Johnson protest 2022.
86. Corrigan M. Let the people see": it took courage to keep Emmett Till's memory alive. NPR. 2018. Available at: https://www.npr.org/2018/10/30/660980178/-let-the-people-see-shows-how-emmett-till-s-murder-was-nearly-forgotten. Accessed March 17, 2022.
87. Trayvon Martin's mom: 'We are never going to recover from this'. ABC News. 2020. Available at: https://abcnews.go.com/GMA/News/trayvon-martins-mom-recover/story?id=71715637. Accessed March 19, 2022.
88. Sforza T. A year after her "spectacular prom," girl dies in care of controversial Murrieta foster home. Orange County Register. 2019. Available at: https://www.ocregister.com/2019/04/30/a-year-after-her-spectacular-prom-16-year-old-dies-in-care-of-controversial-murrieta-foster-home/. Accessed March 17, 2022.
89. Robinson C. He was sunshine": 15-year-old boy dies by suicide after he was bullied for being gay. WXII News. 2019. Available at: https://www.wxii12.com/article/he-was-sunshine-15-year-old-boy-dies-by-suicide-after-he-was-bullied-for-being-gay/27255723#. Accessed March 17, 2022.
90. Cineas F. Reckoning with the theft of native American children. Vox. Published july 27. 2021. Available at: https://www.vox.com/22594144/native-american-boarding-schools-children. Accessed June 24, 2022.
91. Kaba M. We do this' til we free us: Abolitionist organizing and transforming justice. Chicago, IL: Haymarket Books; 2021.

718   Legha & Gordon-Achebe

92. Ford CL, Airhihenbuwa CO. Critical Race Theory, race equity, and public health: toward antiracism praxis. Am J Public Health 2010;100(Suppl 1):S30–5.
93. Fellner KD. Returning to our medicines: Decolonizing and Indigenizing mental health services to better serve Indigenous communities in urban spaces. University of British Columbia; 2016. Available at: https://open.library.ubc.ca/collections/83l/24/items/1.0228859.

Cultural Considerations in Working with Arab American Youth

Rana Elmaghraby, MD[a,b,*], Magdoline Daas, MD[c,d],
Alaa Elnajjar, MD[e], Rasha Elkady, MD[f]

KEYWORDS

- Middle East and North Africa (MENA) • Arab American • Youth • ARAB culture
- Discrimination • Mental illness • Special considerations

KEY POINTS

- Arab Americans are a heterogeneous group with different ethnic, religious, and cultural backgrounds.
- Arab American youth are particularly vulnerable to mental illness because of prejudice, stereotyping, macroaggressions, and bullying.
- Seeking care for mental illnesses can be challenging in the Arab American communities due to the stigma associated with mental illness.
- Mental health professionals must provide culturally sensitive care and educate themselves on key cultural considerations when working with Arab Americans.

INTRODUCTION

Arab Americans are a heterogeneous group of people who live in the United States and come from 22 different countries. Arab Americans are one of the most diverse ethnic groups in the United States[1] with roots in a variety of ancestral nations, cultures, beliefs, and migratory patterns.[2]

The first wave of Arab Americans to come to the United States occurred in the 1800s, followed by the second wave in 1940 around World War I, the third wave

[a] Sea Mar Community Health Centers, 14508 NE 20th Avenue, Suite #305, Vancouver, WA 98686, USA; [b] University of Washington, Seattle, WA, USA; [c] Community Health Network Indianapolis, 6950 Hillsdale Court, Indianapolis, IN 46250, USA; [d] Osteopathic Medical School-Marian University, 6950 Hillsdale Court, Indianapolis, IN 46250, USA; [e] Bradley Hospital, Alpert Medical School of Brown University, 5775 Post Road, #297, East Greenwich, RI 02818, USA; [f] University of Missouri School, of Medicine, One Hospital Drive, DC 067.00, Columbia, MO 65212, USA
* Corresponding author. Sea Mar Community Health Centers, 14508 NorthEast, 20th Avenue, Suite #305 Vancouver, WA 98686
E-mail address: relmaghrabymd@gmail.com

Child Adolesc Psychiatric Clin N Am 31 (2022) 719–732
https://doi.org/10.1016/j.chc.2022.06.007
1056-4993/22/© 2022 Elsevier Inc. All rights reserved.

around and after 1965 with the passing of the National Act, and the fourth wave in 2010 and after the Arab Spring.

Even though Arab migration to the United States began in the 1880s, they are frequently misunderstood, unjustly represented, and hated.[3]

Arab immigrants in the United States had an uncertain, if not confusing, status before the 1940s.[4] In the 1940s, the Census Bureau decided that Arab Americans should be treated in the same way as other European immigrants. According to the US government's Office of Management and Budget, Arab Americans fall into the "White" racial category, with origins in the Middle East.[5]

Arab American organizations and members of the community began lobbying for the special Middle East and North African (MENA) identifier on the US census in the 1990s.[6] Despite several attempts to add MENA as a category, officials decided not to add it to the US Census in 2020.

According to the Arab American Institute, the United States has about 3.7 million Arab Americans. The majority of Arab Americans live in 10 states: California, Michigan, New York, Florida, Texas, New Jersey, Illinois, Ohio, Pennsylvania, and Virginia. Orthodox Christianity, Catholics, Coptic Christianity, Islam, and Judaism are among the religions practiced by Arab Americans.[7]

Arab American Youth

The majority of adolescent Arab Americans are second-generation Arab Americans, having been born in the United States to immigrant parents. Adolescent immigrants generally grasp acculturation before their parents do. When parents rely on their children to communicate with others, role reversal may develop. Arab American youth typically rely on support from their family and communities.[8] Family support and religious beliefs are important for Arab American adolescents' mental health and well-being. Arab American youth are particularly vulnerable to mental illness consequent to prejudice, discrimination, bullying, stereotyping, and macroaggression.

Building positive relationships with Arab American youth and encouraging them to speak up about their issues could lead to more successful solutions.[9]

ARAB CULTURE

Religion, morality, honor, generosity, education, hospitality, respect, and the role of the family are some of the important values of Arab culture. The father is regarded as the family's leader. Although there has been a departure from this conventional role in recent years, the mother's duty has typically been that of raising and teaching her children. In Islam, the mother holds a sacred position; elders are highly respected; and the sons carry the family name. Boys usually are expected to protect their sisters. In Muslim Arab Americans, there is a strong emphasis on modesty from all genders. Premarital sex is forbidden in Islam. Most Arabs report that religion is very important to them and plays an important role in their lives. Arab Americans–whether Christian, Muslim, or Jewish–tend to value spirituality.

Many Arab Americans work to balance their traditional values with American values, which can be challenging. It is common for Arab Americans to prioritize their familial membership over their individuality.[10] Further, the family is often an individual's primary source of support.[11,12] As a representation of one's identity, the family is one social unit. The concept of preserving the family refers to the familial relationship that is at the heart of Arab culture. Arab societies are more concerned with preserving the community's identity as a whole rather than focusing on a single individual. This value is unique to the Arab world.

While living in America, which is known for its individualism, the Arab diaspora may find it difficult to reconcile their traditional values of communal responsibility and cohesion with the individualism that is cherished in American culture. Individualism can also be difficult to assimilate into a culture that emphasizes the value of the community link.

There is strong support from extended family. The individual's or family's conduct and activities are heavily influenced by the spouse, children, and relatives. All big decisions are discussed frequently with the rest of the family. Individual, familial, and cultural values all have an impact on the assessment of patients' needs and the delivery of medical treatment. Members of two or three generations live in a single household in Arab civilization, or a family compound in affluent families. This extended family is made up of a married man, his adult sons, and their families. In some cases, a grandparent may live with the family. Several brothers and their families may live in a compound with a grandma and other elderly relatives as a variant of this familial structure.

The extended family that makes up a single household is only found among recent immigration among Arab Americans. Families tend to create nuclear families as they acculturate and assimilate, with the odd addition of an old grandmother and an unmarried adult kid. Adult married children from less assimilated families establish a home near their parents and married siblings. This arrangement allows extended family networks to be maintained while still reaping the benefits of living in a nuclear family.

In many Arab families, honor is just as important as family values. Maintaining family honor inspires principles such as "hard work, thrift, and conservatism" and consequently, the pursuit of higher education and economic status.[13]

According to Amer and Awad,[11] honor can affect young people in areas of development that non-Arab peers do not, such as dating limitations, educational aspirations, and marital and family issues. Because familial issues are supposed to stay inside the family, protecting family honor may be jeopardized by discussing family problems with outsiders.[14] Honor is linked to mental health stigma and can influence young Arabs' help-seeking behavior.

When people have mental health problems, gender has an impact on how they seek treatment. Young women are expected to seek help from elderly women, whereas young men are supposed to seek help from elderly men. Young Muslim Arab women, for example, may be required to avoid dating, social activities, and living independently,[15] whereas young men, particularly eldest sons, may be expected to assume the role of the household head.

Arab culture values emotional secrecy and discourages the verbal expression of feelings, particularly among women and girls. As a result, religious explanations for psychological symptoms are popular, and psychological suffering is frequently communicated via physical symptoms.[16]

It is vital to be mindful of gender disparities that may exist in more traditional representations of Arab culture. A provider may feel uncomfortable or behave improperly if he or she is unaware of gender standards for young Arab Americans.

The comparatively high usage of religious leaders as sources of support by Arab Americans contributes to their low utilization of mental health treatments.[17-20]

According to research, Arab American children are less likely to seek the psychological assistance they require.[21] They are cautious to express their feelings because they are scared that doing so will reflect negatively on them and their society. It can take a little longer for them to trust their doctor. Furthermore, some Arab Americans prefer to work with a provider of their gender.

Many Arab Americans strive to strike a balance between traditional and American ideals, which can be difficult. Owing to cultural characteristics and the stigma around mental illness in Arab American communities, seeking help for mental illnesses and discussing sensitive subjects (sex, addiction, and so forth.) can be difficult. Therefore, mental health providers need to provide culturally sensitive care to Arab American youth with emphasis on the American Academy of Child and Adolescent Psychaitry (AACAP) parameter.[22]

Acculturation

Although there is a lot of research done to examine the effect of acculturation on the mental health of immigrants of different ethnic groups, little research was done on Arab Americans and how they are affected by acculturation despite their vulnerability as a minority, diverse ethnic group.

Using a sample of 1016 participants, Aprahamian and colleagues[23] investigated the relationship between acculturation and mental health among Arab immigrants. The study discovered that "faith, discrimination experiences, and age" all have an impact on Arab Americans' mental health (p 88). This implies that societal bias and discrimination hurt this group's mental health. Other predictors of Arab immigrants' mental health are "income level, age, gender, length of time in the United States, and discrimination experiences." [24]

According to Jadalla and Lee,[25] Arab immigrants who accept the dominant American culture as a whole are more likely to drink, have better physical health, and have worse mental health. Research supports that immigrants who experience trauma are at high risk for developing depression, anxiety, and post-traumatic stress disorder (PTSD).[26]Language barriers are another important factor that can add to the risk of developing mental illness in Arab Americans.

Britto and colleagues[27] emphasized that Muslim Arab American youth must navigate a complex ethnic identity as members of a cultural group that is sometimes at odds with the mainstream Western world on a sociopolitical level, and they are sometimes viewed with skepticism by mainstream American culture, which can affect their daily interactions and complicate their adjustment at home and school.

The value of cultural resources in the lives of teenagers who suffer discrimination and acculturative stress[28] indicated a favorable correlation, which confirmed prior studies.[29,30] Adolescents with a stronger ethnic identification and religious support were less likely to experience distress.

These findings highlight the importance of taking into account the current sociopolitical environment in which Arab Americans live, as well as the effect of discrimination and acculturative stress in the post-9/11 era of racial profiling, cultural stigma, and social marginalization due to ethnic minority status, religion, and, in some cases, immigration and language. Access to culturally relevant resources may help to reduce the likelihood of Arab American teenagers experiencing psychological discomfort.

DISCRIMINATION TOWARD ARAB AMERICAN

Arab Americans have experienced structural racism, discrimination, and exclusion in the United States for as long as the country has existed. Incidents of racism affecting Arab Americans have drastically increased since September 11, 2001, making it difficult for them to completely assimilate into American society.[31,32] Furthermore, recent political upheavals, such as the "Arab Spring," have caused a lot of anxiety and stress among Arab Americans.

Arab Americans are often portrayed as violent, backward people who are inflexible, and oppressive toward their women. Arab Americans are usually depicted in the media as unprogressive in their civilization and technology in addition to Middle Eastern countries often displayed as desert land that is sandy and hot, full of tents for housing, and camels as means of transportation.

This discrimination and stereotyping of Arab Americans continued throughout the centuries with different political actions between the United States and the Middle East. During the Trump era, with the implementation of the travel ban, the stereotype and discrimination toward Arab Americans continued and got worse. For the longest time, Arab Americans were viewed and continue to be viewed as a monolithic group that is a security threat to the United States.

Consequent to decades of discrimination toward Arab Americans, they have been exposed to their own kind of trauma for being marginalized and viewed as "terrorists" for decades. In fact, anyone that looks like an Arab American would also be discriminated against. This perpetuates the generational trauma that is present in most Arab American families as they try to fight the stereotypes against them. This further impedes their ability to seek mental health treatment, as it is often difficult to trust a system that caused the trauma.

Discrimination, stereotyping, bullying, Islamophobia, as well as anti-Arab prejudice, have all been connected to poor mental health outcomes.[33,34] Depression, anxiety, substance misuse, and suicidal thoughts are common among Arab American youth.[17,35–37]

Arab American youth are a vulnerable group that struggles with formulating their identity while being American. Discrimination toward Arab American youth can be conducted by peers or adults, and it can range from name-calling to violence, and it can happen in schools or other public places. Arab American youth may be bullied at school and discriminated against. Some Arab American youth may change their names to a more common American name to avoid prejudice and unfair treatment toward them. Arab American youth can be bullied based on media stigmatization and being of a religious minority.[1] A study looked at Arab American adolescents (12–16 years old) who were recruited from a community and mosque setting in Michigan and found that bullying resulted in adverse health outcomes for those adolescents independent of psychosocial stressors.[38]

Assumptions and Stereotypes: Case Examples

The following are the most common stereotyped notions presented as case examples:

1. assumption about family: A teenage boy is ridiculed by his friends and asked if his dad has multiple wives and is oppressive toward them. This makes him receive more judgments and gets bullied by his friends. When the reality is that his father is a physician who immigrated to the United States at an older age and is now working minimum wage jobs to provide for his family.
2. assumption about the choice of clothing: A young 17-year-old Arab girl comes in wearing her hijab (head scarf) and is believed to be oppressed and forced to wear this. The treatment team is confused as to how to treat her and if they should even allow her to wear her head cover in the inpatient unit. There are premade judgments and beliefs about her. The truth was she chose to wear it and enjoys the colorful scarves that she gets to wear as she practices her religion freely.
3. assumption about identity: A young Arab man who has a beard and dark hair comes in psychotic and agitated. As part of his altered mental status exam, he mutters words in Arabic that the staff felt they heard the word "Allah." The staff gets worried that he is a terrorist and their safety is at risk. They immediately detain him physically and chemically and there are five security guards standing outside

his door. Again, there was a preconceived prejudice that this young man looked like what the media depicts so he must be a terrorist. When the truth is, he had encephalopathy that resulted in delirium and he was uttering random Arabic words as a result of his altered mental status.

ARAB AMERICAN YOUTH IDENTITY

Youth in Arab American families have an important role in maintaining family honor by working hard, succeeding in school, and practicing their culture and religious beliefs. Regarding Arab American youth's role and identity, the expectation is unconditional respect and obedience without questioning. It is not acceptable to blame parents or to be loud or disrespectful toward them, regardless of what actions they take. American culture prepares and encourages youth to be independent from parents by age 18. In contrast, in Arab American families, it is usual for young adults past the age of 18 years to continue living with their parents.

It is of great value that clinicians appreciate the intersectional identities of Arab American youth. "Identity versus role confusion" is the fifth stage of psychosocial development.[39] During this period, an adolescent's developmental task is to develop a sense of self- and personal identity. The child begins to practice moving into adulthood and separating from the mother or disengaging from the primary loved object.[40] Such disengagement, Akhtar[41] wrote, can be significantly compromised during immigration. This could cause the adolescent to struggle with regulating strong emotions and feel confused regarding his or her identity.

Another component that Arab American teens face with defining their identity is their consistent catering to two distinct cultures. One involves honoring and respecting their home culture, religion, and traditional values. The second displays itself as they fit into the receptive culture and blend in with their peers in school. Biculturalism holds them to two different normative expectations. Gender segregation and dressing modestly are norms in Arab cultures, which limit participation in school social events, such as prom or school dances, in many Arab families. Sleepovers are rare occurrences. Family communication about taboo topics, such as sex is minimal to nonexistent. And if it does exist, it is usually unspoken and enforces abstinence. Premarital sex, especially for females, and homosexual relationships are strongly stigmatized.[42,] Seeking birth control or sexually transmitted disease testing is not well perceived by Arab parents. There is a myth that safe sex education encourages kids to have sexual encounters early in their youth.[43]

MENTAL ILLNESS AMONG ARAB AMERICAN YOUTH

Arab American youth have unique risk factors predisposing them to psychiatric disorders. Simply announcing their names in public that they are Arab and/or Muslims, or even wearing their traditional clothing (hijab or headscarf) makes them more targeted for bullying and discrimination. Further, 56% of Arab immigrants have faced persecution in their home country, and 54% of those who reported an adverse event had symptoms, such as a PTSD diagnosis.[44] PTSD rates have reached alarming numbers in Arab youth, whose lives were wrecked by war–in some reports up to 35%–50%.[44]

Arab American youth are at high risk of getting bullied and face victimization both within and outside of the classroom.[20,35] In a large sample of Arab American youths, Ahmed and colleagues[17] discovered a strong relationship between discrimination and poor mental health. In 2007, Amer and Hovey[45] found that discrimination based on religious affiliation or ethnicity may lead to some Arab American Muslim youth trying to hide their identity. Ajrouch and colleagues[46] found a link between stereotypes and internalized prejudice about Arab Americans and low self-esteem and pessimism. Also, personal experiences with prejudice and acculturative stress, in particular, hurt the developmental outcomes of young Arabs.[47]

In a study by Jaber and colleagues, 98 adolescents aged 12–17 years from Dearborn, which has the largest population of Arab Americans in the country, were surveyed. Their findings showed that 14% of the subjects surveyed reflected moderate-to-severe depression. At the same time, only 2% of the subjects reported a formal diagnosis of depression by a mental health professional.[21] In a similar study, it was postulated that Arab Americans commonly conceptualized illness using spiritual models, such as evil eye and black magic, possession by spirits or Jinn, personal shortcomings that cause depression, and encouraging nearness to God to be protected from depression. Smith and colleagues[48] reported that Arab Americans frequently displayed psychological distress as physical symptoms, such as somatization and conversion disorders because the biological model was commonly reported for illness conceptualization.

Smoking cigarettes and hookah, alcohol use, and substance use are a concern among Arab American youth. Tobacco use is frequent among Arab American teenagers, especially in the form of hookah.[49] Because of religious prohibitions against substance use, the use of alcohol and drugs is considered disgraceful in many Arab households, particularly Muslim families. Parents' displeasure and the stigma associated with substance abuse and mental health care may discourage children from getting help.

Other topics that Arab Americans youth may be hesitant to address include intimate relationships and sex. They keep their dating and relationships under wraps. The youth's guilt and concealment may cause them to continue in an abusive relationship, as well as sadness and suicidal thinking. Instead of sharing their pain with their family, the teenager may opt to suffer alone and in silence.

While it does seem that many factors hinder Arab American youth's mental health access, they do have many protective factors. Family and community network support, resilience, adaptability, and religious coping are protective against distress, substance abuse, suicide, depression, and PTSD.[50]

TREATMENT AND SERVICE UTILIZATION

Arab Americans can be at risk of not getting the mental health care that they need. There are various factors at play but most significantly: stigma and negative stereotypic presentation of Arab Americans. Arab Americans may worry that by seeking mental health care, they are going to be judged. Likewise, clinicians may have an implicit bias toward Arab Americans seeking care. One of the best ways a clinician can support an Arab American is to not only have awareness of Arab culture but also understand the challenges of the negative stereotypes toward Arab Americans. It is particularly important to understand how Arab American youth struggle with positive self-identity and the role that plays in various mental illnesses.

Sue and colleagues[51] pointed out the three domains of cultural competencies, which include clinicians' awareness of their own assumptions, values, and implicit biases; understanding the patient's experience; and using culturally competent tools in assessment and treatment. Thus, with Arab American youth it is important to be aware of biases toward them, understand their experience growing up in a world where there is a negative stereotype toward their race, and provide interventions that are based on cultural competence.

Understanding the family background and values that an Arab American youth comes with is critical and is an important part of the three domains of cultural competence. For example, a child of Lebanese origin might have different challenges and family expectations compared to a child of Saudi origin.

One important barrier to care that is shared by all Arab Americans despite their ethnic background is the stigma to seek mental health care as well as the presentation of mental health illness. It is more common for Arab American families to present with somatic complaints than mental health symptoms. Additionally, families may try to avoid their child from getting mental health care or hide that their child is. Many Arab American families fear being judged or labeled as "crazy" for seeking mental health care. It tends to be done in secrecy.

ASSESSMENT/EVALUATION

With Arab American youth, certain areas that mental health providers need to keep in mind while assessing psychosocial stressors, such as the intersectionality between cultural, spiritual, religious, and sexual identities and the impact of this on parent–child relationship development. Providers may use these supplementary modules in two ways: (1) as adjuncts to the core cultural formulation interview (CFI) for additional information about specific aspects of illness affecting diverse populations and (2) as a tool for in-depth cultural assessment independent of the core CFI. Clinicians may administer one, several, or all modules depending on what areas of an individual's problems they would like to elaborate on.[22]

Case Example

Mo is 16 years boy, domiciled with both parents in Brooklyn with two younger siblings. Mo was born in New York. His parents are immigrant Muslims from Jordan, who speak Arabic. Mo is identified as a first-generation American, dual language speaker (Arabic and English). Mo presented to the outpatient clinic for evaluation after a recommendation from the school counselor for hopelessness and low energy to finish school assignments. During the intake session, he reported feeling sad for the last 6 months after his father was deported back to Jordan. He reported feeling guilty about his father leaving the country as it happened after the teacher reported to child protective services his absence from school for 5 days for getting sick with COVID. He referred to himself as now being "the man of the house." He has been more irritable with his younger 15-year-old sister, especially when she asks her mother to go out with her friends. He identifies his primary current problem as losing interest in things that he used to enjoy; for example, he felt guilty about not being able to fast Ramadan like the rest of his family this year. In interviewing his mother, she reported feeling overwhelmed with work since her husband left the country as she used to be a stay-home mother and was forced to start working as an Uber driver to provide for her three kids. Mo, as the oldest son, became more responsible for extra errands at home, but she noticed in the last few months, that he is sleeping more often and it is hard for him to take care of his hygiene. He has been eating more junk food and gained about 20 lb in the last 3 months. His mother also reported her suspicion that he started smoking Hookah but was not sure how to ask him about this. At the end of the evaluation, mom asked if he needs to be on medications and if he can be treated without them.

Clinical Questions

1. What is your understanding about your current mental health?
2. How do you cope with your current mental challenge?

3. What does fasting Ramadan mean to you? And how does your family celebrate it?
4. Can you elaborate more on your feelings regarding how your father was deported?
5. What role does culture play in your family life?

Clinical Discussion

Multiple cultural considerations should be included in the biopsychosocial formulation of this case and explored from different aspects for further assessment. First, trying to understand the bicultural identity (Arab and American) of the patient, and also exploring whether the social network is stress or a buffer. Second, the patient is going through a major traumatic event (father's deportation). This major change in this family dynamic, not just losing a major family member from an immigrant family, but what the father figure means to him as part of Arab culture and what their relationship growing up, and what it would mean for the patient to now be the paternal figure of the house. Third, and most importantly, understanding the impact of stigma on readiness to seek help and acceptance of different therapeutic interventions. So, for example, in this case, is being diagnosed with depression considered as bringing shame to the family? Is taking medication considered somehow an affront to God's will?

RECOMMENDATIONS

It is recommended to apply the AACAP practice guidelines when working with Arab American youth. The following are some of the recommendations illustrated from the earlier discussed case example:

1. Identify and address barriers that may prevent youth from obtaining mental health services: someone else in the family can also be an undocumented immigrant and avoid help if she/he/they are afraid of getting deported like Mo's father.
2. Conduct the evaluation in the language in which the child and family are proficient, by using a proper interpreter. As the Arabic language has multiple dialects, this family may prefer the Jordan dialect. It would be helpful to note that with the interpreter's request.
3. Understand the impact of dual language competence on the child's adaptation and functioning: Even if the mother speaks the same language as the clinician, some parents feel ashamed for not being fluent in the language of the country they immigrated to and would shy away from asking for an interpreter if it was not offered.
4. Be cognizant of your own cultural biases and address them: Mo carries the risk of being discriminated against for being part of minority groups in the United States.
5. Apply knowledge of cultural differences in development, idioms of distress, and symptomatic presentation to clinical formulation and diagnosis: Mo reported guilt around not being able to fast Ramadan which is a holy month in the Islamic religion. Confirm depression is a differential diagnosis for this case. His guilt about his inability to practice it can be exaggerated as a depression symptom.
6. Assess the history of immigration-related loss or trauma and community trauma and address them in treatment: There are two important stages in this family's immigration timeline. First is the time Mo's parents immigrated to the United States, which may have a gradual traumatic impact on them especially if the father has been undocumented for a while. The second is the time his father got deported suddenly. This presents acute stress for the whole family with the mother having to take the father's role as a working parent while dealing with the sudden loss of her husband.

7. Evaluate and address acculturation stress and intergenerational acculturation family conflict: Ask for a deeper understanding for how it was like to be born in the United States in a family from a Middle East background. Smoking Hookah can be culturally not accepted in some Arab families, which could explain how the mother has a suspicion about Mo smoking but may be afraid to ask about that.

8. Evaluate and utilize the child and family's cultural strengths in treatment interventions. Some of the following themes could be considered strengths for this family: acceptance of psychiatric referral by the school counselor, the ability of the mother to adjust rapidly to the loss of the father and starting to work, and the patient was articulate and open about certain fears and guilt.

9. Support parents to develop appropriate behavioral management skills compatible with their cultural values and beliefs. In this case, explaining what confidentiality means to the parent as this is their first interaction with the mental health system and taking the time to understand their expectations during the process of assessment and treatment.

10. Use evidence-based psychological and pharmacological interventions specific to the child and family's ethnic/racial population: Explaining to the family the demographics of the patients in the studies that are used to guide the clinical decisions regarding treatment of both depression symptoms and trauma-related symptoms, and share if any data included patients from similar backgrounds as Mo.

FUTURE DIRECTIONS

There is a scarcity of literature and research on Arab American youth mental health in general and in particular on the importance of cultural competence when working with Arab American youth.[52,53] As a result, additional research, education, and training for mental health providers to provide culturally sensitive care are critical. This will help providers improve their abilities in building strong therapeutic rapport, doing stronger assessments, and comprehensive treatment planning.

CONCLUSION

This article provides an overview of the Arab Americans/MENA and Arab American youth demographics, migration, traditional culture and values, Arab American youth identity, acculturation and acculturation stress, and the impact of discrimination on Arab American youth all discussed in detail. It also sheds light on mental illness in Arab American youth, therapy, and cultural variables in seeking help, suggestions, guidelines, and cultural considerations when working with Arab American youth, all of which could help clinicians become more aware of and better equipped to work with this unique group.

CLINICAL PEARLS

When meeting an Arab American youth for the first time, be mindful of the cultural sensitivities that can be at interplay during the session. Stigma can affect a family's willingness to participate in treatment. Clinicians should take advantage of the first time a patient arrives because it may be their only chance to deliver psychoeducation to the patient and family before they drop out of treatment.

When explaining mental health to Arab American families, do not dismiss the role of an imam or priest in treatment. A lot of Arab families, particularly Muslim families, will rely on their religious leader. Involving the religious leader would ensure the most success for the youth.

When assessing Arab American families, be mindful of the value of honor as an integral part of Arab culture. Don't forget to ask about different roles the youth has within the household as responsibilities can be gender-based.

When treating Arab American youth, take into consideration generational trauma, particularly the negative stereotype they have been facing for decades. Be mindful of your own implicit bias and prejudice when treating them.

When formulating cases for Arab American youth, be conscious of the impact of discrimination on their mental health. Understanding how discrimination and racism affect psychological functioning would be beneficial.

When formulating a case and implementing treatment strategies, be mindful of acculturative stress among Arab American youths, as it plays a key role in their mental health.

When treating Arab American teenagers, be aware of intergenerational family strife and assist the family in resolving these conflicts. Teenagers frequently disagree with their parents regarding clothing, relationships, schooling, and careers.

DISCLOSURE

The authors have nothing to disclose. The authors did not recieve funding or grant support for this work.

REFERENCES

1. Abuelezam NN, El-Sayed AM, Galea S. The health of Arab Americans in the United States: an updated comprehensive literature review. Frontiers in public Health 2018;6:262.
2. Awad GH, Nguyen H, Castellanos F, Payne T, Hashem H. Mental health considerations for immigrants of Arab/MENA descent. In: Mental and Behavioral Health of Immigrants in the United States. Academic Press; 2020. p. 201–15.
3. Tehranian J. The last minstrel show? Racial profiling, the war on terrorism and the mass media. Papers.ssrn.com. 2022. Available at: https://papers.ssrn.com/sol3/papers.cfm?abstract_id=1312941. Accessed March 15, 2022.
4. Calendar.rgj.com. Available at: http://calendar.rgj.com/cgibin/open/file.php?title=race+and+arab+americans+before+and +after+9+11+from+invisible+citizens+to+visible+subjects+pdf& id=8aa59b18ab2060f0b8ebbd03db2da82e. Accessed March 15, 2022.
5. Office of management and Budget | the white house. The White House; 2022. Available at: https://www.whitehouse.gov/omb/. [Accessed 15 March 2022]. Accessed.
6. Census Bureau may count arab-Americans for the first time in 2020. PBS news hour. 2022. Available at: http://www.pbs.org/newshour/rundown/census-bureau considering-new-category-arab-americans-2020-count. Accessed March 15, 2022.
7. Demographics 2021. Arab American Institute. Available at: http://www.aaiusa. org/demographics. Accessed April 22, 2022.
8. Fakih RR. Ethnic identity among Arab Americans: An examination of contextual influences and psychological well-being. Wayne State University; 2013.
9. Borup I, Holstein BE. Schoolchildren who are victims of bullying report benefit from health dialogues with the School Health Nurse. Health Educ J 2007;66(1):58–67. https://doi.org/10.1177/0017896907073787.
10. Budman CL, Lipson JG, Meleis AI. The cultural consultant in mental health care: the case of an Arab adolescent. Am J Orthop 1992;62(3):359–70.

11. Amer M, Awad G. Handbook of arab american psychology. New York: Routledge Taylor & Francis Group; 2016.

12. Beitin BK, Aprahamian M. Family values and traditions. In: Nassar-McMillan S, Ajrouch K, Hakim-Larson J, editors. Biopsychosocial perspectives on Arab Americans. Boston, MA: Springer US; 2014. p. 67–88.

13. Erickson CD, Al-Timimi NR. Providing mental health services to Arab Americans: recommendations and considerations. Cultur Divers Ethnic Minor Psychol 2001; 7(4):308–27.

14. Abudabbeh N, Nydell MK. Tanscultural counseling and Arab Americans. 2nd. Akexandria, VA.: American Counseling Association; 1993. p. 261–84.

15. Springer PR, Abbott DA, Reisbig AMJ. Therapy with muslim couples and families: basic guidelines for effective practice. Fam J 2009;17(3):229–35.

16. Al-Krenawi A, Graham JR. Culturally sensitive social work practice with arab clients in mental health settings. Health Soc Work 2000;25(1):9–22.

17. Ahmed S, Reddy LA. Understanding the mental health needs of american muslims: recommendations and considerations for practice. J Multicultural Couns Develop 2007;35(4):207–18.

18. Al-Krenawi A. Mental health practice in Arab countries. Curr Opin Psychiatry 2005;18(5):560–4.

19. Hamdan A. Arab muslim women in Canada: the untold narratives. J Muslim Minor Aff 2007;27(1):133–54.

20. Youssef J, Deane FP. Factors influencing mental-health help-seeking in Arabic-speaking communities in Sydney, Australia. Mental Health. Religion Cult 2006; 9(1):43–66.

21. Jaber RM, Farroukh M, Ismail M, et al. Measuring depression and stigma towards depression and mental health treatment among adolescents in an Arab-American community. Int J Cult Ment Health 2014;8(3):247–54.

22. Pumariega AJ, Rothe E, Mian A, et al. Practice parameter for cultural competence in child and adolescent psychiatric practice. J Am Acad Child Adolesc Psychiatry 2013;52(10):1101–15.

23. Aprahamian M, Kaplan D, Windham A, et al. The relationship between acculturation and mental health of Arab Americans. J Ment Health Couns 2011;33(1): 80–92.

24. Berry JW. A psychology of immigration. J Soc Issues 2001;57(3):615–31.

25. Jadalla A, Lee J. The relationship between acculturation and general health of Arab Americans. J Transcult Nurs 2012;23(2):159–65.

26. Abuelezam NN, El-Sayed AM, Galea S. The health of Arab Americans in the United States: an updated comprehensive literature review. Front Public Health 2018;6:1–18. https://doi.org/10.3389/fpubh.2018.00262.

27. Britto PR. Who Am I? Ethnic identity formation of arab muslim children in contemporary U.S. society. J Am Acad Child Adolesc Psychiatry 2008;47(8):853–7.

28. Ahmed S, Kia-Keating M, Tsai K. A Structural model of racial discrimination, acculturative stress, and cultural resources among Arab American adolescents. Am J Community Psychol 2011;48(3–4):181–92.

29. Sellers RM, Shelton JN. The role of racial identity in perceived racial discrimination. J Pers Soc Psychol 2003;84(5):1079–92.

30. Wong CA, Eccles JS, Sameroff A. The influence of ethnic discrimination and ethnic identification on African American adolescents' school and socioemotional adjustment. J Personal 2003;71(6):1197–232.

31. A_Structu ral_Model_of_Racial_Discrimination_Acculturative_Stress_and _Cultur-al_Resources_Among_Arab_American_Adolescents. Available at: https://www.researchgate.net/publication/49803976_. Accessed March 15, 2022.
32. Ibish H, Stewart A. Report on hate crimes and discrimination against Arab Americans: the post-September 11 backlash, September 11, 2001–October 11, 2002. Washington, DC: American-Arab Anti-Discrimination Committee; 2003.
33. Moradi B, Hasan NT. Arab American persons' reported experiences of discrimination and mental health: the mediating role of personal control. J Couns Psychol 2004;51(4):418–28.
34. Tabbah R, Miranda AH, Wheaton JE. Self-concept in Arab American adolescents: implications of social support and experiences in the schools. Psychol Schools 2012;49(9):817–27.
35. Albdour M, Lewin L, Kavanaugh K, et al. Arab American adolescents' perceived stress and bullying experiences: a qualitative study. West J Nurs Res 2016; 39(12):1567–88.
36. Balaghi D, Oka E, Carter Andrews D. Arab American adolescents' responses to perceived discrimination: a phenomenological study. J Muslim Ment Health 2021. https://doi.org/10.3998/jmmh.131.
37. Kumar R, Warnke JH, Karabenick SA. Arab-American male identity negotiations: caught in the crossroads of ethnicity, religion, nationality and current contexts. Social Identities 2013;20(1):22–41.
38. Albdour M, Hong JS, Zilioli S, et al. Self-reported physical and psychological symptoms among victims and perpetrators of bullying in Arab American Adolescents. J Child Adolesc Psychiatr Nurs 2020;33(4):201–8.
39. Reports — library — arab American Institute. Arab American Institute. 2022. Available at: https://www.aaiusa.org/library/category/Reports. Accessed March 15, 2022.
40. Blos. The adolescent passages. New York: International Universities Press; 1979.
41. Akhtar S. Immigration and identity: turmoil, treatment, and transformation. North-vale, NJ: Jason Aronson; 1999.
42. Ikizler AS, Szymanski DM. A qualitative study of Middle Eastern/Arab American sexual minority identity development. J LGBT Issues Couns 2014;8(2):206–41. https://doi.org/10.1080/15538605.2014.897295.
43. Widman L, Evans R, Javidi H, et al. Assessment of parent-based interventions for adolescent sexual health: a systematic review and meta-analysis. JAMA Pediatr 2019;173(9):866–77. https://doi.org/10.1001/jamapediatrics.2019.2324.
44. Reimann JO, Rodriguez-Reimann DI, Ghulan M, et al. Project salaam: assessing mental health needs among san diego's greater middle eastern and East african communities. Ethn Dis 2007;17(2):39.
45. Amer MM, Hovey JD. Socio-demographic differences in acculturation and mental health for a sample of 2nd generation/early immigrant Arab Americans. J Immigrant Minor Health 2007;9(4):335–47.
46. Ajouch KJ, Hakim-Larson J, Fakih RR. Youth Development: An Ecological Approach to Identity. In: Amer M, Awad G, editors. Handbook of Arab American Psychology. Windsor, Canada: University of Windsor; 2016.
47. Rasmi S, Chuang SS, Hennig K. The acculturation gap-distress model: extensions and application to arab Canadian families. Cultural diversity and ethnic minority psychology. Advance online publication; 2014. https://doi.org/10.1037/cdp0000014.
48. Smith J. Removing barriers to therapy with Muslim-Arab-American clients. New England: Antioch University; 2011.

49. Kulwicki A, Hill Rice V. Arab American adolescent perceptions and experiences with smoking. Public Health Nurs 2003;20(3):177–83.
50. Abu-Ras W, Abu-Bader S. Risk factors for posttraumatic stress disorder (PTSD): the case of Arab- & Muslim-Americans, post-9/11. J Immigrant Refugee Stud 2009;7(4):393–418.
51. Sue DW. Multidimensional facets of cultural competence. Couns Psychol 2001; 29(6):790–821.
52. Goforth AN, Pham AV, Chun H, et al. Association of acculturative stress, Islamic practices, and internalizing symptoms among Arab American adolescents. Sch Psychol Q 2016;31(2):198–212.
53. Soheilian SS, Inman AG. Competent counseling for middle eastern american clients: implications for trainees. J Multicultural Couns Develop 2015;43(3):173–90. https://doi.org/10.1002/jmcd.12013.

Cultural Considerations in Working with Black and African American Youth

Check for updates

Qortni Lang, MD[a],*, Toya Roberson-Moore, MD[b],
Kenneth M. Rogers, MD, MSPH, MMM[c], Walter E. Wilson Jr, MD, MHA[d]

KEYWORDS

- Systemic racism • Black and African American • Mental health • Healthcare equity

KEY POINTS

- Black children and adolescents experience more poverty, discrimination, marginalization, and racism compared with their White counterparts in the United States. These are factors that greatly impact the mental health of this population.
- Black youth are less likely to be diagnosed with mental illness and receive adequate timely treatment, despite significant prevalence of disease.
- It is important to understand that owing to the institutionalized beliefs and attitudes regarding race, African Americans, Native Americans, and other people of color are still dealing with the trauma and discrimination every day.

INTRODUCTION

According to the most recent US Census Bureau data (2020),[1,2] individuals identifying as Black or African American make up 12.4% of all individuals living in this country (41.1 million), and when including those who identify as Black in combination with another race group this number increases to 14.2% of the population (46.9 million). The Black community in the United States is incredibly diverse and represents not a monolith but a group with members who are descendants of slaves as well as those who are more recent immigrants. We appreciate the nuances and both shared and distinct backgrounds for this community. For the purpose of this article, we use the terms Black and African American interchangeably in reference to members of the Black Diaspora, which is individuals with ancestry tracing to Africa, living in the United States.

[a] NYU Grossman School of Medicine, NYU Langone Health, NYC Health + Hospital - Bellevue Medical Center, One Park Avenue, 7th Floor, New York, NY 10016, USA; [b] University of Illinois at Chicago College of Medicine, ERC Pathlight Mood and Anxiety Center, Shine Bright Child and Adolescent Behavioral Health, 333 North Michigan Avenue Suite, 2107, Chicago, IL 60601, USA; [c] South Carolina Department of Mental Health, 2414 Bull Street, Suite 321, Columbia, SC 29201, USA; [d] HealthPoint Family Care, Inc., 1401 Madison Avenue, Covington, KY 41011, USA
* Corresponding author.
E-mail address: qortni.lang@nyulangone.org

Child Adolesc Psychiatric Clin N Am 31 (2022) 733–744
https://doi.org/10.1016/j.chc.2022.05.003
1056-4993/22/© 2022 Elsevier Inc. All rights reserved.
childpsych.theclinics.com

Non-Hispanic Black youth make up approximately 14%, or just over 10 million, of the youth population in the United States. This is a number that has remained relatively the same over the last decade, although there has been a slight, gradual decline.[2] For these youth, mental health is a critical factor in development that significantly impacts how they view themselves, calibrate their own self-worth, determine their place in society, and interact with the world around them. The mental, behavioral, and emotional well-being of Black youth is incredibly important to cultivate in a healthy way for the advancement and continued evolution of the Black community in the United States.

Data have emerged recently that there has been an alarming increase in suicide rates for Black children and adolescents over the last generation. This is important to recognize as it challenges the historical narrative of Black children being at decreased risk of suicide. According to the Congressional Black Caucus Emergency Task Force on Black Youth Suicide and Mental Health Black boys, less than 13 are twice as likely to die by suicide compared with their White peers. The task force also found that despite the alarming statistics, limited research dollars have been committed by organizations such as National Institutes of Health and National Institutes of Mental Health to further investigate causes, prevention, or treatment for Back youth suicide and mental health.[3]

According to Bitsko and colleagues,[4] there are several indicators to help inform parents on whether or not their child is experiencing positive mental health which can differ depending on the specific age group being studied. According to a parental survey report administered from 2016 to 2019, the following were identified as being qualities demonstrated by children with positive mental health:

- Children ages 3 to 5 years: positivity (98.7%), affection (97.0%), curiosity (93.9%), and resilience (87.9%)
- Children ages 6 to 11 years: curiosity (93.0%), persistence (84.2%), and self-control (73.8%)
- Children ages 12 to 17 years: curiosity (see 86.5%), persistence (84.7%), and self-control (79.8%)

In children, the most commonly diagnosed mental disorders are Attention Deficit Hyperactivity Disorder (ADHD) (9.8%), anxiety (9.4%), behavioral problems (8.9%), and depression (4.4%), with these top four mental health conditions accounting for approximately 20 million children nationwide.[4] Furthermore, many of these conditions, as we know, often occur together. More specifically, children with depression most commonly suffer from another mental disorder such as anxiety (73.8%) and almost half of these children also demonstrated behavioral difficulties (47.2%).[5] In addition, children with anxiety demonstrated behavioral problems (37.9%) as well as depressive symptoms (32.3%), and children with behavioral problems primarily also experienced anxiety (36.6%) and depression (20.3%).[5] These statistics clearly demonstrate that as clinical providers, a multifaceted approach to children's mental health is not only often important but also necessary.

Equally as concerning, depression and anxiety among US children has seemed to increase in prevalence over time. For example, among children aged 6 to 17 years, 5.4% identified as being diagnosed with anxiety in 2003 which is a number that increased to 8% in 2007, although the rates of depression increased from 5.5% to 6.4% in the 5-year span from 2007 to 2012.

When evaluated closely, it becomes evident that not only do various mental and behavioral conditions begin in very early childhood but also the treatment rates and prevalence of specific mental disorders in youth seem to change with age. For example, behavioral dysregulation seems to peak and become more common from age 6 to 11 years, although the diagnoses of ADHD, depression, and anxiety seem to increase in frequency as young children progress into adolescence.[5] Unfortunately, for children aged 3 to 17 years, only 78.1% eventually receive treatment for their depressive symptoms, whereas a mere 59.3% and 53.5% of children in this age group received treatment for their anxiety and behavior disorders, respectively.[5] Current statistics also highlight the importance of early intervention for mental health providers as one in six US children ages 2 to 8 years, or approximately 17.4%, have been diagnosed with a behavioral, mental, or developmental disorder.[5] There is also evidence of gender differences regarding diagnosis in youth as, among children aged 2 to 8 years, boys seem to be more likely than girls to suffer from behavioral, developmental, and mental disorders.[6]

Many social factors, collectively known as the social determinants of mental health, also play a significant role in the development of healthy mental well-being for youth in the United States, particularly for Black youth development. Generally speaking, the social determinants of health framework focuses on understanding health outcomes in the context of the circumstances in which people live and work.[7] Some of the social determinants of mental health include food insecurity, poorly built environment, housing insecurity, adverse early life experiences, discrimination/social exclusion, poor education, poverty/income inequality, and unemployment/underemployment in job insecurity.[8] Many, if not all, of these social factors disproportionately impact youth of color in the United States.

Black children and adolescents experience more poverty, discrimination, marginalization, and racism compared with their White counterparts in the United States.[9] These are factors that greatly impact the mental health of this population. More specifically, 39% of African American children live in poverty, as compared with 14% of non-Latino, White, and Asian children and adolescents.[37] With regard to racism, perceived discrimination has been shown to contribute to mental health disorders among racial/ethnic groups such as Asian Americans and African Americans.[10] Unfortunately, less than half of Black teens suffering with depression actually receive treatment[11] which is extremely concerning given recent data suggesting that suicide attempts for Black adolescents increased by approximately 73% between 1991 and 2017.[12,13] Causing further disparity, there are studies that suggest Black youth and their families may be less likely to identify mental health symptoms when they manifest.[14] In addition, unconscious bias and outright discrimination have also played a significant role in access to care for Black youth. White teens are more likely to be treated with beneficial psychiatric medications when mental illness is identified than Black adolescents, and Black youth are more likely to be involuntarily hospitalized for psychiatric illness than their White counterparts.[15] Discriminatory treatment of Black youth is further evidenced by the fact that Black youth with psychiatric disorders are more likely than White youth to be referred to the juvenile justice system rather than to appropriate mental health treatment.[15] Regardless of the underlying reason, it is clear that Black youth lag behind other ethnic/racial groups when it comes to receiving timely mental health diagnoses, having equal access to care and engaging in evidence-based mental health treatment once connected to care.

DEFINITIONS
What Is Race?

- Race is the idea that the human species is divided into distinct groups by *inherited physical and behavioral differences*.

- Genetic studies in the late twentieth century refuted the existence of biogenetically distinct races
- Scholars now argue that "races" are cultural inventions reflecting specific attitudes and beliefs that were imposed on different populations in the wake of western European conquests beginning in the fifteenth century.

Race as a Construct

How has this construct developed and influenced race relations in North America?

"Racial classifications appeared in North America and in many other parts of the world as a form of social division predicated on what were thought to be natural differences between human groups. Analysis of the folk beliefs, social policies, and practices of North Americans about race from the eighteenth to the twentieth century reveals the development of a unique and fundamental ideology about human differences. This ideology or "racial worldview" is a systematic, institutionalized set of beliefs and attitudes that includes the following components:

- All people of the world can be divided into biologically separate, discrete, and exclusive populations called races. A person can belong to only one race.
- Phenotypic features, or visible physical differences, are markers or symbols of race identity and status. Because an individual may belong to a racial category and not have any or all of the associated physical features, racial scientists early in the twentieth century invented an invisible internal element, "racial essence," to explain such anomalies.
- Each race has distinct qualities of temperament, morality, disposition, and intellectual ability. Consequently, in the popular imagination, each race has distinct behavioral traits that are linked to its phenotype.
- Races are unequal. They can, and should, be ranked on a gradient of inferiority and superiority. As the nineteenth-century biologist Louis Agassiz observed, since races exist, we must "settle the relative rank among [them]."
- The behavioral and physical attributes of each race are inherited and innate— therefore, fixed, permanent, and unalterable.
- Distinct races should be segregated and allowed to develop their own institutions, communities, and lifestyles, separate from those of other races.

These are the beliefs that wax and wane but never entirely disappear from the core of the American version of race differences. From its inception, racial ideology accorded inferior social status to people of African or Native American ancestry. *This ideology was institutionalized in law and social practice, and social mechanisms were developed for enforcing the status differences.*[16]

People argue that slavery was abolished more than 100 years ago, so African Americans should no longer be affected by those atrocities. It is important to understand that owing to the institutionalized beliefs and attitudes regarding race, African Americans, Native Americans, and other people of color are still dealing with the trauma and discrimination every day.

Dr Joy DeGruy, PhD, coined the term Post-Traumatic Slave Syndrome (PTSS) to help explain the consequences of multigenerational oppression from centuries of chattel slavery and institutionalized racism and to identify the resulting adaptive survival behaviors. PTSS differs from post-traumatic stress disorder (PTSD), which results from a single trauma experienced directly or indirectly. "When we look at American chattel slavery we are not talking about a single trauma; we are talking about multiple traumas over lifetimes and over generations. ...Living in Black skin is a whole other level of stress."[17]

Implicit Bias

- In the United States, racial health care disparities are widely documented, and implicit race bias is one possible cause.
- Implicit bias is an unconscious thought process and decision-making can affect the provider–patient interaction, therapeutic options, diagnoses, and other areas of health care.

According to a systematic review by Fitzgerald and Hurst, health care professionals exhibit about the same levels of implicit bias as the general population does, and evidence indicates that biases are likely to influence diagnosis and treatment decisions in some circumstances.[18] Mental health professionals had better approach emotions, expressing more compassion, sadness, interest, and acceptance than non-professionals and medical students toward patients with mental illness, but both groups held negative implicit bias attitudes toward the mentally ill.[19–21]

Health Care Equity

As we all know, Emancipation was only one battle won in the centuries-long struggle for Black Civil Rights—a struggle that is far from over. Racism continues to rear its head in every aspect of American life. Income and housing inequality, police brutality, voter suppression, hate speech, and political bigotry are just a few of the forms that racism still takes.

One important racial justice issue that does not always get discussed nearly as much as it should is health care equity. According to the Centers for Disease Control and Prevention (CDC), African American adults and youth are less likely to see a doctor due to high costs, lack of accessible care, or other barriers. Stigma around mental health in the Black community also contributes to a reluctance to recognize the need for the help of a physician or therapist. Institutional racism means the health concerns of Black patients are often taken less seriously than Caucasian American patients, and serious health issues are often diagnosed later. As noted in the American Association of Medical Colleges (AAMC) article, how we fail Black patients in pain[22] inadequate treatment of pain because of a patient's race or ethnicity happening in 2020 and is simply unacceptable. The CDC reports that African Americans ages 18 to 49 years are twice as likely to die from heart disease than Caucasian Americans, and African Americans ages 35 to 64 years are 50% more likely to have high blood pressure than Caucasian Americans. They are also more likely to suffer from conditions such as diabetes and strokes at an earlier age, as experiences of racism in health care often deter people of color from getting the preventative screenings needed to catch the warning signs of these issues. Subsequently, we have seen that Black individuals have suffered disproportionately due to COVID-19.

These health inequalities are also pronounced in the Black lesbain, gay, bisexual, transgender, queer or questioning (LGBTQ) community. Black gay and bisexual men are more affected by human immunodeficiency virus (HIV) than any other group in the United States; in 2018, they accounted for 26% of total new HIV diagnoses and 37% of new diagnoses among all gay and bisexual men, according to the CDC. Queer women, and in particular Black queer women, are less likely to have regular preventative care such as mammograms and cervical cancer screenings. Black transgender women experience profound health and wellness inequality. An estimated 44% of Black transgender women are living with HIV. Transgender women of color are also disproportionately targeted in violent hate crimes and make up most of the transgender murder victims (Fenwayhealth.org).

Impact on Mental Health

An example of how ethnicity influences specific psychiatric diagnosis is that African American patients have been found to be diagnosed with schizophrenia spectrum disorders more frequently and depression less frequently during routine clinical assessments compared with similar Caucasian patients. Furthermore, this apparent misdiagnosis of schizophrenia may lead to inadequate recognition and treatment of mood disorders, which in turn results in the lower use of mental health treatment of mood disorder among African Americans.

With regard to children and adolescents, research shows that even after controlling for important socio-demographic variables and functional status, race and ethnicity still influenced the diagnosis and clinical characteristics of children in treatment[23] When the mental health needs of minority children are poorly understood, these children and adolescents are likely to be inadequately served by systems of care.[24,25] There is little research on the psychiatric diagnoses of racially and culturally diverse youth as compared with Caucasian youth despite the growth in population of racially and ethnically diverse children! There is a limited understanding of the influence of ethnicity on diagnosis, and we know the differences in assessment and diagnosis in minority children have important implications for treatment and outcomes. Inaccurate assessment and diagnosis may lead to inappropriate treatments and subsequent disparities in care for ethnically and racially diverse children and their families.

For example, African American youth are more likely than Caucasian youth to be given a diagnosis of ADHD and less likely to have been given the diagnosis of mood disorders.[26] In a retrospective chart review of hospitalized adolescents, African American youth were more commonly diagnosed with conduct disorder than Caucasian youth.[27]

In another study, although African American and Native Hawaiian children were more likely to have been diagnosed with disruptive behavioral disorders, there was no corresponding elevation in scores on the caretaker-derived Child Behavioral Checklist externalizing subscale. This inconsistency may be explained by culturally based differences in clinician and caretaker perspectives or may also indicate the possibility of clinician bias in assigning diagnosis.

Most research has been done in children showing a misdiagnosis of children with disruptive behaviors who have mood disorders. So, what contributes to the misdiagnosis?

Clinician factors that influence diagnosis include:

- Ratings of child problem behavior are a function of the observer and child ethnicity
- Clinician perception of the child based on his or her own cultural frame of reference
- Cultural variations in attitudes toward interpretations of children's behaviors
- Culturally based differences in clinician and caretaker perspectives
- Clinician bias in assigning diagnosis

The aforementioned points are evidence for the necessity for cultural competency training for mental health providers. As clinicians, we know that misdiagnosis leads to unnecessary overprescribing of antipsychotic medication, resulting in unnecessary increased risk for development of metabolic syndrome in children and adults.

Protective Factors

Although there are challenges in the Black community, it is important to also consider protective factors and strengths. Religion and more broadly speaking spirituality are frequently important parts of Black communities. The participation in organized religion, belonging to a community and attending services, has been correlated to decreased suicide risk in African American groups.[28] Family support, community support, and feelings of connectedness have been shown to be protective factors in Black youth in preventing suicidal behavior and mitigating symptoms of depression.[29] It is important for clinicians to be open to and explore nonclinical sources of support in patient's lives, such as community groups, houses of worship, and community leaders outside the medical model. In addition, research focusing on protective factors and strength-based interventions are needed.

Lack of Representation in Providers

According to data from the AAMC, Black or African Americans make up only 5% of the US physician workforce.[30] Even when considering the upstream contributors, the disparities persist; the rate of Black or African American males matriculating into medical school has actually decreased since 1978. When looking specifically at psychiatry of the 41,000 psychiatrists in the United States, only 2% are Black or African American. Psychology has a similar limited diversity composition with Black or African Americans making up only 4% of active US psychologists.[9]

Although there has been increased attention on this issue with creation of various pipeline programs which may increase the readiness of someone for medical training, the reality is that physicians from racial and ethnic minority groups often face bias and racism from superiors and peers in addition to patients.[31,32] Black or African American physicians are more likely to treat patients from their own ethnic group and also more likely to provide care in underserved communities.[33] This reality makes it easy to see how the decreased number of minority mental health practitioners compounds health care disparities.

Applications

As mental health care providers, we have an obligation and opportunity to better educate ourselves and others in the field on specific needs in Black communities. Countless studies have shown that implicit bias affects the quality of patient care. We provide services to a diverse population of patients, so understanding implicit bias is especially important in providing individualized quality care. Unconscious thought processes and decision-making can affect the provider–patient interaction, therapeutic options, diagnoses, and other areas of health care. A 2017 systematic review revealed that health care professionals exhibit about the same levels of implicit bias as the general population does, and evidence indicates that biases are likely to influence diagnosis and treatment decisions in some circumstances. Even professional clinicians with a lot of experience interacting with diverse groups have implicit biases. A 2015 study by Kopera and colleagues showed that mental health professionals had better approach to emotions, expressing more compassion, sadness, interest, and acceptance than nonprofessionals and medical students toward patients with mental illness, but both groups held negative implicit bias attitudes toward the mentally ill.[33]

Cultural humility and structural humility are two related concepts that can serve as a useful perspective for well-intentioned clinicians seeking to provide affirming care to Black children. Cultural humility is related to cultural competence and expands on the concept by calling for a lifelong commitment to self-evaluation and self-critique and not to be seen as obtaining a fixed set of knowledge.[34] Although there is clear information to be learned to better understand the lived experience and historical context for Black children in America, the reality is that given the diversity of experience a cultural humility orientation can place clinicians in a better position. Metzl defines structural competence as "structural competency as the trained ability to discern how a host of issues defined clinically as symptoms, attitudes, or diseases also represent the downstream implications of several upstream decisions about such matters as health care and food delivery systems, zoning laws, urban and rural infrastructures, medicalization, or even about the exact definitions of illness and health.".[35,36] Metzl positions structural humility as a component of structural competence that recognizes the limitations of the practice. A clinician seeking to provide the best care to their patients should prioritize learning about the structural factors that may be at play not just in their patient's lives but in the larger societal context. Learning about structural racism and the downstream effects leading to health care disparities can be a step toward creating equity for our patients.

Case Example

Johnny is a 16-year-old African American boy who has been detained for the past 6 months in a local juvenile justice facility for assault and battery. The incident occurred during a fight at school. Several youths were making inappropriate comments to his mother as she was working in the yard. These youths have also been harassing him at school.

Johnny's older brother, Charles, was a member of a local gang, but had never had any arrests or disciplinary problems at school. He was an excellent student and starting guard on the school's basketball team. Charles was on track to play college basketball at a Division 1 school. He was shot and killed 1 year ago. A Black sport utility vehicle (SUV) drove past his house, whereas Johnny and his family were working in the yard. Gunshots were fired from the SUV striking and mortally wounding Charles who died in Johnny's arms. Johnny did not receive mental health care following the incident. He continued to attend school where he was an A/B student and a starting guard on the high school basketball team.

On the day of the incident that led to Johnny's arrest, the school resource officer is called to break up a fight between Johnny and another youth. This youth was suspected to be one of the individuals riding in the SUV on the day that Charles was killed. This was the first disciplinary referral that Johnny has had during his entire school career. His teachers describe him as an exemplary student-athlete who is mild mannered and respectful.

Johnny's mother and father have been married for 22 years and have lived in the same community for their entire lives. The current home is the only one where Johnny and Charles have ever lived along with their younger sister. Johnny and Charles shared a room and a close relationship with each other. They attend the same schools that their parents attended.

During his initial evaluation at the juvenile justice facility, Johnny was diagnosed with major depressive disorder, PTSD, and cannabis use disorder. Despite being present at the time of his brother's death, Johnny did not endorse symptoms of PTSD, including the experiencing of a traumatic event. During the entire initial evaluation, he continued to deny that his brother's death has affected him. He states that he misses his big brother and laments that fact that he cannot play basketball with him or even talk about the future with him anymore. He states that he worries more about his parents, especially his mother, than he worries for himself.

Case takeaways

1. Mental health treatment services were never identified or initiated by the school or by the juvenile justice system. School based mental health treatment services were available at the school and evidence-based services were available for PTSD and grief counseling; however, a referral was never made likely based on the perceived behaviors of

the youth and the fact that he stated that he was "ok". This lack of referral likely related to implicit bias that was present. Although implicit bias is generally discussed in the context of race, this is a youth that lived in a predominantly African American neighborhood and attended a school with similar demographics. In this case, there seemed to be bias because of perceived gang membership and behavioral issues.

2. The school where Johnny attended did not have a policy in place for protecting victimized youth for perpetrators of violence. In this case the school had knowledge that gang member were targeting the brother of a murder victim, yet there was no intervention and a decision to arrest Johnny as he attempted to protect himself. This again seems to be related to bias that the youth had behavioral issues, despite all objective measures pointing otherwise.

3. Despite all of the markers that would generally ensure success, two parent family, good grades, home ownership, financial stability, and parental involvement/support, one son was murdered and a second is now in a juvenile detention center. As is frequently the case, many African American youth grow up in toxic neighborhoods where the deck is stacked against them. In these situations, governmental and community intervention is required beyond what mental health providers are able to offer.

SUMMARY

In 1863, slavery was abolished in the United States and in 1954, 91 years later, segregation was ruled unconstitutional. Today, in 2022, there is still so much work to be done. True racial justice cannot exist, whereas these barriers to health and wellness still exist. Although recent injustices are currently plaguing the minds of many of us, they are only a fraction of the various racial injustices Black youth may deal with on a daily basis that are barriers to obtaining health and wellness. One important initiative we can do as mental health providers is to begin with self-reflection and work toward becoming more aware of our own implicit biases. What are some prejudices that you might hold that you are not aware of? Taking time to better understand our patients through a lens that recognizes their home, family, community, and larger societal context. We all can have a role to play in making this better, and with more implicit bias training and a more culturally inclusive assessment process, we are hopeful that it can happen!

CLINICS CARE POINTS

- Systemic racism and social determinants of health impact the mental health of Black youth and their families. These impacts are multifactorial and may represent generations of cumulative impact.

- What is known as the African or Black Diaspora is incredibly diverse and made up of multiple ethnicities, clinicians should be open to exploring their own biases.

- Clinicians should maintain a posture of humility as they learn more about the experiences of Black patients and keep an awareness of both individual and structural factors that may contribute to clinical presentations.

DISCLOSURE

Q. Lang reports no financial relationships or interests. T. Roberson-Moore reports no financial relationships or interests. K.M. Rogers reports no financial relationships or interests. W.E. Wilson reports no financial relationships or interest.

REFERENCES

1. American Psychological Association. Ethnic and racial minorities & socioeconomic status. Washington: American Psychological Association; 2017. Available at: https://www.apa.org/pi/ses/resources/publications/minorities. [Accessed 10 April 2022].
2. US Census Bureau, Population Division (2020).
3. Watson Coleman B. A Report to congress from the congressional Black Caucus emergency task force on Black youth suicide and mental health. 2019. Available at: https://watsoncoleman.house.gov/uploadedfiles/full_taskforce_report.pdf. Accessed March 1, 2022.
4. Bitsko RH, Claussen AH, Lichtstein J, et al. Surveillance of children's mental health – United States, 2013 – 2019. MMWR 2022;71(Suppl-2):1–42.
5. Ghandour RM, Sherman LJ, Vladutiu CJ, et al. Prevalence and treatment of depression, anxiety, and conduct problems in U.S. children. J Pediatr 2019; 206:256–67.e3.
6. Cree R, Bitsko R, Robinson L, et al. Health care, family, and community factors associated with mental, behavioral, and developmental disorders and poverty among children aged 2–8 Years — United States, 2016. MMWR Morb Mortal Wkly Rep 2018;67(50):1377–83.
7. Marmot M. Social determinants of health inequalities. Lancet 2005;365(9464): 1099–104.
8. Compton M, Shim R. The social determinants of mental health. Focus 2015;13: 419–25.
9. American Psychological Association. Demographics of the U.S. Psychology workforce: findings from the 2007-16 American community survey. Washington, DC: American Psychological Association; 2018. Available at. https://nces.ed. gov/FCSM/pdf/F3_Lin_2018FCSM.pdf. Accessed March 1, 2022.
10. Jang Y, Chiriboga D, Kim G, et al. Perceived discrimination in older Korean Americans. Asian Am J Psychol 2010;1(12):129–35.
11. Jon-Ubabuco N, Dimmitt Champion J. Perceived mental healthcare barriers and health-seeking behavior of African American caregivers of adolescents with mental health disorders. Issues Ment Health Nurs 2019;40(7):585–92.
12. Lindsey M, Sheftall Arielle H, Xiao Yunyu, et al. Trends of suicidal behaviors among high school students in the United States: 1991–2017. Pediatrics 2019; 144(5):e20191187.
13. Mak W, Rosenblatt A. Demographic influences on psychiatric diagnoses among youth served in Californa systems of care. J Child Fam Stud 2002; 11(2):165–78.
14. Alegría M, Lin J, Green J, et al. Role of referrals in mental health service disparities for racial and ethnic minority youth. J Am Acad Child Adolesc Psychiatry 2012;51(7):703–11.e2.
15. Breland-Noble A. Mental healthcare disparities affect treatment of black adolescents. Psychiatr Ann 2004;34(7):534–8. Available at: https://journals.healio.com/doi/abs/10.3928/0048-5713-20040701-14.
16. Smedley A, Wade P, Takezawa YI. Race. Chicago: Encyclopedia Britannica; 2020. Available at: https://www.britannica.com/topic/race-human. [Accessed 1 April 2022].
17. DeGruy J. Post traumatic slave syndrome: America's legacy of enduring injury and healing. Milwaukie: Uptone Press; 2005.

18. Fitzgerald C, Hurst S. Implicit bias in healthcare professionals: a systematic review. BMC Med Ethics 2017;18(1):19.

19. Kopera M, Suszek H, Bonar E, et al. Evaluating Explicit and implicit stigma of mental illness in mental health professionals and medical students. Community Ment Health J 2015;5:628–34.

20. Lavner JA, Hart AR, Carter SE, Beach SRH. Longitudinal effects of racial discrimination on depressive symptoms among Black youth: between- and within-person effects. J Child Adolesc Psychiatry 2022;61(1):56–65.

21. Liang J, Matheson BE, Douglass JM. Mental health diagnostic considerations in racial/ethnic minority youth. J Child Fam Stud 2016;25(6).

22. Sabin Janice A. 2020. Available at: https://www.aamc.org/news-insights/how-we-fail-black-patients-pain.

23. Nguyen L, Huang LN, Arganza GF, et al. The influence of race and ethnicity on psychiatric diagnoses and clinical characteristics of children and adolescents in children's services. Cultur Divers Ethnic Minor Psychol 2007;13: 18–25.

24. Gibbs JT, Huang LN, editors. Children of color: Psychological interventions with culturally diverse youth. San Francisco: Jossey-Bass/Wiley; 2003.

25. Hoffman K, Trawalter S, Axt J, et al. Racial bias in pain assessment and treatment recommendations, and false beliefs about biological differences between Blacks and Whites. Proc Natl Acad Sci U S A 2016;113(16):4296–301.

26. Yeh M, McCabe K, Hurlburt M, et al. Referral sources, diagnoses, and service types of youth in public outpatient mental health care: a focus on ethnic minorities. J Behav Health Serv Res 2002;29:45–60.

27. Delbello M, Lopez-Larson M, Soutullo C, et al. Effects of race on psychiatric diagnosis of hospitalized adolescents: a retrospective chart review. J Child Adolesc Psychopharmacol 2001;11(1):95–103.

28. Taylor R, Chatters L, Joe S. Religious involvement and suicidal behavior among african americans and Black caribbeans. J Nerv Ment Dis 2011;199(7):478–86.

29. Matlin SL, Molock SD, Tebes JK. Suicidality and depression among african american adolescents: the role of family and peer support and community connectedness. Am J Orthopsychiatry 2011;81(1):108–17.

30. American Association of Medical Colleges. Fostering diversity and inclusion. Washington: AAMC; 2019. Available at: https://www.aamc.org/data-reports/workforce/interactive-data/fostering-diversity-and-inclusion. Accessed March 10, 2022.

31. American Association of Medical Colleges. Altering the course: Black males in medicine. Washington: AAMC; 2015. Available at. https://store.aamc.org/downloadable/download/sample/sample_id/84/. Accessed March 1, 2022.

32. Association of American Medical Colleges. Diversity in medical education: facts and figures 2019. Washington, DC: Association of American Medical Colleges; 2019. Available at. https://www.aamc.org/data-reports/workforce/report/diversity-medicine-facts-and-figures-2019. Accessed March 1, 2022.

33. Komaromy M, Grumbach K, Drake M, et al. The role of Black and Hispanic physicians in providing health care for underserved populations. N Engl J Med 1996; 334(20):1305–10.

34. Tervalon M, Murray-García J. Cultural humility versus cultural competence: a critical distinction in defining physician training outcomes in multicultural education. J Health Care Poor Underserved 1998;9(2):117–25.

35. McLaughlin KA, Hilt LM, Nolen-Hoeksema S. Racial/Ethnic differences in internalizing and externalizing symptoms in adolescents. J Abnorm Child Psychol 2007; 35(5):801–16.
36. Metzl JM, Hansen H. Structural competency: theorizing a new medical engagement with stigma and inequality. Soc Sci Med 2013;103:126–33. https://doi.org/10.1016/j.socscimed.2013.06.032. Available at:.
37. https://datacenter.kidscount.org/data/tables/44-children-in-poverty-by-race-and-ethnicity (Accessed 1 April 2022), 2020.

East Asian Population

Shinnyi Chou, MD, PhD[a],[*], Crystal Han, MD[b],
Jessica Xiaoxi Ouyang, MD[c], Annie Sze Yan Li, MD[d]

KEYWORDS

- Acculturation • East Asian • Mental health • Model minority myth • Systemic racism

KEY POINTS

- Asian Americans (AA) represent the fastest-growing racial group in the United States, with East Asian Americans (EAA) representing approximately 40% of this group.
- Systemic racism toward East Asians (EA) in the United States, in the form of xenophobia, the model minority myth, perpetual foreigner stereotype, and the silencing of Asian American and Pacific Islanders (AAPI) history, has persisted since the 1800s, culminating in heightened discriminations during the COVID-19 pandemic.
- EAA children and adolescents, balancing the complexities of acculturative stress, endured additional hardships during this period as they navigated societal changes amid the pandemic while facing overt racism toward themselves and their adult caretakers, leading to increased mental health distress.
- Numerous grassroots and organizational interventions arose during this period as ways to foster resiliency and empower agency in EA youths, including those emphasizing destigmatization of mental illness and mental health service utilization.

INTRODUCTION

A series of unprecedented recent events has warranted special considerations in addressing the mental health needs and concerns of youths and families in the Asian American and Pacific Islanders (AAPI) community. The AAPI community is the fastest growing minority group in the United States. In recent years, AAPI garnered greater representation in sports, films, and literature, facilitating dialogues about shared experiences that could be articulated and processed. Opportunities arose to chip away the stigma that often stifled conversations on mental wellness among AAPIs. Then came the onset of the COVID-19 pandemic in early 2020, a time when xenophobia and

[a] University of Pittsburgh Medical Center, 3811 O'Hara Street, Pittsburgh, PA 15213, USA;
[b] University of Maryland Medical Center, 701 West Pratt Street, Baltimore, MD 21201, USA;
[c] Georgetown University School of Medicine, MedStar Georgetown University Hospital, 2115 Wisconsin Avenue Northeast, Suite 200, Washington, DC 20002, USA; [d] NYU Grossman School of Medicine, NYU Langone Health, NYC Health + Hospital–Bellevue Medical Center, NYU Child Study Center, One Park Avenue, 7th Floor, New York, NY 10016, USA
* Corresponding author.
E-mail address: chous@upmc.edu

Child Adolesc Psychiatric Clin N Am 31 (2022) 745–763
https://doi.org/10.1016/j.chc.2022.05.006
1056-4993/22/© 2022 Elsevier Inc. All rights reserved.
childpsych.theclinics.com

blame for the origin of the coronavirus resulted in the targeting of AAPI populations. Racism, discrimination, and acts of hate escalated at a time when the world collectively experienced significant disruption to functioning and routines, losses of family and friends, apprehension to falling ill, and for some, recovering from COVID-19. Sadly, such acts of hate, especially in the form of verbal and physical assaults happening in public spaces, have not subsided.

To talk about AAPI mental health at this moment requires understanding the lived experience of AAPI through the COVID-19 pandemic. Open discussion about AAPI mental health is currently plagued by barriers of stigma, scarcity of AAPI mental health professionals, and low mental health literacy and utilization. Ushering in an era of healing, as we reckon with racial injustice and advocating at the height of a national child and adolescent mental health crisis, requires a commitment of building resilience, embracing cultural values, and celebrating differences in the attributes of a heterogenous group that comprises the East Asian (EA) population.

BACKGROUND

The term "Asian American" evokes an array of associations, connotations, perceptions, and emotions (**Box 1**). There is a fundamental complexity to being an Asian American (AA) because of the heterogeneous cultures with different histories, strengths, identities, and needs. This complexity is why this volume is intentional regarding the article divisions, knowing the content of this article only begins to scratch the surface of this topic. Issues such as colorism, classism, and inequity within the AAPI diaspora[1–3] intersect with racism and acculturation to shape children and adolescent identity development for this unique population.

As of 2019, there are approximately 22.9 million AAPI in the United States,[4] representing the fastest-growing race between 2000 and 2019 at 82% growth,[5] with individuals under the age of 24 years representing 7% of total youths in the United States.[6] Among AAPI, the Chinese and Chinese American population is the largest at 5.2 million as of 2019.[4] Individuals from East Asia, defined geographically and culturally, include China, Taiwan, Japan, Mongolia, and North and South Korea,[7] make up approximately 40% of the Asian population within the United States.[8]

Box 1
Definitions of common terminologies used in this article

Terms and definitions
- Asian American (AA)/Asian American Pacific Islander (AAPI): Used interchangeably; umbrella terminology used to describe people who identify with and/or have ancestry in more than 50 Asian ethnic and Islander groups, with 100+ languages and dialects.
- East Asian (EA): People groups from China, Japan, Mongolia, North Korea, South Korea, Taiwan.
- East Asian American (EAA): People groups from East Asia living in the United States.
- First generation: The first of a generation of immigrants to settle in the United States, who were born outside the United States.
- Second generation: Individuals born in the United States with at least 1 parent who was born outside the United States.
- Multiracial East Asian American: Individuals with 2 or more ethnic heritages, with at least 1 part of the ancestry tracing back to East Asia in the previous generation.
- LGBTQIA+: Lesbian, gay, bisexual, trans-, questioning, intersex, asexual, and other sexual/gender minorities.
- Xenophobia: The fear or hatred of what is perceived to be foreign.

In US history, AAPI communities have experienced systemic racism and oppression since the 1800s. They survived against these odds because of their capacity to build community with mutual aid, organization, and unrelenting resistance against oppression and silencing.[9] The need for understanding AAPI experiences and mental health has gained prominence in recent years given the increase in anti-AAPI attacks amid the COVID-19 pandemic, yet the longstanding systemic racism against AAPI communities is often disavowed but plays a significant role in perpetuating the mental health inequities experienced by AAPI communities. Indeed, anti-AAPI racism is woven into the fabric of the United States (**Table 1**) and manifests overtly during major crises, such as the COVID-19 pandemic.[10] Jose Rizal, a Filipino nationalist and author, writes,

Table 1
A brief history of anti-Asian racism in the United States

Date and Major Initiatives/Events	Event Details
1790—Naturalization Act	The act barred naturalization of any non-white person
1854—People vs Hall	California's Supreme Court ruled an Asian person could not testify in court against a white person
1871—Chinese massacre in Los Angeles	Following the shooting of a white man killed in cross fire of rival Chinese gangs, hundreds of white and Hispanic people attacked the Los Angeles' Chinese community on October 24, 1871. Nearly 20 Chinese people were lynched or shot dead, the largest mass lynching in US history
1875—Page Act	Designed to prohibit women who had "lewd and immoral purposes" from entering the United States, the Page Act was enforced mostly against Chinese women, most of whom were attempting to join Chinese men working in the country
1882—Chinese Exclusion Act	The law banned immigration of Chinese laborers, the first law that excluded an entire ethnic group. It was not repealed until 1943, 61 y later, when forces were needed during World War II
1922–1923—Supreme Court on citizenship	In separate cases in 1922 and 1923, the Supreme Court ruled that a Japanese-born man and an Indian-born man were not white and ineligible for naturalization
1924—Johnson Reed Act	The law effectively blocked immigration from Asia and drastically cut the number of immigrants allowed to enter the United States
1942–1945—Japanese internment	During World War II, the United States forced >100,000 people of Japanese descent, most of whom were US citizens, into internment camps
1960s—Immigration and Nationality Act of 1965	Resulted in much higher numbers of AAPI immigration; AAPI student activists created the term "Asian American" to increase political visibility
1982—Murder of Vincent Chin	Two white men in Michigan assaulted and killed Vincent Chin, a 27-y-old Chinese American man, blaming him for the success of the Japanese auto industry. They served no jail time
2020—Anti-Asian hate crimes surge	Reporting forum Stop AAPI Hate has received >10,000 incidents of anti-Asian hate crimes since March 2020
2021—Atlanta shootings	On March 16, 2021, shootings at 3 spas near Atlanta, Georgia resulted in the murder of 6 Asian women

"Know History, Know Self. No History, No Self."[11] Knowing where one comes from gives one grounding in discovering self-context, history, identity, and sense of self. Similarly, knowing the sociopolitical history of the AAPI community is integral in understanding the current climate in which mental health providers serve the AAPI population.[9]

COVID-19 AND OTHER HISTORICAL CONSIDERATIONS

The COVID-19 pandemic, declared in March 2020, impacted AAPI in unique ways. From a health equity lens, data indicate that AAPIs experienced nearly double the rates of COVID-19–related hospitalization and deaths compared with the white population.[12]

Racism

From a racial inclusivity lens, the pandemic not only accentuated the perpetual foreigner sentiment, but also generated overt xenophobia,[13] an outcome partially owing to US leaders' misrepresentations and blaming of Asians as the source of the COVID-19 spread.[14] A disturbing statistic noted a 150% increase in anti-AAPI racism.[13] Understandably, studies indicate that greater than half of AAPI survey participants believed the country has become more dangerous for their ethnic groups, with more than 40% of those surveyed believing that social media contributed to the bias leading to this hostility, and greater than 30% feeling worried that others may think they have COVID-19 owing to their race or ethnicity.[15]

The ways in which systemic racism manifests against AAPI communities take many forms, including xenophobia historically referenced as the "yellow peril," the model minority myth (MMM) (**Table 2**), the perpetual foreigner stereotype, and the silencing and erasure of AAPI experiences, voices, and contributions in multiple facets of society.[18] Other examples include lack of AAPI representation in the media, in positions of leadership across various industries, lack of access to translation services in health care and beyond, and lack of data collection in multiple realms of society on individual AAPI subethnicities.

The MMM engenders resentment of AAPI from both white and communities of color. It also facilitates scapegoating of AAPI when the dominant population who holds power is not held accountable to systemic flaws that perpetuate AAPI disparities. This unique intersection of sociopolitical historical dynamics sets AAPI communities up to be attacked, to be seen as perpetual foreigners that need to be exterminated, harkening back to the "yellow peril," which informs the anti-Asian attacks in the present day.[9]

In the perpetual foreigner stereotype, ascribing the American identity to white European American results in the "othering" of ethnic minorities, preventing individuals, even those born in the United States, from being acknowledged and embraced as American. This construct heightens acts of microaggressions that questions birth citizenship and English proficiency and conveys messages of exclusion and inferiority, consciously or not. In one study, awareness of the perpetual foreigner stereotype significantly predicted identity conflict, lower sense of belonging to the American culture, lower hope, and decreased life satisfaction for AAPI.[19]

Invisibility of AAPI issues is reflected in the absence of AA history in educational curriculum, as well as lack of attention and funding in research, community programs, and other avenues of support (**Box 2**).[20] Silence of AAPI is also noted in the binary nature of racial discourse in America as black and white, with AAPI as neither. This may lead to a lack of understanding, confidence, sense of belonging, and compromised sense of self.[9,20]

Table 2 The model minority myth	
MMM Component	**Definitions**
Function	• Positions "well-behaved, obedient, hardworking" Asians in opposition to black communities' rising social justice activism • Serves to keep AAPI communities pigeonholed within certain stereotypes, such as politically silent, quiet, and not fit for leadership
History	• Began to be perpetuated in the 1960s, when AAPI comprised 0.2% of the population and had experienced 5 y of Japanese internment, 2 decades of surveillance/deportation, and the terrorizing of Chinese Americans during the Cold War and were not in a position to push back on the narrative • New immigrants who arrived did so due to the extremely selective 1965 Immigration Act, only allowing wealthy and educated AAPI, with resources and positions garnered in their own societies, not from US resources
Myth 1: AAPI are monolithic and homogenous	• Portrays the AAPI community as a monolithic and homogenous group, when it is composed of >50 different countries and languages each with its own complex history and cultures • Paints AAPI as academically and economically successful and "well-behaved" immigrants • In truth, AAPI has the widest wealth gap among its subgroups compared with other minority populations. For example, the average poverty rate is <5% for Japanese and South Asian/Indian communities but >15% for Hmong, Nepalese, and Burmese communities[16]
Myth 2: AAPI are not a real minority	• Erases, makes invisible, and delegitimizes Asian struggles and individual differences, portraying AAPI communities as "not a real minority," and thus perpetuating the idea that AAPI do not experience issues such as racism or mental health disorders • This myth is often internalized by AAPI communities, creating a barrier in seeking help[17]
Myth 3: If AAPI can succeed, others can too	• Used as a wedge, making a flawed comparison between AAPI and other groups, particularly black Americans, to argue that racism, including more than 2 centuries of black enslavement, can be overcome by hard work, education, and strong family values • Ignores the powerful systemic ways racism functions to maintain oppression • Falsely conflates anti-Asian racism with anti-black racism—these groups all experience racism but in different ways, which ultimately distracts communities of color from striving in solidarity toward equity for all

Research shows a well-established relationship between racial discrimination and adverse mental health symptoms. More is being written on race-based traumatic stress (depression, anxiety, hypervigilance, avoidance, and negative cognitions owing to racism) and minority stress.[21] One recent study noted that racial microaggressions predicted suicidal ideation in young adults of color, mediated through depressive symptoms, anxiety, trauma symptoms, somatic symptoms, and medical sequelae, including heart disease and diabetes.[22,23] Although AAPI are not predisposed to mental illness, the oppressive systems they navigate have the capacity to serve as a combination of predisposing, precipitating, and perpetuating factors,[24] and more research is needed to detail how systemic, institutional, and individual racism impacts AAPI mental health.

Box 2
Examples of systemic invisibility of Asian American and Pacific Islanders

Systemic invisibility of AAPI
- Since 1996, the National Institutes of Health has spent only 0.17% of their total budget for clinical research on AAPI.
- In 2017, AAPI made up 13.5% of New York City's population, but AAPI organizations were granted only 1.4% of total spending for social service contracts despite having the highest poverty rate in the city.
- In June 2021, the National Institutes of Health revealed a new initiative known as "UNITE" to address structural racism but neglected to specifically include AAPI communities.
- As of 2022, 3% of Congress and 3.7% of senior executive services are represented by AAPI individuals.

Education

Children and youths bore the burden of peer discriminations in the school setting during the COVID-19 pandemic.[25] Not only did statistics indicate that one in 4 AAPI children reported experiencing racism throughout the pandemic,[26] but also they reported being afraid of race-related harassment in the public setting.[27] Notably, these factors contributed to more Asian children and youths opting to avoid returning to in-person school, disrupting important cognitive and social development and identity formation.[28] For transitional age youths (currently defined as 16–25 years old[29]), one study suggests that more than a quarter reported experiencing COVID-19–related racial/ethnic discrimination,[30] with these experiences being associated with 2 times greater odds ratio of meeting criteria for clinically significant depression, anxiety, and suicidal ideations, and one and a half greater odds ratio of engaging in binge alcohol use and nonsuicidal self-injuries.

The disruption in education is particularly salient for the AAPI population in the COVID-19 era given the emphasis and pressure on academic success for AAPI youth and their families. The family structure, parenting values, cultural mindset, political influences, and the MMM work together to create an environment in which youth are expected to devote great effort and time into their studies. To illustrate, *Sky Castle*, a 2018/2019 South Korean television series, captures the near-obsession of South Korean families with academic success at all costs. Parental expectations and immigration status play a significant role in creating a mindset of academic achievement in EAA youth. It becomes clearer when examined in the context of the 1965 Immigration and Naturalization Act, where previous limitations of Asian immigrants were removed and immigrants with a high level of education and skill were encouraged to further develop them in the United States.[31] The "new immigrants" thus became parents who themselves greatly valued education and expected the same from their children, seeing education as the only path to success. However, the afterschool tutoring, academic coaching, and hours of studying decreased time for socialization and relationship building. Specifically, EAA youth, among all Asians, have more conflict with parents, less time with friends, and lower positive feelings toward self.[31] Although the stereotype of Asians achieving academically may provide some advantages, for those not fitting the stereotype, identity and purpose are often questioned, leading to psychological struggles, such as shame and even suicide attempts.[32] The long-term effects of the pandemic on not only AAPI, but all youth education are yet to be fully understood.

Family

Compounding personal racially stigmatizing experiences for Asian children and youths during the pandemic was their vicarious trauma through discriminations against their adult caregivers, attributable to racism, language barriers, and economic hardship.[33] Notably, nearly half of all Chinese parents in a survey study experienced online or in-person COVID-19 racial discrimination,[25] which was negatively associated with psychological well-being and positively associated with anxiety and depressive symptoms.

AAPI have long placed high priority on family, parenthood, and successful marriages.[34] Although diverse practices exist across various Asian cultures and generations of immigrants in the United States, traditional AAPI families typically uphold the patriarchal lineage. Historically, women marry into the husbands' households, and families live together in a multigenerational system, thus creating a family village to raise children.[34] The cultural duty to care for the elderly, termed *filial piety*, is a core EA belief thought to be originally influenced by Confucius. A surface level understanding of *filial piety* is that children honor their parents and their years of sacrifice by involving them in major life decisions, caring for their activities of daily living as needed, and often living together in multigenerational households once their parents are more elderly. On a deeper level, such practices can often help to foster intergenerational relationships and pass on traditions and values.[35] The multigenerational household, or at least the ability to visit and offer tangible help to one another, allows for economic stability, social support, and fulfilling *filial piety*. However, second-generation EAA often find themselves caught between traditional EA family values and Western cultural values experienced outside of the home (**Table 3**). These intergenerational cultural and value differences among the EAA families may often be a source of tension between first-generation parents and second-generation children. Even so, the extended family can be a tremendous source of strength and resilience for the EAA youth, with multiple generations invested in their success.

During the pandemic, this source of strength and resilience from the extended family was visibly absent, with family members having to distance themselves from each other through both self- and government-imposed quarantines.[38] This disrupted the multigenerational home structure in AAPI families in 2 ways. First, physical distancing to reduce risk of exposure separated many families, creating a distinct challenge to honor and fulfill the duty to care for the elderly. Second, in families without financial resources who continued to live in multigenerational homes, the risks for exposure and more serious illnesses in the elderly were increased, against the backdrop of already escalated levels of worries and distress from COVID-19. Arguably, even worse was the increase of anti-Asian hate during this time, adding another layer of fear among the AAPI community; this time, it was for their psychological and physical safety, their sense

Table 3 Comparison of East Asian and East Asian American family values[36,37]	
Traditional EA Family Values	**EAA Family Values**
Collectivism	Individualism
Duty/responsibility	Autonomy
Self-control	Pursuit of happiness
Respect for authority	Democratic relations
Reverence for elderly (filial piety)	Psychological well-being
Educational achievement	Emotional expressiveness
Honor	Open and honest communication
Patriarchal gender roles	Flexibility

of identity and belongingness in this country not only for elderly parents and grandparents but also for themselves and their children.[39] Not all, but many AAPI families may experience a distinct grief for those who lost family members during this period, ranging from guilt related to the inability to honor filial piety, to a deep sense of isolation stemming from the permanent rupture of generational structures, although more rigorous studies may be necessary to expand upon qualitative reports.[38]

Religion

Outside of the home, shutdowns of local areas that served as social anchors, such as business districts in Chinatowns, as well as ethnic temples and churches across the country, led to further weakening of communities.[33] A national survey of AAs found that among US AAPI adults, Christians are the largest religious group, and the unaffiliated (agnostic, atheist, not affiliated with a religious group) are second (**Fig. 1**).[34] Upon examining disaggregated data, it may be surprising to find that there are differences among the EAA groups. Specifically, Japanese Americans were nearly an even mix of Christians, Buddhists, and the unaffiliated. Most Korean Americans identified as Protestant, and about a quarter identified as unaffiliated. Among the Chinese Americans, over half are unaffiliated, whereas Christians make up almost one-third.

Despite the quarantining mandates of the pandemic, churches pivoted to holding virtual meetings for members and delivered meals and other basic items to those in need. For AA, ethnic churches not only are centers to celebrate and teach culture and language but also often provide for the livelihood needs of the community, including social services, citizenship education, English classes, and socialization.[37] The development of one's identity and close relationships for children and teens often takes place at the church for a subset of EAA. In particular, the church often is a "home-base" where

Religious Affiliation of Asian Americans

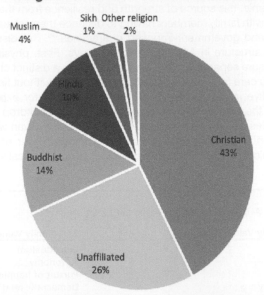

Fig. 1. Self-reported religious affiliations of AA adults. *Data from* The Rise of Asian Americans. Pew Research Center. 2013; Washington, D.C. Accessed April 1, 2022. https://www.pewsocialtrends.org/wp-content/uploads/sites/3/2013/04/Asian-Americans-new-full-report-04-2013.pdf

people can come together to provide and receive help of all kinds, especially for the Korean immigrant population, as they largely identify as Christian Protestants.

IDENTITY FORMATION FOR EAST ASIAN AMERICAN CHILDREN AND ADOLESCENTS

How do we as providers promote healthy integration of cultural identities for EAA children and adolescents undergoing identity formation during this period, shaped not only by family influences, ethnic identification, nationality, socialization, and religious values (**Box 3**) but also by societal unrests during the pandemic?

AAPI and non-AAPI individuals must see value, meaning, and respect placed on both cultural identities—by what is reflected back to them in their homes, community, and school—and be given the opportunity to practice and develop both identities. Considering the process of assimilation, when systems fail to uplift, represent, and incorporate students' bicultural identities and cultures, students will assimilate by default to white, Western culture (ie, with high American identity, low AAPI identity). AAPI cultures are then minimized and erased as it is made invisible, and AAPI communities are forced to give up their heritage and adjust to survive.[40]

A sense of belonging is the experience of personal involvement in a system or environment so that individuals feel themselves to be an integral part of the system or environment. A low sense of belonging is a predictor of depression.[41] For example, in school curricula, if one's identity is not represented in the materials students consume, it is internalized that "people who look like me don't write books or if they did, they are not good enough to make it into our syllabi." In the field of self-psychology, Kohut[42] posits that the elements outlined in **Box 4** are required to integrate the development of self and identity, fully participate in life, and develop resilience.

SPECIAL CONSIDERATIONS: A BRIEF OVERVIEW OF EAST ASIAN INTERSECTIONAL POPULATIONS
Multiracial East Asian Americans

The 2020 Census reported a sharp increase in multiracial children and people in the United States, from 2.9% (9 million) to 10.2% (33.8 million) in the span of a decade (**Table 4**). Although Asian populations grew 35.5% between 2010 and 2020, Asian mixed-race population grew by 55.5% at the same time.[43] Specifically, the white and Asian population increased by 1.1 million or by 65.8% over the last 10 years. In short, Asians and mixed Asian races are among the fastest growing populations in the United States. Nevertheless, like other areas of AA studies, multiracial youth

---

Box 3
Factors affecting identity formation of East Asian American children and adolescents[34,37]

Factors affecting identity
- Parent/family identity and influences
- Parent and child phenotype
- Children's age (impacts children's understanding of identity)
- Family relationships
- Educational status
- Generational status
- Acculturation status
- Socioeconomic status
- Community demographics
- Experiences (eg, of discrimination)
- Intergenerational trauma or racism
- Religion and faith community

> **Box 4**
> **Elements required for integrated development of self and identity[42]**
>
> - Mirroring: Reflecting back value to the facets of identity from individuals and other aspects of society.
> - Twinship: A sense of likeness seen in aspects of society leading to sense of belonging.
> - Idealization: Sources of comfort and calm, as well as objects whom one aspires to emulate.

understanding is limited. The American Psychological Association reports that active "socialization" of children in multiracial families is rare.[44] Despite the visible differences in phenotypes and appearances of mixed-race young people, explicit conversations about racial and ethnic identities are not common. Furthermore, parents of mixed-race children often avoid conversations about race, citing the lack of skills to start the conversation, having underdeveloped racial awareness and a sense of protection toward their children, which fueled "compounded societal invisibility" wherein multiracial AA lack a central community of support, leading to internalized oppression and belief of oneself's inferiority."[45] Future research must invite collaborations with patients and families to share and explore together the identities and needs of this growing population.

East Asian American Adoptees

Among the EAA population is a group raised in transracially adopted families, usually by white families. AA transracial adoptees, like multiracial AAs, are underrepresented, and their experiences are not well understood in the United States. Small studies attempting to fill the knowledge gap have found that South Korean adoptees internalized less ethnic identity than US-born or immigrated Korean/Korean Americans,[46] that Asian adoptees struggled with processing the surge of anti-Asian hate during the pandemic owing to never feeling like they truly belong in either the AA community or white America, and that "colorblind" parenting contributes to children internalizing that the exploration of their identity and culture is less important.[47,48] Commonalities found included the struggle of balancing Asian and white identities and the need to know how to access supports and resources who may share a similar origin story. It is important to not generalize each person's lived experiences, but rather, seek to understand each individual adoptee's strengths and challenges. Child and adolescent psychiatrists (CAP) can advocate for and facilitate parent communication workshops to help families address potential discriminations their children may face, which are not often directly experienced by adoptive parents.

Lesbian, Gay, Bisexual, Trans-, Questioning, Intersex, Asexual, And Other Sexual/Gender Minorities

As with other AA populations, literature is scarce with AA lesbian, gay, bisexual, trans-, questioning, intersex, asexual, and other sexual/gender minorities (LGBTQIA+). It appears that although the younger generation tends to be more accepting of LGBTQIA+, older Asian generations feel less comfortable. This can lead to internal conflict for the EAA youth, especially when family values differ from that of the individual, including traditional marriage and child rearing. AAPI LGBTQIA+ students experience an increased sense of victimization, discrimination, and a decreased sense of support beyond those experienced by white LGBTQIA+ youths.[49] The perceived and explicit trauma, coupled with a lack of belongingness, can be striking in this population, who

Table 4
Key considerations in special Asian American and Pacific Islanders populations

Intersection Population	Key Considerations
Multiracial	• Other terms include *hapa* in Hawaii/Pacific Islands, and *hafu* in Japan • An increasing population with heterogeneous experiences in the United States • Underdeveloped racial awareness, lack of established community, and societal invisibility
EA Adoptees	• Many struggled with being able to identify with and process through anti-Asian hate sentiments • Conversations about race, racism, discrimination between adoptee and adoptive families are less common and needed
LGBTQIA+ and sexual/gender minorities	• Difficult to be accepted from a more traditional EA family value system • Increased discrimination in the LGBTQIA+ space
EAA children with disabilities	• Increased level of caregiver stress and anxiety during the pandemic • Disruptions in behavioral health care, even among well-resourced families

identify as minorities in multiple domains (AAPI, multiracial, sexual minority to name a few), as studies indicate that racial and ethnic identity can modify the levels of distress and well-being within the LGBTQIA+ space. As with all AAPI population health and well-being, further research and advocacy work are needed to better understand the full scope of this issue and equip our providers, families, and youth for a stronger future together.

East Asian American Children with Disabilities

The impact of the COVID-19 pandemic on parents and caregivers for children with disabilities has been found to be higher than that of parents with neurotypical children.[50] A small study of AAPI parents in Maryland noted concerns related to school and clinic closures, resulting in disruption and cessation in some cases of therapies, recreation and social skills training, and other social activities necessary for children with developmental disabilities, such as autism spectrum disorder.[51] The pause in therapy frequently led to increased behavioral challenges and parental stress, as many families went through quarantine periods with their children. Unfortunately, not all agencies are able to provide interpreters for appointments or therapies for EAA families. As we move away from COVID-19 and its restrictions, providers can invite these families to share and process through the emotional journey, including experiences of discrimination.

HOW DO WE ADDRESS THE NEEDS FOR EAST ASIAN AMERICAN YOUTHS AS WE HEAD OUT OF THE PANDEMIC?

It is important to remember that the higher rates of mental illness within AAPI communities are not due to a higher predisposition to mental illness but rather to the oppression and stigma within the systems in which they are forced to navigate (**Table 5**).

AAPI communities have higher rates of depressive symptoms and suicide attempts but are among the least likely to receive treatment.[52] AAPI college students reported

Table 5
Factors contributing to mental health treatment barriers in Asian American and Pacific Islanders communities

Structural Factors	Cultural Factors
• Financial barriers • Language barriers • Lack of access or awareness of mental health resources • Lack of culturally sensitive services • Mental health interventions not adapted for diversity with provider, diagnostic and systemic bias	• Stigma against mental illness • Beliefs that psychiatric symptoms reflect weak character • Emotional inhibition • Low awareness of services and treatment options

more concerning psychiatric symptoms than their white counterparts and were 1.6 times more likely to be considering suicide, but received half the number of diagnoses.[53] Other studies suggest AAPI communities were 2 to 3 times less likely to seek treatment and more likely to rate psychiatric services as unhelpful.[32]

The discriminations experienced by many during the pandemic years were faced with an equally resilient force of activism and advocacy. Experts and community leaders leveraged the ubiquitous nature of virtual platforms to empower AA.[54,55] Educators also encouraged youths and young adults to discover their own resiliency through the humanities, such as the "Through Our Eyes, Hear Our Voices" photovoice project, which poignantly showcased examples of college students embracing strengths through proactively dispelling the MMM and engaging in political rights.[33] Importantly, health care providers may collaborate with AA youth grassroots organizations, such as AAPI Youth Rising,[56] Project Lotus,[57] and faith organizations, to dialogue and foster greater cultural understanding and disseminate reliable health information.

Other ways to address the issues detailed above include self-reflecting questions that providers and institutions may use to promote racial healing and representation (**Table 6**), and many other innovations currently underway (**Box 5**). Of note, training psychiatrists in structural competency and cultural humility is more predictive of positive patient outcomes than ethnic matching.[64] Ultimately, acknowledgment of lessons learned from these difficult experiences may lead to improved mental health care for our children and youths.[65]

SYNTHESIS AND SUMMARY

Multimodal approaches are necessary to meet AAPI youth and families where they are. To start, (1) focus on wellness and mental health prevention, (2) advocate for policies and education within AA communities, and (3) equip health care providers with the necessary cultural awareness and cultural humility tools in approaching EAA families and communities. EAs and EAAs tend to value a strong work ethic, education, intergenerational relationships, honor and respect for the family and elders, and commitment to their communities. Despite these, there is notable heterogeneity when it comes to socioeconomic status, religion and faith, and cultural identification, among others. Therefore, it is of utmost importance to ask, not assume, what is important and what the values are for the EAA family and patients before us in the office. There is also a need to facilitate dialogue between children and family, and between families and other community organizations, including schools and churches, in as

Table 6
Considerations in addressing Asian American and Pacific Islanders racial healing, mental health disparities, and representations[58]

Promoting Racial Healing	Questions to Help Address Disparities in AAPI Mental Health Care	Questions to Help Increase AAPI Representation
Naming, acknowledging, and validating experiences, including discrimination, microaggressions, examples of systemic racism and oppression, and racial socialization	How does my work environment foster understanding and acceptance of cultural differences?	Do program leaders value ethnoracial equity and model a shared commitment to dismantling anti-AAPI racism?
Preparation for racism and racist experiences	How do patient materials accurately represent the histories, experiences, and contributions of various cultural groups?	In teaching and learning, is the curriculum being used to challenge racial inequity and strive for cultural humility?
Promoting social support, empowering individuals, families, and communities, encouraging sense of agency	How do my assessment methods reflect the diversity of patient experiences, languages, and cultures?	Do AAPI students, staff, and faculty feel valued, safe, and respected?
Promoting cultural, racial, and ethnic pride	How does my work tap into patients' families, languages, and cultures as foundations for healing?	Are AAPI trainees, students, and faculty well-being being seen as a priority, and are there supportive spaces and mentorship that exist for AAPI in the program?
Facilitating cross-racial relationships, coalitions, and solidarity Giving permission to pause and rest Healing beyond just coping, including encouraging development of efficacy and agency, collective and authentic spaces, creativity and dreaming, and self-determination	Beyond just fostering coping skills, what are providers and institutions doing to make racial healing and coping safe, normative, accessible, and health promoting?	

many domains as possible. CAPs are well positioned to create opportunities beyond the office and clinical setting, like in education and advocacy within our communities, at churches and temples, schools, and local and federal governments through our professional organizations. In this way, CAPs can create the change we hope to see with and for our communities through partnerships and collaborations.

Policy and education matters. New Jersey recently joined Illinois as the second state in the United States to require public schools to teach students about the history and contributions of AAPI to the United States.[66] The integration of AAPI history and lived-experiences in all levels of education, as well as making the time and space to talk about race in schools, health care settings, and within the community matter.

> **Box 5**
> **Examples of interventions to support Asian American and Pacific Islanders youths**
>
> - Affinity groups for AAPI identifying individuals to build community in all realms of society (school, religious institutes, health centers for patients, trainees, and faculty).
> - Support groups for intersectional AAPI demographics, such as international students, LGBTQIA+ individuals, adopted individuals, multiracial individuals, and so forth.
> - Supporting legislation to mandate teaching of AAPI history in educational curricula.
> - *Let's Talk! Professional Conference:* A conference especially designed for educators and mental health clinicians who support Asian and AA students in K–12 schools, in higher education, and in the community.[59]
> - *Stanford CHIPAO (Communication Health Interactive for Parents of Adolescents and Others):* Workshops run by faculty, staff, and students from the Stanford department of psychiatry to help families communicate more effectively about difficult topics and improve the well-being of AAPI families.[60]
> - *Compassionate Home, Action Together:* AAPI storytellers and mental health professionals create narratives that address the dynamics of AAPI family life through stories and skits to bring compassion and harmony to AA families.[61]
> - *United Chinese Americans:* A nationwide nonpartisan nonprofit coalition, empowering Chinese Americans, protecting civil rights, engaging, and serving the next generation.[62]
> - *The Georgetown Consortium Program:* A yearlong virtual institute that helps staff support international students through monthly lectures on cross-cultural student mental health, private 1:1 clinical case consultations, case series discussions, a peer community of like-minded educators, and exclusive services for schools, students, and parents.[63]

Funding matters. More federal, local, and private investments for AAPI health research are critical to enable data collection to better characterize and understand AAPI health disparities.

More studies are needed to explore the ways in which systemic racism impacts mental health disparities, and the intersections in which systemic racism and cultural differences converge to perpetuate these inequities. Research has shown that non-white communities have lower access to mental health treatment; AAPI communities access mental health resources even less than black and Latino communities.[67] Even fewer studies exist on in-depth understanding of the access to and quality of mental health treatments, especially for the intersectional AAPI populations. Broader work-force goals include the standardization and expansion of culturally and structurally humble curricula in psychiatric training, implementation of culturally sensitive clinical supervision, and increase in culturally sensitive inclusion in research to make lasting structural changes.

CLINICS CARE POINTS

- Systemic racism against Asian American and Pacific Islanders includes the model minority myth, perpetual foreigner stereotype, and erasure of Asian American and Pacific Islander experiences, which contribute to disparities in Asian American and Pacific Islander mental health.
- Traditional East Asian values, such as those of educational achievement and collectivism, may conflict with Western ideals and require a merging of Western and Eastern values within the Asian American family system.

- Healthy integration of Asian American and Pacific Islanders cultural identities requires AAPI experiences and histories to be taught in schools and shared in collective safe spaces.

- East Asian Americans encompass heterogenous identities, values, and beliefs. It is important for providers to approach each patient with humility and seek clarifications rather than assume.

DISCLOSURE

S. Chou reports no financial relationships or interests. C. Han reports no financial relationships or interests. J.X. Ouyang reports no financial relationships or interests. A.S. Li reports the following conflict of interest: chapter coauthor for *Cultural Psychiatry in Children Adolescents and Families*, American Psychiatric Publishing, 2021.

REFERENCES

1. Yi SS, Ali SH, Chin M, et al. Contrasting the experiences for high- and low-income Asian Americans during COVID-19. Prev Med Rep 2021;24.
2. Ahmmad Z, Wen M, Li K. Self-rated health disparities among Asian Americans: mediating roles of education level and household income. J Immigr Minor Health 2021;23(3):583–90.
3. Lee HY, Rhee TG, Kim NK, et al. Health literacy as a social determinant of health in Asian American immigrants: findings from a population-based survey in California. J Gen Intern Med 2015;30(8):1118–24.
4. Asian American and pacific islander heritage month: May 2021. United States Census Bureau. 2021. Available at: https://www.census.gov/newsroom/facts-for-features/2021/asian-american-pacific-islander.html. Accessed April 1, 2022.
5. A more Diverse Nation. United States Census Bureau. Available at: https://www.census.gov/library/visualizations/2021/comm/a-more-diverse-nation.html. Accessed April 1, 2022.
6. American Community Survey S0201, selected population profile in the United States. United States Census Bureau. Available at: https://data.census.gov/cedsci/table?q=ACSSPP1Y2019.S0201&t=031%20-%20Asian%20alone%20or%20in%20combination%20with%20one%20or%20more%20other%20races. Accessed April 1, 2022.
7. East Asia | RAND. Rand Corporation. Available at: https://www.rand.org/topics/east-asia.html. Accessed April 1, 2022.
8. Asian and pacific islander population in the United States. United States Census Bureau. 2020. Available at: https://www.census.gov/library/visualizations/2020/demo/aian-population.html. Accessed April 1, 2022.
9. Jean Yu-Wen Wu. Know History, Know Self: To Be Grounded In Our Critical Histories. In: Let's Talk! Professional Conference; 2021.
10. Boodhoo N. The centuries-long history of anti-Asian racism and violence in the U.S. Published March 21, 2021. Available at: https://www.axios.com/anti-asian-racism-violence-history-1ecd62dc-1219-4dff-aac5-70f1af0118f6.html. Accessed April 1, 2022.
11. No history, No self — FIND, Inc. Available at: https://www.findinc.org/findink/2017/10/30/no-history-no-self. Accessed April 1, 2022.
12. Rubin-Miller L, Alban C, Artiga S, et al. COVID-19 racial disparities in testing, infection, hospitalization, and death: analysis of epic patient data – issue brief

– 9530 | KFF. Kaiser family foundation. 2020. Available at: https://www.kff.org/report-section/covid-19-racial-disparities-in-testing-infection-hospitalization-and-death-analysis-of-epic-patient-data-issue-brief/. Accessed April 1, 2022.

13. The Lancet. Racism in the USA: ensuring Asian American health equity. Lancet 2021;397(10281):1237.

14. Hswen Y, Xu X, Hing A, et al. Association of "#covid19" versus "#chinesevirus" with anti-Asian sentiments on twitter: March 9-23, 2020. Am J Public Health 2021;111(5):956–64.

15. COMPASS brief report. COMPASS. Available at: https://compass.ucsf.edu/. Accessed April 1, 2022.

16. Poverty by detailed group (National) – AAPI data quick stats. Available at: https://aapidata.com/stats/national/national-poverty-aa-aj/. Accessed April 1, 2022.

17. Kim PY, Lee D. Internalized model minority myth, Asian values, and help-seeking attitudes among Asian American students. Cultur Divers Ethnic Minor Psychol 2014;20(1):98–106.

18. Chung Allred Nancy. Asian Americans and affirmative action: from yellow peril to model minority and back again. Asian Am L J 2007;14(1):57.

19. Huynh QL, Devos T, Smalarz L. Perpetual foreigner in one's own land: potential implications for identity and psychological adjustment. J Soc Clin Psychol 2011;30(2):133–62.

20. Hyeouk Chris Hahm. How We can prevent history from repeating itself: addressing anti-asian discrimination and supporting asian youth. In: Let's talk! Professionals conference; 2021.

21. Carter RT. Racism and psychological and emotional injury: recognizing and assessing race-based traumatic stress. Couns Psychol 2007;35(1):13–105.

22. O'Keefe VM, Wingate LR, Cole AB, et al. Seemingly Harmless racial communications are not so harmless: racial microaggressions lead to suicidal ideation by way of depression symptoms. Suicide Life Threat Behav 2015;45(5):567–76.

23. Torino G. How racism and microaggressions lead to worse health. Los Angeles, CA: Center for Health Journalism; 2017. Available at: https://centerforhealthjournalism.org/2017/11/08/how-racism-and-microaggressions-lead-worse-health. Accessed April 1, 2022.

24. Gee GC, Ro A, Shariff-Marco S, et al. Racial discrimination and health among Asian Americans: evidence, assessment, and directions for future research. Epidemiol Rev 2009;31(1):130.

25. Cheah CSL, Wang C, Ren H, et al. COVID-19 racism and mental health in Chinese American families. Pediatrics 2020;146(5):2020021816.

26. They blamed Me because I Am Asian: Findings from youth-reported Incidents of anti-AAPI hate. 2020. Available at: http://www.asianpacificpolicyandplanningcouncil.org/wp-content/uploads/Stop-AAPI-Hate-Youth-Campaign-Report-9.11.20.pdf. Accessed April 1, 2022.

27. Beers LS, Szilagyi M, Seigel WM, et al. Immunizing against hate: Overcoming asian american and pacific Islander racism. Pediatrics 2021;148(1). https://doi.org/10.1542/PEDS.2021-051836/179714.

28. Mitchell C. Asian American students face threat of harassment, attacks – Center for Public Integrity. Washington, D.C: The Center for Public Integrity; 2021. Available at: https://publicintegrity.org/inside-publici/newsletters/watchdog-newsletter/asian-american-students-threat-harassment-attacks/. Accessed April 1, 2022.

29. Kozloff N, Shapiro G, Larson J, et al. Frequently asked questions for child, adolescent, and adult psychiatrists and other professionals working with

transitional age youth with substance Use Disorders. 2017. Available at: https://www.aacap.org/App_Themes/AACAP/Docs/clinical_practice_center/systems_of_care/sud-tay.pdf. Accessed April 1, 2022.
30. Zhou S, Banawa R, Oh H. The mental health impact of COVID-19 racial and ethnic discrimination against Asian American and Pacific Islanders. Front Psychiatry 2021;12. https://doi.org/10.3389/fpsyt.2021.708426.
31. Hsin A, Xie Y. Explaining Asian Americans' academic advantage over whites. Proc Natl Acad Sci U S A 2014;111(23):8416–21.
32. Kisch J, Leino EV, Silverman MM. Aspects of suicidal behavior, depression, and treatment in college students: results from the spring 2000 national college health assessment survey. Suicide Life Threat Behav 2005;35(1):3–13.
33. To PDN, Huynh J, Wu JTC, et al. Through our eyes, hear our stories: a virtual photovoice project to document and archive asian American and pacific islander community experiences during COVID-19. Health Promotion Pract 2022;23(2):289–95.
34. The rise of Asian Americans. Washington (DC): Pew Research Center; 2013. Available at: https://www.pewsocialtrends.org/wp-content/uploads/sites/3/2013/04/Asian-Americans-new-full-report-04-2013.pdf. Accessed April 1, 2022.
35. Lim AJ, Lau CYH, Cheng CY. Applying the dual filial piety model in the United States: a comparison of filial piety between Asian Americans and Caucasian Americans. Front Psychol 2022;12:6607.
36. Family & home AAPI. Available at: https://aapi.umhistorylabs.lsa.umich.edu/s/aapi_michigan/page/family-and-home. Accessed April 1, 2022.
37. Asian-American families - religion and cultural values - family, development, social, and ethnic - JRank articles. Available at: https://family.jrank.org/pages/104/Asian-American-Families-Religion-Cultural-Values.html. Accessed April 1, 2022.
38. Gunawan J, Juthamanee S, Aungsuroch Y. Current mental health issues in the era of Covid-19. Asian J Psychiatry 2020;51. https://doi.org/10.1016/j.ajp.2020.102103.
39. Pan D. Asian Americans who experienced COVID-related racism report increased levels of anxiety, depression, and PTSD. The Boston Globe. 2021. Available at: https://www.bostonglobe.com/2021/06/06/metro/asian-americans-who-experienced-covid-related-racism-report-increased-levels-anxiety-depression-ptsd/. Accessed April 1, 2022.
40. Josephine M. Kim. The role of schools and educators in the identity development of bicultural Asian American students. In: Let's talk! Professionals conference. 2021.
41. Allen KA, Arslan G, Craig H, et al. The psychometric evaluation of the sense of belonging instrument (SOBI) with Iranian older adults. BMC Geriatr 2021;21(1). https://doi.org/10.1186/S12877-021-02115-Y.
42. Heinz K. The Restoration of the self. Madison, CT: International Universities Press; 1977.
43. Jones N. Marks R. Ramirez R. Census Illuminates racial and ethnic Composition of the country 2020 2021. Washington, D.C, United States Census Bureau. Available at: https://www.census.gov/library/stories/2021/08/improved-race-ethnicity-measures-reveal-united-states-population-much-more-multiracial.html. Accessed April 1, 2022.
44. Kasuga-Jenks S. Racial and ethnic socialization within interracial Asian and White families: a summary. Washington, D.C: American Psychological Association; 2013. Available at: https://www.apa.org/pi/families/resources/newsletter/2013/08/asian-white-socialization. Accessed April 1, 2022.

45. Chang SH. Raising mixed race: multiracial Asian children in a post-racial world. 1st edition. Routledge; 2015. https://doi.org/10.4324/9781315658254/RAISING-MIXED-RACE-MULTIRACIAL-ASIAN-CHILDREN-POST-RACIAL-WORLD-CHANG-SHARON.

46. Lee RM, Yun AB, Yoo HC, et al. Comparing the ethnic identity and well-being of adopted Korean Americans with immigrant/U.S.-Born Korean Americans and Korean International Students. Adopt Q 2010;13(1):2.

47. Westerman A. Am I asian enough?" adoptees struggle to make sense of spike in anti-asian violence : NPR. National public radio. 2021. Available at: https://www.npr.org/2021/03/27/981269559/am-i-asian-enough-adoptees-struggle-to-make-sense-of-spike-in-anti-asian-violenc. Accessed April 1, 2022.

48. Mcdermott FE. Understanding the lived experiences of Asian American transracial adoptees in college. University of Northern Iowa ScholarWorks. 2021. Available at: https://scholarworks.uni.edu/hpt. Accessed April 1, 2022.

49. Truong NL, Zongrone AD, Joseph Kosciw MG. Erasure and resilience: the experiences of LGBTQ students of color Asian American and pacific Islander LGBTQ youth in U.S. Schools. 2020. Available at: www.glsen.org/research. Accessed April 1, 2022.

50. Willner P, Rose J, Stenfert Kroese B, et al. Effect of the COVID-19 pandemic on the mental health of carers of people with intellectual disabilities. J Appl Res Intellect Disabil 2020;33(6):1523–33.

51. Dababnah S, Kim I, Wang Y, et al. Brief report: impact of the COVID-19 pandemic on Asian American families with children with developmental disabilities. J Dev Phys Disabil 2021. https://doi.org/10.1007/s10882-021-09810-z.

52. Han B, Hedden SL, Lipari R, et al. Receipt of services for behavioral health problems: results from the 2014 national survey on drug use and health. SAMHSA Center for Behavioral Health Statistics and Quality. 2015. Available at: http://www.samhsa.gov/data/. Accessed April 1, 2022.

53. Chen JA, Stevens C, Wong SH, et al. Psychiatric symptoms and Diagnoses among U.S. College students: a comparison by race and ethnicity. Psychiatr Serv 2019;70:442–9.

54. American Psychological Association. Use Your WITS: How Asian Americans can Respond to Covid-19 discrimination. 2020. Available at: https://www.youtube.com/watch?v=UijL-kXgojU. Accessed April 1, 2022.

55. American Psychological Association. Acknowledge, Validate, Reframe: How Asian Americans can Respond to Covid-19 discrimination - YouTube. 2020. Available at: https://www.youtube.com/watch?v=iQaD8-6cluU. Accessed April 1, 2022.

56. AAPI Youth Rising. AAPI youth rising. Available at: https://aapiyouthrising.org/about/. Accessed April 1, 2022.

57. Project Lotus. Project Lotus. Available at: https://www.theprojectlotus.org/. Accessed April 1, 2022.

58. Alvin Alvarez. Asian American racial trauma: it isn't fair. In: Let's talk! Professionals conference; 2022.

59. Let's talk! Let'S talk! Professional conference. 2022. Available at: https://www.talkhgse.org/. Accessed April 1, 2022.

60. Home | stanfordchipao. Stanford CHIPAO. 2019. Available at: https://www.stanfordchipao.com/. Accessed April 1, 2022.

61. Compassionate home, action together - mental health, Asian Americans. Yale CHATogether. 2021. Available at: https://chatogether.org/. Accessed April 1, 2022.

62. United Chinese Americans – serve | lead | inspire. United Chinese Americans. 2022. Available at: https://ucausa.org/. Accessed April 1, 2022.
63. vande Berg M, Connor-Linton J, Paige RM. The Georgetown Consortium project: interventions for student learning abroad. Interdiscip J Study Abroad 2009; 18(1):1–75.
64. Kirmayer LJ, Eric Jarvis G. Culturally responsive services as a path to equity in mental healthcare. Healthc Pap 2019;18(2):11–23.
65. Cheng TL, Conca-Cheng AM. The pandemics of racism and COVID-19: danger and opportunity. Pediatrics 2020;146(5). https://doi.org/10.1542/peds.2020-024836.
66. Bellamy-Walker T. Schools are starting to mandate Asian American studies. More could follow suit. NBC News. 2022. Available at: https://www.nbcnews.com/news/asian-america/schools-are-starting-mandate-asian-american-studies-follow-suit-rcna11118. Accessed April 1, 2022.
67. Substance Abuse and Mental Health Services Administration, Racial/ Ethnic Differences in Mental Health Service Use among Adults. HHS Publication No. SMA-15-4906. Rockville, MD: Substance Abuse and Mental Health Services Administration, 2015.

Beyond Children's Mental Health

Cultural Considerations to Foster Latino Child and Family Mental Health

Barbara Robles-Ramamurthy, MD[a],*, Jessica F. Sandoval, MD[a],
Amalia Londoño Tobón, MD[b], Lisa R. Fortuna, MD, MPH, MDiv[c]

KEYWORDS

- Latino children's mental health • Latinx mental health • Latino family mental health
- Diversity • Mental health equity • Structural competence • Racism
- Developmental psychology

KEY POINTS

- Promoting Latino children's mental health requires clinicians to adopt frameworks that extend outside of traditional clinical practice or the medical model and include sociopolitical frameworks that incorporate the whole family's well-being.
- Structural humility and competence and anti-racism are foundational tools that all clinicians must embrace to reduce harms perpetuated by traditional mental health care models.
- Clinicians can promote family engagement to improve Latino children's engagement, retention, and response in mental health treatment.

Promoting Latino children's mental health requires that clinicians understand social systems and structures impacting the child's well-being and engage in a therapeutic approach that considers and respects the child's cultural identity and family cultural values. Hence, this article not only focuses on Latino children's mental health but also informs clinicians seeking to embrace and apply a developmental framework that incorporates cultural, environmental, and sociopolitical dimensions into their clinical practice.

---

[a] Department of Psychiatry and Behavioral Sciences, University of Texas Health San Antonio, 7703 Floyd Curl Drive, MC 7792, San Antonio, TX 78229, USA; [b] National Institutes on Minority Health and Health Disparities, 6707 Democracy Boulevard, Suite 800, Bethesda, MD 20892-5465, USA; [c] Department of Psychiatry and Behavioral Sciences, University of California in San Francisco, 1001 Potrero Avenue, 7M16, San Francisco, CA 94110, USA
* Corresponding author.
E-mail address: roblesramamu@uthscsa.edu

Child Adolesc Psychiatric Clin N Am 31 (2022) 765–778
https://doi.org/10.1016/j.chc.2022.05.005
1056-4993/22/© 2022 Elsevier Inc. All rights reserved.

childpsych.theclinics.com

The Latino population is the largest and one of the fastest growing "minority" group in the United States combined, people of diverse Latin American heritage, including from the Caribbean, Central, and South America.[1] In the United States, this population has historically been labeled Hispanic for census and research purposes. In the early 1980s, the United States began using the term Latino in the census, yet as of 2010, books were still using the term "Hispanic Americans."[2]

Both terms, Hispanic and Latino, carry historical ties to colonial violence, sparking ongoing debate about their use. The term Latino has conferred some separation from Spain and its violent overtaking of indigenous and native civilizations. Although the term Latino connects more than 20 Latin American countries, a 2019 survey from the Pew Research Center showed that most Latinos would rather be called by the name associated with their family's country of origin (ie, Mexican, Cuban, and so forth).[3] For some, the terms Hispanic and Latino still inspire feelings of disconnection within this group; therefore, research findings should not be generalized when they do not offer clarity regarding the specific groups studied.

Regarding its highly gendered nature, the Spanish language has been experiencing a transformation. Women and activists have been pushing to decenter patriarchal domination in the Spanish language by trying to find more female-empowering ways of describing groups of people or items.[4] This translates to the most current push to transition away from Latino and into the use of Latinx or Latine as a gender-neutral term that is more inclusive of all genders. In this article, the terms Latino and Hispanic are used interchangeably to maintain uniformity with their use in the cited research. The term Latinx is increasingly being used in the scientific literature when describing gender-heterogeneous or gender nonbinary groups.

With these clarifications in mind, this article aims to expand the knowledge and expertise of clinicians working with Latino children by embracing empowering frameworks that destigmatize children's behavior, are family-centered and incorporate intergenerational conceptualizations that include a consideration of immigration histories, loss of language and culture, and other important socio-ecological factors. Conceptualization of care also includes considering the ongoing victimization due to systemic racism and violence frequently inflicted on Latino groups, especially indigenous and Afro-Latino people.

SOCIOCULTURAL CONCEPTS PERTINENT TO LATINO FAMILY MENTAL HEALTH

Clinicians working with Latinos will find it useful to understand well-known concepts in Latino mental health literature described in the following sections. These terms *should not* be used as generalizations that perpetuate stereotypes and instead as constructs that can guide inquiry about family values and cultural identities. In general, the scientific literature shows these concepts have both positive and negative effects on Latino mental health.

Acculturation, Enculturation, and Ethnic Identity

The terms Hispanic and Latino are considered an ethnicity as opposed to a racial group, though some scholars suggest that the hybrid term "ethnoracial" may be a more inclusive and representative term that reflects these intersectional social constructs. Although there are many factors that may contribute to the study of ethnic identity, acculturation, *the process of cultural and psychological change that follows intercultural contact,* is one of the most important processes studied in immigrants and their future generations.[5]

Many studies suggest that with increasing acculturation and time in the United States, immigrants and their families have worse mental health outcomes and second-generation youth have worse mental health than first-generation immigrant youth.[6] However, it is important to identify the ways that youth and their families adapt resiliently during the acculturation process.[7] The concept of acculturation has evolved into a multidimensional construct where individuals who are *bicultural,* which is the ability to incorporate both their heritage *and* host cultures into their own, have the most adaptive, positive outcomes.[8,9] An expanding consideration of how enculturation and adaptive acculturation may contribute to positive mental health outcomes is emerging.[10,11]

Ethnic identity refers to the sense of belonging, pride, and attachment to ethnic group membership.[12] Rather than emphasizing the designation that others attribute to the individual, this construct represents the individual's subjective feelings toward their self-ascribed identity. A positive ethnic identity has been associated with prosocial behaviors, positive self-esteem, and fewer internalizing and externalizing symptoms. In young adult samples, strong ethnic identity has been found to be protective against hopelessness in the face of acculturative stress and discrimination, buffering vulnerability to depression and suicidal ideation.[13] Other factors such as social position, experiences of social support versus social exclusion, and language competency and ability can all also influence mental health and the impact of acculturative stress. Exploring how these factors intersect allows clinicians to consider cultural nuances and adaptations from a resilience framework and not solely in terms of risk.[14]

Familismo

Familismo is a cultural concept that highlights the centrality of nuclear and extended family to the individual via importance of filial piety, family support (cohesion and loyalty), obedience, respect (particularly toward adults and elderly family members), and the role of obligation to family.[15] This framework may be woven throughout decisions and behaviors seen throughout development. As child psychiatrists and mental health professionals practicing in a society that emphasizes the individual, we could instead consider the benefits of a developmental framework that emphasizes and understands the role of collectivism.

A systematic review found familismo protective for depression, suicide, and internalizing behaviors.[16] There may be benefits to mental health across members; familismo may predict lower levels of depression for both youth *and their parents.*[17] Family support can uniquely buffer negative effects of acculturation stress and depressive symptoms.[17,18] An association of stronger familism values with higher self-esteem, fewer internalizing, and depressive symptoms has been previously described.[19,20] However, in samples with heavy parental alcohol use, these beneficial associations were no longer present.[19] Overall, familism is central to Latinos and protective for mental health in the context of family cohesion, and it can be a source of vulnerability in the context of high intrafamilial conflict and distress.

Developmental considerations in Latino family mental health

It is important to consider the sociocultural concepts discussed above in the context of developmental phases for Latino children and their families.

PREGNANCY, INFANCY, AND EARLY CHILDHOOD

Although all phases of childhood development are sensitive to environmental changes, pregnancy and early childhood periods are particularly sensitive to environmental perturbations.[21] Disruptions during this period can have lasting impacts through adulthood and intergenerationally. This is particularly important for Latino families in the United States who, as a whole, have been shown in epidemiologic surveys to have intergenerational progressive decline in health.[22] Biological embedding of stressors (eg, acculturation stress, other psychological stress, food insecurity/ diet, housing insecurity, discrimination) via fetal programming (changes in gene expression that affect fetal growth and physiologic parameters that are reset by environmental events and can endure over the lifespan) has been proposed as a mechanism for the observed intergenerational transmission of adverse health outcomes in US Latino families.[23,24]

Acculturation is associated with morbidity and mortality during the perinatal period for Latino families. Multiple studies have shown that birth outcomes such as higher birth weight, lower infant mortality, and higher rates of breastfeeding are associated with lower acculturation in Latinos.[22,25,26] In addition, studies show higher risk of perinatal depression and anxiety disorders in Latina mothers who are more acculturated. Less is known about the role of acculturation and other values in Latino father's risk for perinatal mental illness. Overall, focusing on parental mental health during the perinatal and early childhood period is of utmost importance, as it is highly linked to development and psychopathology risk in children.[27,28]

The perinatal period may result in increased intensity of intergenerational conflict between new parents and their family of origin. Beyond the contextual stress of pregnancy and childbirth, additional acculturation and intergenerational conflict may serve as stressors for Latino families impacting attachment and child-rearing practices (e.g., feeding, sleeping, childcare arrangements, discipline practices, instillment of language and cultural values).[29,30] Conflicting viewpoints and parenting approaches may be offered by the US health care providers and family members, possibly resulting in excessive anxiety for new parents.

For example, a new mother who expresses feelings of depression may be encouraged to not complain and to fulfill her role with appreciation *como una mujer buena* (like a good woman). This example captures how the concept of marianismo could impact the gender role expectation of Latina women to be dedicated primarily to the family by the way of providing childcare, loyalty, and submissiveness to her husband and withstanding sacrifices and suffering for the sake of the family.[31,32] Deviation from traditional cultural roles and expectations may result in psychological distress attributable to the conflict that it creates with family and peers; although it has been less frequently studied in fathers, clinical experience and conceptual frameworks highlight this experience is pertinent to both mothers and fathers.[31,33]

Overall, it is important to note that gender role expectations vary by level of acculturation, specific national origin, nativity, and other factors. The interaction of these variables has differential effects on parental and child mental health and well-being in the perinatal and early childhood years. A study including Mexican and Dominican immigrant families demonstrated a relationship between maternal-reported level of familismo and acculturation on preschool children's externalizing and internalizing psychopathology symptoms that varied by child gender, family income, and cultural identity.[34] Therefore, when working with Latino families during this period, it is crucial that clinicians seek to understand specific nuances rather than generalize this knowledge.

Middle Childhood and Early Adolescence

For many Latino families navigating acculturation stressors, children as young as 8-year old are placed in a unique position of cultural brokerage.[35] Although sometimes reduced to mean a child helping their parents by assisting with interpretation of language, this role of interpreting and translating language may evolve into different forms of mediation as they assist in education, medical, commercial, employment, financial, and even legal settings. Mixed data show both positive and negative effects of this childhood experience, so the pros and cons in these roles must be considered for each individual child.

These role-reversals have been postulated to put more strain on families, resulting in less effective parenting methods and in deferring to children to make important decisions. Families in a study with higher language brokering burdens had higher levels of family stress, lower levels of parenting effectiveness, poorer adolescent academic functioning, and more substance use than those with lower burdens.[36] When youth who reported ethnoracial discrimination brokered more frequently, there was an increase in depression and social anxiety symptoms.[37] A longitudinal study of early adolescents found that perceiving language brokering as a burden was associated with increased acculturation stress, subsequently increasing the risk of marijuana and alcohol use. However, when the child perceived it as a positive experience was confident in their skills and the activity was normalized among their peers, there was no significant association with substance use.[38]

Some researchers argue that culture brokers may be in a unique position that allows them to empathize with the life experiences of their parents which may improve their relationships. This role may also help them build independence, maturity, and self-esteem as they build new skills and competence while promoting both acculturation and enculturation. Mental health clinicians should work with families to understand their child's social, emotional, and cognitive maturity to navigate the brokerage position, while connecting families to local resources that may help minimize the burden on the child.

Adolescence

As youth transition to adolescence, it is not uncommon for conflict to exist between youth and their parents as they begin to explore their identity, autonomy, and independent appraisal of values and goals. Adolescents become more reliant on their community and peers. During this time, generational "gaps" may develop when the youth acculturates more quickly than their parents.[39] This can contribute to intergenerational conflict and poorer mental health outcomes if changing values, together with communication difficulties, arise and result in cycles of distress and conflict.[40] These conflicts can exacerbate the impacts of discrimination as was found in a study where parent–child conflicts mediated the relationship between acculturation conflicts and perceived discrimination on internalizing symptoms.[20]

This is referred to as the "acculturation gap-distress" model, which has been studied in broad measures of internalizing and externalizing symptoms, self-esteem, prosocial and antisocial behaviors, and use of substances. In a meta-analysis of 61 research reports, acculturation mismatches mildly correlated with intergenerational cultural conflict, and this was negatively correlated with offspring mental health.[41] The literature on the impact of acculturation and acculturation dissonance in parent–child dyads on mental health outcomes has overall been mixed, likely due to broad methodology.

Sibling relationships may also impact mental health outcomes. In adolescent sibling dyads of Mexican descent, sibling dyads who endorsed strong familism values and sibling intimacy had lower rates of depressive symptoms and higher rates of positive values, such as the importance of service to other or develop healthy habits. The younger siblings of these dyads were found to have less risky sexual behaviors as teenagers *and* into young adulthood.[42] Latino siblings who were more enculturated described more sibling positivity during COVID-related school closures.[43]

Ethnic identity in adolescence and mental health

Although younger children may recognize the ethnic labels that society assigns to them, adolescents begin to contemplate what being Latino means as a self-determined identity. Enculturation in this stage of development may be protective. Stronger ethnic identity is associated with multiple positive outcomes such as higher self-esteem, lower depressive symptoms, and healthier diets.[44–46] Latino adults with stronger ethnic identity are less likely to perceive discrimination relative to those with lower levels of ethnic identity.[47]

Everyday experiences of discrimination have been reported by up to 30% of US Latinos in adult samples, and these may impact mental health outcomes directly and indirectly.[47] Discrimination experienced by Latino adolescents and young adults is associated with higher depressive symptoms, lower levels of self-esteem, decreased life satisfaction, and in small pilot studies with greater physiologic reactivity.[20,46,48,49] Male Latino adolescents exhibiting a combination of stronger identification with their host culture and a *weaker ethnic identity* are at higher risk of discrimination-associated depressive symptoms and poor self-esteem. Females, however, were at risk of these negative impacts regardless of their identity strengths and compared with their male peers had higher levels of depression and lower self-esteem. Latinas with low family cohesion experience higher depression and anxiety symptoms. There are several cultural considerations for why Latina adolescents may be more at risk for experiencing internalizing symptoms as compared with their male counterparts. Further empirical investigation that includes an examination of the associations of intersecting identities, minoritized, and family stress with mood disorders is needed.[50]

Young Adulthood

A distinct developmental phase termed "emerging adulthood" is defined as the time between ages 18 and 25 years and is of particular interest to youth mental health in Western cultures, including the United States. During this time, young people can maximize their independence and exploration of their identities in the areas of love, work, and worldviews. This may not be applicable across all cultural and socioeconomic groups; some may not be able to defer adult responsibilities (e.g., financially contributing to family) to fully explore other life possibilities. Latinos in this age range are more likely than their White peers to continue to live at home. This has been attributed to both financial circumstances and attitudes about when it is appropriate for adult children to leave the home, factors that may be mutually reinforcing, particularly for communities with limited socioeconomic resources.[51]

Family obligations are central to decision-making regarding pursuits after high school. A family may depend on the young adult's support financially and to care for the house, siblings, or elders.[52] Owing to a lack of generational wealth, Latino young adults are less likely to have sufficient funds to live independently as compared with their White non-Latino counterparts. How this relates to mental health outcomes can vary. Young adults of Central American origin experienced less negative self-image when they took personal responsibility for meeting familial expectations and needs. Meeting the family's academic expectations was associated with both positive self-image and less negative self-image.[53] In a mixed gender sample, provision of emotionally supportive caretaking was associated with greater depressive symptoms when the youth endorsed average to high levels of familism, leading the authors to summarize "for children of immigrants, the burden of tasks that require them to be emotional supports for the family is magnified by the sense that it is their responsibility as a member of the family."[54] As youth begin to approach mid-to-late teens, they may anticipate some of these unique challenges and decisions of emerging adulthood.

IMPROVING SYSTEMS OF CARE FOR LATINO YOUTH AND FAMILIES
Foundational Clinical Skills

Experiencing discrimination in clinical encounters impacts subsequent use of health care services.[55] Black, Latino, and uninsured patients are likely to report discrimination in mental health and substance use treatment, with uninsured patients being seven times more likely to report these experiences.[56] Despite experiencing increased risks for mental illness, Latinos are less likely to receive formal mental health services or receive adequate care and are more likely to terminate services prematurely.[57] Family engagement in mental health treatment has been identified as predictive of youth mental health treatment engagement, retention, and response.[58–60]

Cultural and structural humility are foundational skills highly needed in the mental health system to decrease ongoing harms, disparities, and structural inequities inflicted on patients by traditional care models.[61] This is highly pertinent when discussing opportunities to improve access and quality of care for Latino children and their families. Lack of awareness about the social and structural drivers of health can result in treatment that disregards the patient's current lived experience and results in further shame and stigma when accessing services.

Awareness of how policies and laws can impact Latino youth and family mental health is needed, as studies have shown that families experiencing fear of deportation or had a family member deported or detained have higher rates of heart disease, asthma, diabetes, depression, anxiety, suicidal ideation, externalizing symptoms, and Post Traumatic Stress Disorder. These negative effects impact US citizen children as well.[62] Naturalistic research studies have also demonstrated that passage of laws increasing people's ability to apply for documented status, such as the Deferred Action for Childhood Arrivals, is associated with improved sleep, high school graduation rates and employment outcomes, decreased rates of poverty, lower teen birth rates, and an overall stronger sense of belonging. In contrast, the negative impacts were visible when political rhetoric threatened the discontinuation of this law around the 2016 election, with self-reported worsening of sleep.[63]

CULTURALLY TAILORED EVIDENCE-BASED INTERVENTIONS

Several evidence-based interventions have been adapted and tested with Latino children and families; however, it is important to note that the gold standard for the development of new interventions should integrate Latino youth and family voices to cocreate tailored interventions. Lastly, as with any evidence-based intervention, there is a fine line to balance intervention fidelity with respect for the patient and family's current needs and wishes.

The perinatal and early childhood periods present an opportune and critical time for family interventions with potentially lasting effects on child mental health. Not only is it a biologically salient time, but specific to Latinos, cultural values of familism and views on parenthood may be strong drivers for mental health treatment engagement. Interventions developed or adapted for Latinos and delivered during the perinatal period tend to focus primarily on maternal mental health as opposed to family mental health.[64] Some interventions, including Minding the Baby (MTB), an early home-visiting intervention developed and tested with Latina and Black mother–child dyads, incorporate community participatory strategies and a relational-based approach to improve the intergenerational health and mental health of mother–child dyads. Several studies showed positive MTB intervention effects on child attachment, child health, and parenting at the end of the intervention and even years after the intervention concluded.[65–67] This and other approaches need to be further refined and adapted to include the larger family context.

Familias Unidas uses culturally based parenting strategies to prevent adolescent risk behaviors. The intervention is manualized and includes communication techniques for parents to help protect adolescent risk behaviors. The intervention uses a telenovela series that depicts situations that take place within families and with peers and ways that adolescents can respond. The family sessions include each family's particular needs by allowing them to prioritize family goals. The developers recently created a digital eHealth intervention format.[68]

Measurement-based care (MBC), a client-centered practice of collecting and using client-reported progress data throughout treatment, can inform shared decision-making with minoritized youth and their families and improve engagement, involvement in treatment, satisfaction, and retention in care.[69] MBC offers an opportunity to follow outcomes that are prioritized by families, including individualized measures of symptoms, and sociocultural measures (experiences of discrimination, acculturative stress) as well as monitor and address potential barriers to care that are collaboratively identified and addressed by the family and provider.

Other interventions that have incorporated family involvement to improve Latino child mental health include psychoeducation and accompaniment in advocacy activities. Empowering parents through coaching, co-attending check-in meetings with both the teacher and therapist, and role-playing exercises was found to promote positive skill building in Spanish-speaking Latino parents of children with ADHD.[70] Promising data show that when Latino youth access mental health services in childhood, they are more likely to access services if needed again as young adults.[71] In addition, a randomized controlled trial in primary care that compared Brief Behavioral Therapy (BBT) with Assisted Referral to Treatment found BBT to be an effective tool to engage Latino youth and families in mental health treatment.[72] This has critical implications for the urgency to integrate behavioral health into schools and pediatric practices.

SUMMARY AND CLINICAL TAKEAWAYS

Prioritizing efforts that are centered on equity and justice and aim to improve access to quality care are highly needed to better serve Latino families. As scholars, academicians, mentors, and educators, we encourage all readers to prioritize teaching material, opportunities for learning, and clinical practice that promotes a stronger foundation for this and the next generation of mental health providers serving Latino families.

- Ensure that all mental health trainees have experience using the Cultural Formulation Interview (CFI), which was developed by the American Psychiatric Association to help engage individuals in mental health services. The CFI is a core interview of 16 open-ended questions, with prompts for clinicians to understand the cultural content behind each question and the perspective of the child, youth, caregiver, and family.[73]
- It is important to teach trainees about cultural and structural humility and center these concepts in all clinical formulations and establish a curriculum that explicitly equips and empowers clinicians with the knowledge, vocabulary, and tools to

address racism in mental health care along with family-centered approaches.[61,74,75]

- Structural humility invites clinicians to consider how the current polarized political climate and systemic inequities may impact the transmission of intergenerational trauma to younger generations and encourage incorporation of approaches that nourish ethnic pride and strong ethnic identity as a protective strength for youth and family mental health.
- As youth begin to approach mid-to-late teens, they may anticipate some of the unique challenges of emerging adulthood, including their role in supporting their families, and clinicians should explore these issues in clinical care, especially with depressed youth.
- Clinicians seeking to provide quality mental health services to Latino children and families must embrace skills and practices that allow families to develop trust in their care; discussing socio-political stressors and experiences of discrimination can assist patients to develop trust with clinicians and allow them to describe the extent of their stressors, how these impact their mental health.
- As clinicians working with diverse patient populations, who are navigating highly complex social structures, it is imperative that we engage in our own healing process, incorporating self-reflection about our own biases, lived experiences, and intersectional identities in systems of power and disadvantages. Acknowledging our own healing and humanity will empower us to provide empowering care to the patients we serve.

CLINICS CARE POINTS

- Studies demonstrate the importance of several values in Latino culture that should be considered when caring for children including familism. However, the Latino experience is not monolithic and various levels of acculturation, racial-ethnic identity, intersectionality, and migration patterns need to be taken into account in clinical formulations.

- Use the cultural formulation and other evidence-based practices and nonjudgmental discussion of the interrelatedness of culture and mental health, particularly when these seem to be impacting or interfering with clinical care.

- When treating Latino children, identifying opportunities to strengthen their ethnic and racial identity and pride can be important ways to optimize clinical treatment.

- When serving Latino children in medical settings, educate medical providers about the possible negative impacts of language brokering and the importance of using interpreting services appropriately.

- Perinatal mental health providers, pediatricians, obstetricians, and family practitioners can foster mental health in new Latino parents and improve parent–child relational health by facilitating discussions about how acculturation and intergenerational belief systems may impact their parenting trajectory.

DISCLOSURE

Drs B. Robles-Ramamurthy, J. Sandoval and L. Fortuna have no conflicts of interest to disclose. Dr A. Londoño Tobón is supported by the Division of Intramural Research, National Institute on Minority Health and Health Disparities, National Institutes of Health. The contents and views in this article are those of the authors and should not be construed to represent the views of the National Institutes of Health.

REFERENCES

1. Krogstad J. With fewer new arrivals, Census lowers Hispanic population projections. In Pew Research Center. 2014. Available at: https://www.pewresearch.org/fact-tank/2014/12/16/with-fewer-new-arrivals-census-lowers-hispanic-population-projections-2/#:~:text=The%20Hispanic%20population%20is%20expected%20to%20reach%20about,than%20earlier%20population%20projections%20published%20by%20the%20bureau. Accessed March 20, 2022.

2. Alarcon R, Ruiz P. Hispanic Americans. In: Ruiz P, Annelle BP, editors. Disparities in psychiatric care: clinical and cross-cultural perspectives. Baltimore (MD): LWW; 2010. p. 30–40.

3. Gonzalez-Barrera A. The ways Hispanics describe their identity vary across immigrant generations. In Pew Research Center. Available at: https://www.pewresearch.org/fact-tank/2020/09/24/the-ways-hispanics-describe-their-identity-vary-across-immigrant-generations/. Accessed March 25, 2022..

4. Garcia R. El feminismo y la lengua espanola. Replicante. Available at: https://revistareplicante.com/el-feminismo-y-la-lengua-espanola/. Accessed March 30, 2022.

5. Berry JW, Phinney JS, Sam DL, et al. Immigrant youth: acculturation, identity, and adaptation. Appl Psychol An Int Rev 2006;55(3):303–32.

6. Bekteshi V, Kang SW. Contextualizing acculturative stress among Latino immigrants in the United States: a systematic review. Ethn Health 2020;25(6):897–914.

7. Alegría M, Álvarez K, DiMarzio K. Immigration and mental health. Curr Epidemiol Rep 2017;4(2):145–55.

8. Berry JW. Acculturation as varieties of adaptation. In: Padilla A, editor. Acculturation: Theory, Models and Findings. Boulder: Westview; 1980. p. 9–25.

9. Nguyen AM, Benet-Martínez V. Biculturalism and adjustment: a meta-analysis. J Cross-Cultural Psychol 2013;44(1):122–59.

10. Sun Q, Geeraert N, Simpson A. Never mind the acculturation gap: migrant youth's wellbeing benefit when they retain their heritage culture but their parents adopt the settlement culture. J Youth Adolescence 2020;49(2):520–33.

11. Telzer EH, Yuen C, Gonzales N, et al. Filling gaps in the acculturation gap-distress model: heritage cultural maintenance and adjustment in Mexican–American families. J Youth Adolescence 2016;45(7):1412–25.

12. Phinney J. Understanding ethnic diversity: the role of ethnic identity. Am Behav Scientist 1996;40(2):143–52.

13. Polanco-Roman L, Miranda R. Culturally related stress, hopelessness, and vulnerability to depressive symptoms and suicidal ideation in emerging adulthood. Behav Ther 2013;44(1):75–87.

14. Ruiz JM, Hamann HA, Mehl MR, et al. The Hispanic health paradox: from epidemiological phenomenon to contribution opportunities for psychological science. Group Process Intergroup Relations 2016;19(4):462–76.

15. Stein GL, Cupito AM, Mendez JL, et al. Familism through a developmental lens. J Lat/Psychol 2014;2(4):224–50.

16. Valdivieso-Mora E, Peet CL, Garnier-Villarreal M, et al. A systematic review of the relationship between familism and mental health outcomes in Latino population. Front Psychol 2016;7:1632.

17. Ayón C, Marsiglia FF, Bermudez-Parsai M. Latino family mental health: exploring the role of discrimination and familismo. J Community Psychol 2010;38(6):742–56.

18. Raffaelli M, Andrade FC, Wiley AR, et al. Stress, social support, and depression: a test of the stress-buffering hypothesis in a Mexican sample. J Res Adolescence 2013;23(2):283–9.
19. Salcido VV, Christophe NK, Stein GL. Familism and psychological wellbeing among Latinx youth: the role of parental alcohol use. J Fam Psychol 2021. https://doi.org/10.1037/fam0000924.
20. Smokowski PR, Rose RA, Bacallao M. Influence of risk factors and cultural assets on Latino adolescents' trajectories of self-esteem and internalizing symptoms. Child Psychiatry Hum Dev 2010;41:133–55.
21. Londono Tobon A, Stransky AD, Ross DA, et al. Effects of maternal prenatal stress: mechanisms, implications, and novel therapeutic interventions. Biol Psychiatry 2016;80(11):e85–7.
22. Montoya-Williams D, Williamson VG, Cardel M, et al. The Hispanic/Latinx perinatal paradox in the United States: a scoping review and recommendations to guide future research. J immigrant Minor Health 2021;23(5):1078–91.
23. Fox M, Thayer ZM, Ramos IF, et al. Prenatal and postnatal mother-to-child transmission of acculturation's health effects in Hispanic Americans. J Women's Health 2018;27(8):1054–63.
24. Fox M, Entringer S, Buss C, et al. Intergenerational transmission of the effects of acculturation on health in Hispanic Americans: a fetal programming perspective. Am J Public Health 2015;105(S3):S409–23.
25. Hamilton ER, Langer PD, Patler C. DACA's association with birth outcomes among Mexican-origin mothers in the United States. Demography 2021;58(3):975–85.
26. Bigman G, Wilkinson AV, Pérez A, et al. Acculturation and breastfeeding among Hispanic American women: a systematic review. Matern Child Health J 2018;22(9):1260–77.
27. O'donnell KJ, Glover V, Barker ED, et al. The persisting effect of maternal mood in pregnancy on childhood psychopathology. Dev Psychopathol 2014;26(2):393–403.
28. Mahrer NE, Ramos IF, Guardino C, et al. Pregnancy anxiety in expectant mothers predicts offspring negative affect: the moderating role of acculturation. Early Hum Dev 2020;141:104932.
29. Hwang W. Acculturative family distancing: theory, re- search, and clinical practice. Psychother Res Pract Train 2006;43:397–409.
30. Kiang L, Glatz T, Buchanan CM. Acculturation conflict, cultural parenting self-efficacy, and perceived parenting competence in Asian American and Latino/a families. Fam process 2017;56(4):943–61.
31. Morales A, Pérez OFR. Marianismo. The wiley encyclopedia of personality and individual differences: clinical, applied, and cross-cultural research 2020; 247-251. Available at: https://onlinelibrary.wiley.com/action/doSearch?AllField=marianismo&ContentGroupKey=10.1002%2F9781119547181
32. Castillo LG, Perez FV, Castillo R, et al. Construction and initial validation of the Marianismo beliefs scale. Coun Psychol Q 2010;23:163–75.
33. Arciniega GM, Thomas C, Tovar-Blank ZG, et al. Toward a fuller conception of machismo: development of a traditional machismo and caballerismo scale. J Couns Psychol 2008;55(1):19–33.
34. Calzada EJ, Huang KY, Linares-Torres H, et al. Maternal familismo and early childhood functioning in Mexican and Dominican immigrant families. J Latina/o Psychol 2014;2(3):156.

35. Morales A, Hanson WE. Language brokering: an integrative review of the literature. Hispanic J Behav Sci 2005;27(4):471–503.
36. Martinez CR, McClure HH, Eddy JM. Language brokering contexts and behavioral and emotional adjustment among Latino parents and adolescents. J Early Adolesc 2009;29(1):71–98.
37. Felkey J, Graham S. Racial/ethnic discrimination, cultural mistrust, and psychological maladjustment among Asian American and Latino adolescent language brokers. Cultur Divers Ethnic Minor Psychol 2022;28(1):125–31.
38. Kam JA, Lazarevic V. The stressful (and not so stressful) nature of language brokering: identifying when brokering functions as a cultural stressor for Latino immigrant children in early adolescence. J Youth Adolescence 2014;43: 1994–2011.
39. Costigan CE, Dokis DP. Similarities and differences in acculturation among mothers, fathers, and children in immigrant Chinese families. J Cross-Cultural Psychol 2006;37(6):723–41.
40. Szapocznik J, Kurtines WM. Family psychology and cultural diversity: opportunities for theory, research, and application. Am Psychol 1993;48(4):400–7.
41. Lui P. Intergenerational cultural conflict, mental health, and educational outcomes among Asian and Latino/a Americans: qualitative and meta-analytic review. Psychol Bull 2015;141(2):404–46.
42. Killoren SE, Wheeler LA, Updegraff KA, et al. Associations among Mexican-origin youth's sibling relationships, familism and positive values, and adjustment problems. J Fam Psychol 2021;35(5):573–83.
43. Sun X, Updegraff KA, McHale SM, et al. Implications of COVID-19 school closures for sibling dynamics among U.S. Latinx children: a prospective, daily diary study. Dev Psychol 2021;57(10):1708–18.
44. Rogers-Sirin L, Gupta T. Cultural identity and mental health: differing trajectories among Asian and Latino youth. J Couns Psychol 2012;59(4):555–66.
45. Rogers LO, Meltzoff AN. Is gender more important and meaningful than race? An analysis of racial and gender identity among Black, White, and mixed-race children. Cultur Divers Ethnic Minor Psychol 2017;23(3):323–34.
46. Umaña-Taylor AJ, Updegraff KA. Latino adolescents' mental health: exploring the interrelations among discrimination, ethnic identity, cultural orientation, self-esteem, and depressive symptoms. J Adolesc 2007;30(4):549–67.
47. Pérez DJ, Fortuna L, Alegria M. Prevalence and correlates of everyday discrimination among U.S. Latinos. J Community Psychol 2008;36(4):421–33.
48. Lazarevic V, Crovetto F, Shapiro AF, et al. Family dynamics moderate the impact of discrimination on wellbeing for Latino young adults. Cultur Divers Ethnic Minor Psychol 2021;27(2):214–26.
49. Huynh VW, Huynh QL, Stein MP. Not just sticks and stones: indirect ethnic discrimination leads to greater physiological reactivity. Cultur Divers Ethnic Minor Psychol 2017;23(3):425–34.
50. Zayas LH, Lester RJ, Cabassa LJ, et al. Why do so many latina teens attempt suicide? A conceptual model for research. Am J Orthopsychiatry 2005;75(2): 275–87.
51. Fingerman KL, Yahirun JJ. Emerging Adulthood in the Context of Family: Young Adults' Relationships with Parents. In: Arnett J, editor. Oxford Handbook of Emerging Adulthood. New York, NY: Oxford University Press; 2015. p. 172.
52. Sanchez B, Esparza P, Colón Y, et al. Tryin'to make it during the transition from high school: the role of family obligation attitudes and economic context for Latino-emerging adults. J Adolesc Res 2010;25(6):858–84.

53. Mejia Y, Supple AJ, Plunkett SW, et al. The Role of perceived familial expectations on depressive symptoms and self-esteem in emerging adulthood: a cultural analysis. Emerging Adulthood 2021. https://doi.org/10.1177/21676968211005861.

54. Toro RI, Schofield TJ, Calderon-Tena CO, et al. Filial responsibilities, familism, and depressive symptoms among Latino young adults. Emerging Adulthood 2019;7(5):370-7.

55. Findling MG, Bleich SN, Casey LS, et al. Discrimination in the United States: experiences of latinos. Health Serv Res 2019;54(Suppl 2):1409-18.

56. Mays VM, Jones AL, Delany-Brumsey A, et al. Perceived discrimination in health care and mental health/substance abuse treatment among blacks, latinos, and whites. Med Care 2017;55(2):173-81.

57. Kapke TL, Gerdes AC. Latino family participation in youth mental health services: treatment retention, engagement, and response. Clin Child Fam Psychol Rev 2016;19(4):329-51.

58. Stafford AM, Draucker CB. Barriers to and facilitators of mental health treatment engagement among latina adolescents. Community Ment Health J 2020;56(4):662-9.

59. Corrigan PW, Druss BG, Perlick DA. The impact of mental illness stigma on seeking and participating in mental health care. Psychol Sci Public Interest 2014;15(2):37-70.

60. Waid J, Kelly M. Supporting family engagement with child and adolescent mental health services: a scoping review. Health Soc Care Community 2020;28(5):1333-42.

61. Hansen Helena, Jonathan M, Metzl, editors. Structural Competency in Mental Health and Medicine: a case based approach to treating the social determinants of health. Switzerland AG: Springer; 2019.

62. Zayas LH, Heffron LC. Disrupting young lives: how detention and deportation affect US-born children of immigrants. In American Psychological Association. 2016. Available at: https://www.apa.org/pi/families/resources/newsletter/2016/11/detention-deportation. Accessed March 30, 2022.

63. Giuntella O, Lonsky J, Mazzona F, et al. Immigration Policy and immigrant's sleep. Evidence from DACA. J Econ Behav Organ 2021;182:1-12.

64. Ponting C, Mahrer NE, Zelcer H, et al. Psychological interventions for depression and anxiety in pregnant Latina and Black women in the United States: a systematic review. Clin Psychol Psychother 2020;27(2):249-65.

65. Sadler A, Close SN, et al. Minding the Baby: enhancing reflectiveness to improve early health and relationship outcomes in an interdisciplinary home visiting program. Infant Ment Health J 2013;34(5):391-405.

66. Slade A, Holland ML, Ordway MR, et al. Minding the Baby®: enhancing parental reflective functioning and infant attachment in an attachment-based, interdisciplinary home visiting program. Dev Psychopathol 2020;32(1):123-37.

67. Tobon AL, Condon E, Sadler LS, et al. School age effects of Minding the Baby-An attachment-based home-visiting intervention-On parenting and child behaviors -ERRATUM. Dev Psychopathol 2021;33(1):376.

68. Brincks A, Perrino T, Howe G, et al. Familias Unidas prevents youth internalizing symptoms: a baseline target moderated mediation (BTMM) study. Prev Sci 2021. https://doi.org/10.1007/s11121-021-01247-2.

69. Connors EH, Arora PG, Resnick SG, et al. A modified measurement-based care approach to improve mental health treatment engagement among racial and ethnic minoritized youth. Psychol Serv 2022. https://doi.org/10.1037/ser0000617.

70. Gerdes AC, Kapke TL, Lawton KE, et al. Culturally adapting parent training for Latino youth with ADHD: development and pilot. J Latina/o Psychol 2015;3(2): 71–87.

71. Green JG, Oblath R, DeYoung G, et al. Does childhood mental health service use predict subsequent mental health service use during Latino youth transition to young adulthood? Evidence from the Boricua Youth Study. Soc Psychiatry Psychiatr Epidemiol 2020;55(11):1439–48.

72. Brent DA, Porta G, Rozenman MS, et al. Brief behavioral therapy for pediatric anxiety and depressioon in primary care: a follow-up. JAACAP 2019;59(7). https://doi.org/10.1016/j.jaac.2019.06.009.

73. Lewis-Fernández R, Aggarwal NK, Bäärnhielm S, et al. Culture and psychiatric evaluation: operationalizing cultural formulation for DSM-5. Psychiatry 2014; 77(2):130–54.

74. Structural racism throughout psychiatry. In American psychiatric association. Available at: https://ucsf.app.box.com/s/27h19kd597ii66473parki15u0cgochd. Accessed March 30, 2022.

75. O'Brien M, Fields R, Jackson A. Anti-Racism and Race Literacy: a primer and toolkit for medical educators. University of California Differences Matter Working Group; 2021. Available at: https://ucsf.app.box.com/s/27h19kd597ii66473 parki15u0cgochd. Accessed March 30, 2022.

Evaluating Native Youth
Issues and Considerations in Clinical Evaluation and Treatment

Rebecca Susan Daily, MD[a],*, George 'Bud' Vana, MD, MA[b,c],
Joy K.L. Andrade, MD[d], John Pruett, MD, BCFE[e]

KEYWORDS

- Native • Indigenous • American Indian • Native Hawaiian • Alaskan Native
- Pacific Islander

KEY POINTS

- Give sufficient time between questions and answers—this can include prolonged silences while answers are considered.
- Family consists of everyone considered family by the patient.
- Frequently elders make final decisions about important choices of therapy and medication that can lead to multiple sessions to make the decisions with family consulting elders.
- Abandonment and broken promises by the system have been the general experience so trust has to be earned over time.
- Every tribe is a separate nation with their own traditions and cultural beliefs.

Native America is a broad group consisting of multiple cultures and traditions where one size does not fit all. There are 573 federally recognized tribes with at least as many seeking recognition. Chronically underserved and stigmatized for centuries, these groups tend to be cautious when seeking mental health services and interacting with other outside entities, even when in need of services. Many have recently begun building their own health care resources including hiring and training mental health

Disclaimer: Authors have nothing to disclose.
[a] Behavioral Health, Oklahoma State University-College of Osteopathic Medicine at the Cherokee Nation, Cherokee Nation, PO Box 948, Tahlequah, OK 74465-0948, USA; [b] Department of Integrated Psychiatry, University of Washington; [c] Department of Psychiatry & Behavioral Sciences, University of Washington, 2592 Kwina Road, Bellingham, WA 98226, USA; [d] Department of Psychiatry, University of Hawaii John A. Burns School of Medicine, 1356 Lusitania Street, UH Tower 4th Floor, Honolulu, HI 96813, USA; [e] Bellin Health, Green Bay Wisconsin Bellin Psychiatric Center, 301 East Street Joseph Street, Green Bay, WI 54301, USA
* Corresponding author.
E-mail address: SusanDailyMD@msn.com

Child Adolesc Psychiatric Clin N Am 31 (2022) 779–788
https://doi.org/10.1016/j.chc.2022.06.008
1056-4993/22/© 2022 Elsevier Inc. All rights reserved.

childpsych.theclinics.com

Abbreviations	
NA	Native American
AN	Alaskan Native
NH	Native Hawaiian
PI	Pacific Islander
CBD	Cannabidiol

providers. Even so, there is a severe dearth of mental health services for these populations.

There are basic "ground rules" for approaching, evaluating, and treating members of these communities. This article will focus on initial and general approaches to evaluating Native youth. In the context of this article, Native America consists of individuals of Native American (NA), First Nations, Alaskan Native (AN), Native Hawaiian (NH), and Pacific Islander (PI) heritage from a wide variety of individual nations, tribes, and communities.

COMMON RULES AMONG NATIVE AMERICAN/ALASKAN NATIVE/NATIVE HAWAIIAN/PACIFIC ISLANDER COMMUNITIES

1. Respect elders
2. Continuous direct eye contact from youth is disrespectful
3. Important decisions should not be rushed
4. Family participates in decision making
5. Trust has to be earned
6. All aspects of healing must be considered[1]

ASPECTS OF HEALING WITHIN THE NATIVE DIASPORA

Healing within the Native diaspora is a process including spiritual, physical, and cultural-social interaction with all needing to be in balance for health to occur. Healing may be done on an individual basis but more traditional practice includes ceremonies involving the family and community. Special items are often used such as prayer clothes, shawls, and talismans and Group ceremonies involve anointing, smudging, and spending time in sweat lodges anywhere from days to weeks. Health care professionals should be aware of, and ask about a patient's traditional healing practice. For example, the sweat lodge, where there is exposure to high temperatures and possible dehydration, may interfere with medication effectiveness and safety and require further discussion with a patient and family.

Spiritual well-being is not a question of religion but of faith and belief in existence within and outside of oneself. A wide variety of spiritual practices are common in native communities; a mixture of indigenous and Western belief systems is most common. Some individuals do not knowingly practice any traditional beliefs, whereas others attend traditional ceremony regularly. The Native American Church actively combines traditional and Christian practices. Ceremony is a central component of spiritual practice for many and can include dance, drumming, prayers, forms of meditation, and rituals that may or may not include traditional foods, herbs, or medicine. Sweat lodges and personal spiritual journey experiences are also common.

Physical well-being is perceived as bio-psycho-social functioning always in need of careful balancing. Balancing or centering is a process learned from traditional teachings and includes ceremonies, cleansings, and nourishing body and spirit. All reference a person's place within their natural world with a respect for that world and the inhabitants.[2] Physical exercise, a healthy diet, and use of native plants with knowledge of cyclical rhythms of seasons and life are used to provide balance.

Emotional well-being is closely tied to living in harmony with nature, with the community, with the family, and with one's spirituality. It is addressed through shared experiences such as traditions, ceremonies, and social communication. This is true whether traditional or nontraditional approaches are taken.[3]

TRADITIONAL HEALING

Traditional healing in Native populations uses plants, minerals, and sources of water as well as dietary recommendations. Many Native populations have recently reintroduced traditional diets along with providing seeds and community teaching to address rates of diabetes, heart disease, and other disorders related to diet. Medicinal plants vary with different environments, and specific prayers or rituals often accompany their use. During evaluations, professionals should ask for a list of any traditional medicines, drinks, poultices, or practices the individual or family partake of either regularly or occasionally.

Ceremonies may include a variety of steps, some of which may have an effect on a professional's treatment plan. These may include sweat lodges, fasting, dehydration, dancing for extended periods, smudging (burning of specific herbs/plants), smoking (bathing in smoke), the use of mescaline or peyote, and eating of specific herbs/foods. Ceremony may involve the individual or a small group such as immediate family or the larger community. All are geared toward bringing the individual back into balance.

MEDICINE WHEEL

Medicine wheels appear across myriad cultures around the world and symbolize balance between cycle of life and the beliefs of the specific tribe or tribal group. The specifics of any Medicine Wheel can be extremely complicated but generally, wheels are read in a sun-wise (or clock-wise) direction aligning with the rising and setting of the sun, the earth, and the sky. The directions East, South, West, and North are represented by specific colors (depending on the tribe). The cardinal directions also designate other representations such as stages of life, seasons of the year, natural elements, and ceremonial plants. Medicine wheels are for teaching and learning how to keep balance and harmony (**Fig. 1**).

SYMBOLISM

There are many symbols and customs across the Native diaspora Here are just a few:

Recently shorn hair: Hair is often cut when a loved one dies
White shawls/scarves: Prayer-imbued items worn by a person who is suffering
Regalia: Ceremonial clothing, visual manifestation of heritage, not a "costume"
Gifts: Gifts of food should never be refused, as this is offensive
Sweetgrass: Woven bracelets or items may be made of this sacred grass and
    should be treated with respect

HISTORICAL TRAUMA

NAs, NHs, AN, and PIs have a history interacting with European colonizers over the past 600 years that covers the width and breadth of traumatic experiences including cultural genocide. Early contact brought disease, enslavement, and death.

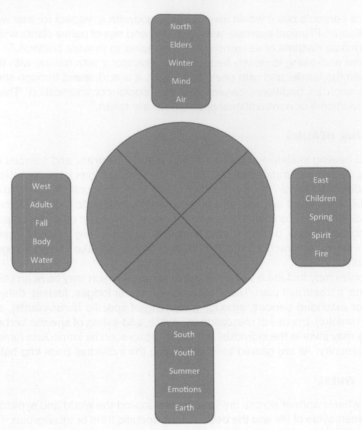

Fig. 1. Medicine wheel.

Progressively stripped of their people, their lands, and their resources as they fled European invaders, many tribes disappeared completely. Cultural genocide manifested through missionaries and boarding schools where children were stripped of their heritage and forced to give up their personal belongings, their hairstyles, their religious beliefs, and their language. Many were abused physically, psychologically, and/or sexually Whole generations lost concepts of healthy parenting leading to intergenerational trauma within families.[4]

Historical trauma continues in the form of discrimination across all areas including education, health care access, social services, criminal justice interactions, and community resources such as employment and housing. NAs experience microaggressions and disproportionate exposure to violence on a personal and community basis as well as high rates of substance abuse, suicide, depression, and stress-related health disorders.[5] Suicide is the second leading cause of death among Native youth at 2.5 times the national rate for all other youth in the United States.[6] Sequelae from historical trauma must be considered in any evaluation.

PSYCHOPHARMACOLOGY

As of this writing, there are no psychiatric medications specifically indicated for NA youth populations. There is research that indicates the effectiveness of naltrexone, buprenorphine-naloxone, methadone for medication assistant therapy for adult indigenous populations to treat substance abuse.[7] There is vast inequity in research among minority populations in the United States.[8] Native people are often cautious about involvement in research due to past mistreatment and harm from research as well as failures of researchers to protect privacy.[9,10]

TELEPSYCHIATRY

Telepsychiatry has been a boon for Native America allowing access to health care in rural areas where before it was almost impossible. Many Native people live on reservations where there may be hundreds of miles between them and a mental health provider. Lack of transportation, lack of money for fuel, and poor roads all affect the ability to access care. Others live where there is a dearth of providers, either rural, suburban, or urban. However, there is also a lack of reliable Internet access to contend with, especially on reservations. Although these barriers exist, studies have shown that there are still opportunities and models to deliver culturally competent care to tribal communities over telepsychiatry.[11]

CASE STUDIES
Native American

A 16-year-old cisgender young man (B) and his mother present for an initial evaluation in person with a non-native child psychiatrist. The patient's reasons for seeking psychiatric care were severe social anxiety, auditory hallucinations, and school avoidance.

Briefly, the patient had been experiencing worsening auditory hallucinations and suicidal ideation for 3 months before seeking psychiatric care. B had left school after experiencing bullying with peers and hearing a teacher make racist statements. He became depressed and more anxious and began working closely with a therapist during this time. After anxiety symptoms persisted he started citalopram, prescribed by his non-native pediatrician at the tribal health center. He never mentioned the auditory hallucinations to his pediatrician because he was both embarrassed and confused by them. After failure to respond to this medication, his pediatrician prescribed sertraline, which worsened B's suicidal ideation leading to an episode where he walked to train tracks with the intent to die by suicide but called his mother before acting. At this time, the family sought psychiatric help.

He and his mother deny other symptoms of agoraphobia, Obsessive Compulsive Disorder, mania or problems with joint attention, social reciprocity or fixed interests. Although B has tried substances like marijuana and CBD to address his symptoms, neither made the problems better so he discontinued them. The mother describes the patient as "an easy gagger" during this time when he ate any new foods.

The patient developed normally and on time with all milestones. During his latency years, his parents became addicted to heroin and the patient and his two siblings stayed with his grandparents (who lived in the same home) while his parents first used substances away from the home and then went away to residential treatment for their addiction. There was no child protective services involved during this time because of his grandparents' intervention. His mother and father came from different tribes; he received his pediatric care at his father's tribe where he was enrolled but received his psychiatric care through his mother's tribe. The patient has no other medical problems aside from a body mass index (BMI) of 35. The family reflected that some of the patient's 'easy gagging' problems had become worse during the family disruption around his parents' substance use treatment.

B's strengths include his love of reading, musical aptitude for playing the guitar, and family support. In terms of the family's spirituality, B denied being religious or following strict tenets of the tribe's religious practices. However, his mother describes that when he was born his great grandmother immediately stated that he would have a gift. The patient's uncle also has a gift and is active in local religious/spiritual traditions. His family members were not taught the local spiritual tradition because his great grandmother had hoped her children would then avoid bullying and abuse should they be taken to boarding schools. Some family members had explored their tribal spirituality in recent times. When asked how the family perceives his gift, both B and his mother agree that he has it, but that he is not quite ready for it to manifest and to control it. They are willing to address it with medication management at this time given the extreme distress it is causing the patient.

Further follow-up appointments were conducted over a secure telemedicine platform because of the patient's home's distance from the clinic. Initially, the child psychiatrist and B trialed aripiprazole to address the auditory hallucinations. After B failed to respond and developed akathisia, the psychiatrist discussed the advantages and disadvantages of lurasidone, which he and his family would prefer given his BMI. When the patient's health insurance would not cover this medication when prescribed to an outside pharmacy without extensive prior authorization, the tribal health center pharmacy was able to order it for him through another funding source. After a slow titration, B's auditory hallucinations resolved completely. His mother described him as more outgoing and willing to engage in psychotherapy. Family therapy conducted with the psychiatrist and in collaboration with his therapist also revealed that the patient's suicidal ideation had increased as he had noticed some relapses in his parents' substance abuse.

B's mother was concerned about addictive properties of the medication, but she and the patient were reassured that prescriptions would be short and this intervention would only be a trial to help B leave his home to enter social situations. He was able to travel with the family to places such as the mall and tolerated a trip to a nearby resort amusement park. At this point, he was re-trialed on an SSRI, was able to tolerate adequate doses of escitalopram to address his social anxiety, and re-engaged in an alternative high school. In time he also approached his uncle to learn more about his perceived spiritual gift and what steps he might take to learn to control it.

This vignette emphasizes the importance of family decision-making and the impact of parental substance abuse on family structure and children's emotional well-being.[9] B's experience with overt racism in school is common for many students in addition to the structural racism that puts them at a disadvantage.[5,9] The family's experience with hearing voices and its cultural and spiritual significance is also nuanced and focused on an improvement in overall functioning rather than only silencing the voices[12] After the historical problems with NA children being adopted out of tribes, families will often organize around parents struggling with substance use or mental health problems so as to avoid Child Protective Services removal.[10,12] For many tribal members the removal of children to boarding schools remains fresh as it continued until the 1980s in some areas.[10] Tribal clinics and pharmacies have different rules and funding streams s than other clinical services or pharmacies; this can limit treatment choices but sometimes allow for other opportunities for treatment that could otherwise be more difficult to procure.

Native Hawaiian

The patient (D) is the child of an NH father from the islands and a White mother who came to Hawai'i looking for a summer vacation but ended up finding her future husband and family. D was raised in a traditional Hawaiian family surrounded by her aunts, uncles, and cousins. The family would come together for holidays, birthdays, and summers. In the summer, everyone would go to the family beach house located on their ancestral ahupua'a (ancient Hawaiian land division system that extended from the mountain to the sea, usually in a pie shape).

Spending summers at the family beach house in their ancestral ahupua'a was a special time for this patient. With her cousins, she would learn about the ocean, how to hunt and gather from the ocean, and most importantly, would hear the stories about her Hawaiian ancestors and the lineage she came from. This time, every year, would teach her about where she came from, strengthening the bonds between her and her extended family and the bond with the 'āina (land). Land, for NHs, is not just a physical piece of earth. Land anchors and connects people to their past and beginning. No matter where they live or travel in the world, Hawaiians will always come back to the 'āina, more specifically their ahupua'a, to remind them from whom and from where they come.

During high school, D's parents divorced. Before her parents' divorce, the patient stated that she knew, starting when she was in middle school, that there were problems in her parents' marriage. What she remembered was her father not being home as much, more fighting between her parents, and her father eventually moving out. Her uncles became like surrogate fathers for her, and her aunts and cousins became her surrogate family as her parents dealt with their divorce. Her extended Hawaiian family were a major stabilizing force for her as she was coping with the loss of her father and her family unit.

Her parents divorced when she was a sophomore in high school. Her mother decided to move with D to another state for a fresh start; however, a fresh start included severing, or in Hawaiian "oki (to cut)," all ties to her Hawaiian family and Hawai'. In therapy, the patient recalled thatwhen she moved away, it was not just cutting ties with her family in Hawai'i, but also severing that part from herself. She felt this way because, as her White stepfather later adopted her, she lost her father's name and changed her Hawaiian birth name to one that sounded American/English so that no one would know she was part Hawaiian. At the time, she wanted to assimilate completely into her new family and community.

Between her sophomore and senior year, she had no contact with her cousins, aunts, uncles and father in Hawai'i. She had nothing to do with Hawai'i, and being part Hawaiian was her past. She focused on creating a "new" person. She did not look mixed ethnicity or Hawaiian, so when she changed her name, "fitting in," especially in high school, became much easier for her.

Despite the changes she made, D described having a hard time assimilating into her new community and with her peers in high school. She did not realize it at the time, but she described that some of the problems she encountered were due to conflict between her Hawaiian values and indigenous person's perspective and the values and perspectives of people in her new community, including her new family and peers, who were predominately White American. She even thought that some of her conflicts with her mother were likely due to this conflict between her Hawaiian values and her mother's White American values.

These internal conflicts in her took a toll on her mental health. She developed symptoms of depression and anxiety. These symptoms progressed to self-cutting and restricting of her food intake. She had intermittent suicidal ideations but never attempted or planned death by suicide. Academically, her grades reflected a progressive decline, to the point where she was barely passing in some classes and failing in others. Being able to graduate on time was in jeopardy because of her poor academics. She stopped cheerleading and stopped caring about her future. Prior, her plans were to go to college and become a lawyer.

Her peer interactions changed to hanging out with older people who, on the surface, appeared to give her the attention and validation that she sought, with limited success, from same-age peers. Most of these older people were in their twenties, but some of them were men much older. It was during her time hanging out with these people that she was introduced to using drugs and to the escort service business. She denied being involved in prostitution. She described her involvement with the escort service as allowing some men to buy her things in exchange for her company. She denied ever trading sex or sexual favors with these men. She described having so much fun, and she did not view what she was doing as dangerous or illegal because everyone in her peer group was doing the same exact things as she was.

The event that changed the course of her life was her mother deciding to send her back to Hawai'i to stay with her relatives during her senior year because she was "out of control." Her mother felt she needed to do something drastic, or her daughter would end up dead. The patient was not joyous about this decision, as she had cut her Hawai'i ties, but she also was not strongly opposed to returning to Hawai'i. She said she somehow knew that this change is what she needed.

The patient came back to Hawai'i during her senior year and stayed with one of her uncles and his family. She thought that it would be a difficult adjustment for her, and she was really worried about not fitting in with her Hawaiian family, as she had aimed to completely disconnect, or *oki,* her ties with Hawai'i and her family, or 'ohana. This feared scenario was the exact opposite of what she experienced.

Her uncle's family home was located on their family's ahupu'a, so she said that when she arrived there, she felt like she was home. She never previously experienced this same sense of home. All of her other relatives also lived close to her uncle's home. Some lived on the same ahupu'a, and others lived on the neighboring ahupu'a.

When she came back, D started going back to the family beach house that she would go to as a child before her parents divorced. At the beach, with her cousins, aunts, uncles and father, she again learned about her lineage, how to forage from the sea, and about her ahupu'a. She realized that returning to Hawai'i, living on her family's ahupu'a, and living with her 'ohana again is what she needed to heal herself.

Moving to Hawai'i physically separated her from a negative peer group and dangerous lifestyle, but the bigger impact was that it healed her by reconnecting her with the Hawaiian part of her. Both D and her mother tried hard to erase her Hawaiian part, which was the part that came from her father who had hurt both of them. From D's perspective, he was the reason their family ended.

In treatment, she started on a low dose of an antidepressant to target depression and anxiety but the key to her treatment was therapy. In therapy, she identified that severing her ties with her Hawaiian side to try to assimilate into her new community was likely the cause of her depression, anxiety, and subsequent dangerous choices in doing drugs and affiliating with negative peer groups to cope. In therapy, she learned how to incorporate her mixed heritage into her identity instead of believing that she had to only identify with one and deny the other part of her heritage.

This vignette illustrates that clinicians working with youth in any setting need to develop a thorough understanding of the family context and the cultures that influenced the youth's development. The clinician's formulation and therapeutic approach needs to consider any disruptions in the youth's development of a healthy self-image and any potential cultural conflicts, tensions, or marginalization resulting from differences in values and perspectives between the patient, family, peers, and others in the community. This vignette also illustrates the need to maintain a broad and inclusive approach to assessing the relationships that influence a person's well-being. These relationships include relationships with the land and physical environment and with living and deceased relatives and others in the spiritual realm. Indeed, clinicians working with indigenous youth may appropriately need to become advocates for a physical and spiritual environment (otherwise vulnerable to destruction through climate change, pollution, and other harms) that allows the development of healthy cultural identification.

Teaching Points

When working with Native peoples, connection, is very important. Why should they trust you? Introduce yourself including your experience and any work with Native peoples you have previously done. Direct eye contact varies among Native peoples; the usual rule is that patients will make less eye contact with physicians as a sign of respect for you and your position. Long periods of silence are normal as most native children are taught to consider answers carefully before replying. Native children are usually more comfortable functioning within a group setting than giving individual input. Elders are consulted with almost all decisions. Family meetings may include quite large numbers as family may include "aunties," "uncles," or "grandparents" who are not directly related. Connection takes time and patience is a definite virtue. Building trust includes openness to traditional practices and belief systems, understanding the local situation (resources, issues), and being patient.

Health care professionals should be well aware of their own cultural and learned expectations regarding Native peoples. Within this group are extensive variations in belief systems and traditions, which are not homogenous or static. Remember the common denominators of trauma and loss, discrimination and oppression experienced by this ethnic community. A good starting place is to familiarize oneself with the tribal beliefs and social interaction (hand gestures and body language) when possible before meeting the patient. Cultural humility is key.

Recommended Screeners

Trauma
Substance abuse
Emotional dysregulation

CLINICS CARE POINTS

- Always be open to conversations about alternative and natural therapies as well as ceremonies.
- Minimal eye contact, long silences, and dropped heads are signs of respect.
- Psychological testing norms are not available for indigenous people so psychological testing must be carefully evaluated.
- Trauma-based evaluations must take into consideration multigenerational trauma including the loss of cultural parenting knowledge through boarding school experiences.

REFERENCES

1. Swinomish Tribal Mental Health Project, Communication Patterns. A gathering of Wisdoms: tribal mental health: a cultural perspective. Mount Vernon (WA): Veda Vangarde; 1991. p. 185–94.
2. Duran E. The healing/therapeutic circle. In: Healing the soul wound. New York: Teachers College Press; 2019. p. 41–9.

3. Koithan M, Farrell C. Indigenous native American healing traditions. J Nurse Pract 2010;6(6):477–8.
4. Walls M, Whitbeck L. The intergenerational effects of relocation poliices on Indigenous families. J Fam Issues 2012;33(9):1272–93.
5. Findling MG, Casey LS, Fryberg SA, et al. Discrimination in the United States: experiences of native Americans. Health Serv Res 2019;54(Suppl 2):1431–41.
6. The Center for Native American Youth, 2300 N Street NW, Suite 700, Washington, DC 20037-1122 Phone: (202) 736-2905, Email: cnayinfo@aspeninstitute.org. Available at: https://www.cnay.org/suicide-prevention/. Accessed March 21, 2022.
7. Venner KL, Donovan DM, Campbell ANC, et al. Future directions for medication assisted treatment for opioid use disorder with American Indian/Alaska Natives. Addict Behav 2018;86:111–7.
8. Gilmore-Bykovskyi A, Jackson JD, Wilkins CH. The Urgency of justice in research: beyond COVID-19. Trends Mol Med 2021;27(2):97–100.
9. Daily, RS, Membership Services Forum 1: Cultural Mentorship Forum 2021: Focus on Disparities, AACAP Annual Meeting 2021. Virtual Meeting (in lieu of COVID), October 25, 2021
10. Weaver H. The Well-being of children and families. In: Trauma and resilience in the lives of contemporary native Americans. New York: Routledge; 2019. p. 71–92.
11. Shore J, Kaufmann LJ, Brooke E, et al. Review of American Indian veteran telemental health. Telemed J E Health 2021;18(2):87–94, 22283396.
12. Swinomish Tribal Mental Health Project. Interacting problems Affecingin mental health of Indian communities. In: A gathering of wisdoms: tribal mental health: a cultural perspective. Mount Vernon (WA): Veda Vangarde; 1991. p. 44–64.

Cultural Considerations for Working with South Asian Youth

Deepika Shaligram, MD[a], Manal Khan, MD[b], Afifa Adiba, MD[c,d],
Seeba Anam, MD[e,*]

KEYWORDS

- South Asian • Mental health • Youth • Children • Racial and ethnic disparities
- Acculturation • Immigrant

KEY POINTS

- South Asian communities are diverse, with a large variance in sociodemographic status, immigration/migration history, premigration stressors, exposure to structural violence, and social determinants of health that impacts the development of mental health concerns in South Asian American (SAA) youth.
- Microaggressions in combination with family, acculturation stressors, and overt discrimination converge during crucial developmental periods and contribute to psychological distress experienced by SAA children; these factors influence the detection and diagnosis of mental health conditions and help-seeking.
- Primary care providers may be the initial point of contact for treatment due to somatic clinical presentation, referral bias, limited perceived need, structural barriers, and mental health-related stigma.
- A nuanced approach to mental health treatment that begins with building a therapeutic alliance, psychoeducation, and harnessing family strengths would help clinicians regardless of background effectively engage SAA youth and families in treatment.
- Culturally responsive approaches for working with SAA youth include eliciting explanatory models and treatment goals, family, and psychotherapeutic interventions that use indigenous terminology and incorporate spirituality and community interventions to raise awareness and address stigma.

[a] Department of Psychiatry and Behavioral Sciences, Boston Children's Hospital/Harvard Medical School, 300 Longwood Avenue, Boston, MA, 02115, USA; [b] Jane and Terry Semel Institute for Neuroscience and Human Behavior, University of California Los Angeles, 760 Westwood Plaza, Suite 37-384, Los Angeles, CA 90024, USA; [c] Sheppard Pratt Health System, 6501 North Charles Street, Baltimore, MD 21204, USA; [d] Yale Child Study Center, Yale School of Medicine, 230 S Frontage Rd, New Haven, CT 06519, USA; [e] Department of Psychiatry and Behavioral Neuroscience, University of Chicago, 5841 South Maryland Avenue, MC 3077, Chicago, IL 60637, USA
* Corresponding author.
E-mail address: sanam@uchicago.edu

Child Adolesc Psychiatric Clin N Am 31 (2022) 789–803
https://doi.org/10.1016/j.chc.2022.06.006
1056-4993/22/© 2022 Elsevier Inc. All rights reserved.

INTRODUCTION

South Asians (SAs) are among the fastest-growing communities in the United States. SA hail from a subset of countries and a global diaspora, associated with distinct languages, religions, cultural traditions, and patterns of migration influenced by colonization. Colonialism involved systematic oppression and exploitation of colonized people and instigation of communal violence as a part of "divide and rule," which cast a long shadow on SA history. British colonial rule terminated with the partition of British India into India and Pakistan in 1947, with Bangladesh following in 1971. This intense period of restructuring of the subcontinent was marked by atrocities committed under colonization, partition, and subsequent wars and armed conflicts.

Although SAs first immigrated to the United States in the 1700s, the South Asian American (SAA) community has grown exponentially in temporal proximity to US immigration policy changes and tremendous shifts occurring in South Asia. SAAs in the United States consist of 80% Indians, 11% Pakistanis, ~ 4% Bangladeshis, and 5% Nepalis, Sri Lankans, Bhutanese, and Maldivians. There are 650 languages spoken and many religions (Buddhism, Christianity, Hinduism, Islam, Jainism, Judaism, Sikhism, and Zoroastrianism) are practiced in South Asia. More than three-quarters of SA residing in the United States are foreign-born, with two-thirds identifying as immigrants.[1,2]

Though the SAA community is heterogeneous, it is frequently lumped together with other Asian American (AA) groups in an aggregate monolith. Grouping AAs into an umbrella category masks distinct patterns and characteristics of AA subgroups in research. Historically, the limited evidence base regarding AA mental health indicated lower prevalence of mental health-related concerns and lower mental health care utilization compared with their non-Asian counterparts. However, recent studies reflect a more complex picture of health inequity among AA subgroups. One study indicated overall rates of psychological distress in AA are notably higher than both rates reported in national samples of the US general population, and those reported in the existing national samples of AAs.[3] SAs are underrepresented in the AA components of national epidemiologic studies that report the low prevalence of mental health conditions and health care utilization in AAs.

Given the paucity of literature on AA mental health, the current evidence base allows for limited characterization of the mental health needs and clinical presentation of SAA youth. However, inferences may be drawn from the growing body of research disaggregating data related to mental health in SAA adults and AA youth.

General Risk and Protective Factors for Mental Health Conditions

Factors affecting mental health in SAA youth include:

1. Acculturation
2. Role of family
3. Role of gender and intersectionality
4. Structural violence and discrimination
5. Social determinants of health

Acculturation

Given that most SAAs are immigrants and most US-born Asians are emerging adults or younger,[1] acculturation-related stressors significantly impact these families. SAA youth face normative challenges of identity development while navigating racial/ethnic socialization and brokering intergenerational cultural conflicts.

SAA youth reported stress related to concealing dating, acculturation, peer acceptance or lack thereof, conflict between autonomy and seeking parental approval and support, and pressures of unmet parental expectations.[4] SAA youth face acculturation stressors parallel to their UK counterparts, including pressure to maintain traditional cultural identity, emphasis on academic and economic success, stigma attached to failure, and demand for deference to elders. These unattainable expectations exacerbate distress for SAA youth.[5] Like other AA youth, as a visible racial-ethnic minority, SAA must balance mainstream and heritage cultures in a racialized society.[6] Immigrant adolescents exposed to acculturative stress showed more withdrawn behavior, somatic, and anxious/depressed symptoms.[7] Acculturation-related stressors affect SAA identity formation and mental health at developmentally sensitive periods.

Role of family

Though SA families diverge in migration histories, historical trauma exposure, and acculturation, they often ascribe to patriarchal family models and authoritarian parenting practices. In seeking to preserve cultural values, first-generation SA parents may prioritize family over individual pursuits. SA immigrant parents may impose "frozen in time" cultural and parenting practices that may be more restrictive than evolving norms in their country of origin. Failure to meet these culturally-prescribed standards and gendered role expectations and internalized parental values may be construed as disobedience or disrespect. Autonomy in sexuality, career choice, and religious practice may generate psychological distress and family conflict.[8] Extended family, including nonbiological "aunties" and "uncles," may be perceived as sources of support and stress, since they may monitor and police youth through adulthood.[9]

Bicultural children act as "go-betweens" or "culture brokers" for parents with limited English proficiency (LEP) or lack of familiarity with American mainstream culture. In particular, 1.5 and second-generation children serve as advocates and cultural interpreters to further their parents' understanding of mainstream American cultural and social norms. This may result in parentification of the child due to role reversal, upending family dynamics, and causing intergenerational conflict. The duality of hyphenated existence for children of immigrants can be isolating. The eldest child may bear the brunt, to protect younger siblings from similar struggles. Mental conditions interfering with academic success may be misattributed to laziness and cause shame, rather than prompt care seeking. Thus, the individualistic versus collectivistic approach may exacerbate acculturative stress, including intergenerational conflict due to differential acculturation between SAA immigrant parents and children.[10,11]

Role of gender and intersectionality

Despite Hindu mythological characters like "Ardhanari" (half-woman) and homo-eroticism in Mughal art, sexuality is predominantly heteronormative and linked to procreation in SA cultures. Though diverse, SA cultures are typically patriarchal, promoting rigid gender roles and social norms. Filial piety, hierarchical deference, centrality of heteronormative marriage, and intimacy exclusively within marriage, are codified through parenting practices and socialization of gender role conformity.[12] These cultural influences inform SAA youths' attitudes toward gender identity, sexuality, and dating. SAA youth may conceal romantic relationships from parents due to stigma, intergenerational differences in values, and an emphasis on academics. Without parental guidance, SAA youth are at risk of dating violence, especially for girls socialized to be deferential and subservient. With respect to parental intimate partner violence (IPV), lack of social support secondary to immigration, cultural factors such as victim-blaming attitudes, the role of women in preserving family dignity, and the stigma of divorce often results in silence,[13] thus unwittingly modeling and reinforcing gender-based power differentials for SAA youth.

Exposure to childhood abuse and/or parental IPV may shape gender norms and perpetuate cycles of intergenerational trauma. Further, corporal punishment, prevalent in SA, may contribute to trauma in SAA children. For SAA children exposed to IPV, extended family factors, bicultural identity, gender, and fear of loss of face impact how trauma is processed.[14]

Of note, lesbian, gay, bisexual, transgender, and questioning (LGBTQ+) youth as well as gender diverse communities within the SAA community are rising. However, LGBTQ + SAA have been largely invisible in the United States, partly due to disclosure stigma associated with cultural and religious values of heteronormativity and its association with familial expectations, honor, and pride. In 2016, only 127,400 AA students identified as LGBT or queer.[15] The experiences of SAA sexual or gender minority youth are understudied.

Intra- and intercommunity social factors contribute to an intersectional experience of marginalization for SAA LGBTQ + youth. These factors have additive and interactive effects on minority stress, driven by discrimination, racism, internalized heterosexism, acculturation, and enculturation.[16] Queer youth of color, including SAA, may be more pathologized than their White counterparts. SAA LGBTQ + youth face additional barriers in reporting sexual violence or receiving services (eg, discrimination in hospital settings due to their intersectional identities[17]). Some SA countries of origin stigmatize, discriminate, and criminalize LGBTQ + individuals, which limits feelings of acceptance and belonging in SAA community spaces.[12,18] In the context of sexual violence, LGBTQ + SAAs may experience a disproportionate health impact due to multiple traumas. This confluence of stressors can significantly elevate risks for depression, anxiety, PTSD, and suicide in these youth.

Structural violence and discrimination

Restrictive policies directed at SA have a long history, starting with the Immigration Act of 1917 restricting Asian immigration and the 1924 Asian Exclusion Act precluding Asian residents from obtaining US citizenship. The US Supreme Court barred SA from naturalization in the *United States v. Bhagat Singh Thind* (1923), because SA were not "White." These policies imposed structural restrictions on economic and social mobility and contributed to the "perpetual foreigner" stereotype for SA. After the Hart-Celler Act of 1965 spurred an influx of SA highly skilled professionals, along with the Immigration Act of 1990 and the 2001 H1-B visa facilitated the immigration of information technology professionals, there was a shift in the racial characterization of SAA as "model minorities."

The "perpetual foreigner myth" implies that SAA do not belong to the broader American fabric. To combat this stereotype and avoid differential treatment by non-SAA peers, SAA youth may code switch—modify speech or language, appearance, behavior, and cultural expression to optimize the comfort of others and better fit in. This concealment results in stress related to devaluing one's authentic self, hypervigilance for discrimination, and distancing in-group members. Immigrant parents may be unaware of these stressors, having been raised in a country where their belongingness was assumed.

"Perpetual foreigner" stereotypes contribute to microaggressions, racialized bullying at school, and discrimination in the larger community. Racism instigated violence in the 1987 murder of Navroze Mody by Dotbusters and the 2012 mass shooting of Sikh Americans. Post-9/11, there was a surge in bias-based bullying and structural racism targeting SAA communities based on assumed religious and ethnic backgrounds. Hate violence targeting SA, Muslim, Sikh, Hindu, Middle Eastern, and Arab American communities increased by 45% in the year after the 2016 election compared with the year before.[19] Perceived Muslim American youth (SAA and non-SAA), in particular, have been targets of xenophobia. Sikh youth wearing turbans reported harassment, mistaken to be Muslim.[20] SAA Muslim females, particularly those whose attire reflects their faith, may be subject to discrimination at the intersection of gender and religion.[21] Perceived discrimination has been linked to overall negative mental health in SAA of Indian origin,[22] and has been linked to depression in SAA.[23] Discrimination related to intersectionality of SAA identity, affiliation with perceived racial/ethnic or religious group, gender, and sexual minorities may compound risks for negative mental health outcomes.

Social determinants of health

SAAs navigate structural barriers and social determinants of health common to other racial minority immigrant communities, but are often overlooked due to the "model minority" myth. The "model minority" stereotype pits SAA against other racial minorities. It also confers pressure to meet unrealistic ideals, while dismissing health disparities, mental health concerns, and structural vulnerabilities. Income inequality, education level, and poverty rates vary widely among AAs, with several SAA communities falling below US national averages.[1] Some SAA immigrants contend with challenges related to unauthorized immigration. These factors counter the narrative of the "model minority" SAA community.

Social determinants of health contributing to underutilization of mental health services by SAAs include poverty, limited access to mental health treatment, lack of culturally informed care, LEP, and discrimination. These determinants increase mental health risk while limiting access to mental health treatment. In addition, health care provider assumptions and limited cultural understanding contribute to referral bias and underutilization of treatment.[24] Structural factors including limited availability of Asian languages in national surveys or accessibility to health care may contribute to the underdetection of mental health needs in Asian communities in research.[3] In addition, health beliefs, stigma, and low perceived need for mental health services in SAA communities contribute to low rates of treatment.

Diagnostic Considerations in Assessment

Depression

Depression in SA communities may present with somatic symptoms, such as fatigue, sleep, or appetite disturbances, which contribute to underdiagnosis and undertreatment in SAA adults.[25] Though most studies examined depression in SAA adults, some identified risk factors including financial stressors, social isolation, prescriptive gender roles, facility with the English language, and younger age at migration may both directly and indirectly pose similar risks to youth.[11,20,26,27,28] Children of Asian immigrant parents had higher levels of internalizing problems and lower levels of interpersonal relationship skills relative to white children.[29] A comparative study of medical students found SAA students, especially females, were more likely to report depression than East AA students and male students.[30] Differential rates of depressive risk were shown in a study of AA communities, with SAs presenting with depressive risk between SEA and EA communities. Indo-Caribbeans showed 2 to 10 times the risk of depression of other SAA subgroups, followed by Bangladeshis, with Asian Indians showing a lower risk of depression than any other SAA or AA communities. The study also found that discrimination had a greater contribution to depressive risk for SAAs than for EA.[20]

Suicidality

SAA youth experienced elevated risks for suicidality related to acculturative stress, discrimination, academic pressure, and family conflict.[31] SA immigrant women had significantly elevated rates of non-suicidal self-injury and suicide, compared with other American women. Risk factors for attempted and completed suicide in young SAA women include conflict with parents and romantic partners, exposure to IPV, and low self-esteem.[32] Among SA immigrants, rates of suicide in Asian Indians aged 15 years or older were higher in the diaspora than in India, especially for girls.[33] Although there is no data specific to school students of SA origin, a study of adolescents in Grades 7-12, showed that African Americans reported relatively high rates of suicidal thoughts and attempts and Southeast Asians reported high rates of suicidal thoughts (34). Young SAA females may be subject to greater risks given rising trends in suicide among preadolescent females in the United States. Middle and high school students of SA and SEA origin experienced higher rates of suicide attempts and suicide than their non-SAA or SEA peers.[34]

Among SAA transitional age youth, hopelessness in Bangladeshi- and Pakistani-American youth was associated with lower levels of suicidal ideation compared with Indian-American peers, possibly due to the protective effects of religious coping in Muslim youth.[35] A model for suicide risk in SA identified family expectations, economic hardships, lack of health insurance, gender, ethnicity, cultural beliefs, cognitive impairment, and mental health conditions as risk factors and cultural and religious sanctions against suicide as protective factors.[36]

Trauma

Many SA families have experienced premigration trauma arising from their colonial past and customs such as the caste system and child marriage. Further, immigration is intrinsically traumatic due to having to start over from scratch, culture shock, identity loss, LEP, loss of social support, and racism. Bhutanese refugees have dealt with oppression, torture, poor living conditions, and general trauma exposure.[36] Thus, historical and pre-immigration trauma compounded with trauma at community, family and individual levels in the United States impact the health of SAA and possibly that of subsequent generations due to downstream effects.

Refugee children from Sri Lanka may experience significant pre-immigration trauma (related to poverty, social, and civil war) and post-migration trauma resulting in high levels of psychological distress. Collective coping through shared goals and female gender may be protective factors in these youth.[37] Treatment considerations in this subgroup include the importance of family involvement, school settings as points of care and services, and timing of care with a focus on the first year of immigration.[38]

Parent trauma was associated with overprotective parenting, family conflict, communication barriers, and role-reversing parenting suggesting intergenerational transmission of trauma in a study of AA that included SAAs.[39] Research in other groups,[40] suggests that greater parental trauma exposure results in higher risk of trauma in children due to (1) maltreatment by parents, (2) difficulties of traumatized parents in relating to and communicating with their children, (3) vulnerability in children's stress responses, and (4) children's susceptibility to stress-related neurobiological abnormalities and genetic modifications[41] (Fig. 1).

Somatization

SA adults with mental health issues commonly interpret their symptoms as physical illnesses (eg, depressive symptoms manifest as pain), "sinking heart" or "heartache," thus contributing to under detection of mental illnesses.[42,43] Somatization among SAs

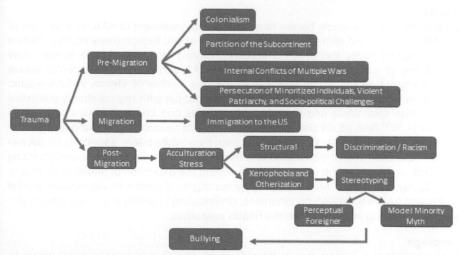

Fig. 1. Migration-related traumatic stressors in South Asian American communities.

may be understood as a function of collectivism.[44] Studies from the SA diaspora indicate that SAA with mental illness are more likely to present with physical symptoms than non-SAA peers. They often underreport depressive symptoms and are less likely to be referred by physicians for mental health services.[45] Shifting family structures, unjust distribution of resources within the family, patriarchy, with an emphasis on family harmony and obedience to elders that disadvantage women and younger family members, may cause unexpressed stress and conflict resulting in a higher prevalence of somatization. Further, collectivism emphasizes the family as the institution of support thus fueling the need to keep "personal problems" private, and viewing mental health services as a last resort when the family has failed to solve the problem.[11]

Psychosis
Explanatory models of psychosis in SAs, included supernatural phenomena like "black magic," "jinns," and "evil eye," psycho-social causes[46] and attribution to moral failure. Hence faith healers were often the first point of contact and many engaged with both faith-based practices (talismans, praying, drinking holy water) and health care providers for treatment. Therefore, psychiatrists need to consider the cultural underpinnings of health beliefs and explanatory models of illness when treating SAA youth with psychosis.

Considerations for Engagement in Treatment

Therapeutic alliance building
Lack of familiarity with SAA culture may result in misinterpretation or miscommunication resulting in misdiagnoses, conflict, fear of judgment, and/or premature treatment termination.[47] When clinicians of all ethnicities practice antiracism by self-assessment for implicit bias, proactive inquiry about discriminatory experiences and expression of allyship, they build trust, invite disclosure, and validate experiences that ultimately facilitate communication and treatment engagement.[48] It is important to elicit and listen to experiences with humility and curiosity, intentionally explore the understanding of illness, treatment goals, sources of resilience and vulnerability, and attitudes toward treatment while being aware of the explicit and/or implicit hierarchy in the physician–patient dynamic. This awareness is especially important in treating SAA, as questioning authority and advocating for self are not normative.

Stigma

Stigma poses a formidable barrier to mental health treatment of SAA. Few studies of mental health-related stigma included subgroups of SA, though many findings have a strong resonance for the SAA community. "Saving face" was found to be a key contributor to mental health-related stigma in AA communities, as mental illness had an impact on the whole family.[49] In the few studies of stigma in SAA adults, SAA showed greater stigma toward families of people with mental illness (affiliative stigma) than their White and East AA counterparts and construed mental illness as weakness.[50,51] SAA adults also showed more stigma toward help-seeking and greater attribution of responsibility for depression than their White peers, especially for SA patients.[52] Concealment of mental illness within families was expected to maintain social standing, avoid burdening family, and preventing the extension of affiliative stigma to other family members.[49] Mental health-related stigma shapes attitudes toward mental illness and treatment in SAA communities, contributing to delays or prevention of help-seeking, resulting in negative mental health outcomes.

Language

Language plays a central role in consideration of culturally tailored approaches to mental health in SAAs. LEP serves as a barrier to health care in many immigrant SAA populations.[1] Conversely, many SA immigrants have high rates of English fluency secondary to British colonization, which may explain the more frequent use of mental health services in Asian Indians in comparison to EA communities.[3] Concerns about confidentiality pose a barrier to mental health treatment in settings where language interpretation is required. If children or other family members serve as interpreters, sensitive mental health history may remain undisclosed. In addition, if interpreters are known community members, concern for privacy and "saving face" may be prioritized over treatment engagement. Further, psychiatric labels may increase mental health stigma and obstruct care seeking. The use of indigenous language like "excessive thinking," reflecting language used by patients, may bolster therapeutic alliance and enhance engagement with SAA youth and parents who are the gatekeepers to treatment.[49]

Psychoeducation

A culturally responsive psychoeducational approach that is exploratory, collaborative, and integrative is a valuable didactic tool and psychotherapeutic intervention. Validation and normalization of experiences can reduce feelings of guilt, shame, self-blame, alienation, and mischaracterization. It can be liberating for patients and their families to understand that their illness is not a character flaw or a fault of their making.

Psychoeducation also offers an opportunity to hold hope, facilitate joining, and a deeper understanding. Emphasizing the mind–body continuum through psychoeducation may enhance help-seeking especially as psychiatric symptoms can be experienced somatically by SAAs. Finally, a holistic approach that inquiries about the concomitant use of indigenous systems of medicine, and discusses the value of nutritional considerations, spiritual practices, and social connectedness in addition to psychotherapy and medication management may be helpful in engaging SAA families[43] (**Fig. 2**).

Family considerations

The family is an important source of support for all children, particularly in collectivistic cultures. Hence family relationships and parent–child communication can be the focus of potential interventions.

Building robust therapeutic alliances and harnessing family strengths helps all clinicians effectively engage SAA youth in treatment. Racially concordant clinicians may be preferred, though confidentiality concerns may emerge. Privacy and confidentiality

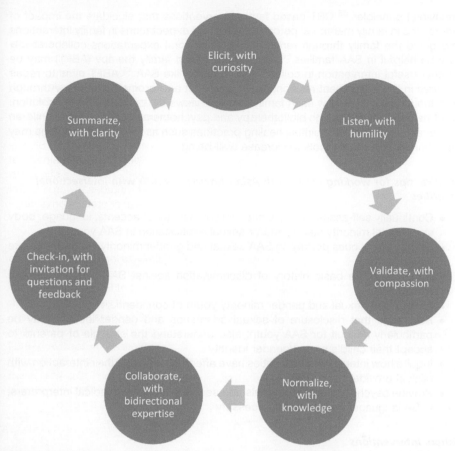

Fig. 2. Psychoeducation.

for the youth and family should be assured at the outset. Youth mental health struggles may be perceived as parental failure, especially for immigrant parents who may have made considerable sacrifices for their children. Recognizing that critical parental attitudes or perceived dismissiveness may mask a sense feeling of parental failure can generate empathy toward parents. Reframing a youth's problems as arising from intergenerational differences in acculturation and differential cultural experiences of parents and youth, may normalize family conflicts and increase parental empathy.[53] When acculturative stress creates an impasse between the different generations, focusing on common goals, building family strengths, and enlisting family support in treatment planning, could be beneficial.[43] Positive aspects of SAA bicultural identities include cross-cultural competency,[9] lower anxiety levels, adaptive emotion regulation strategies, fewer academic problems, and fewer conflicts with parents.[54] To support health, clinicians should encourage families to fortify bicultural identity.

Interventions

Psychotherapy
Psychotherapy may be more culturally acceptable and less stigmatizing than medication in some SAAs, as the Hindu scripture, Bhagavad Gita, is rooted in cognitive–

behavioral principles.[55] CBT-based family interventions that elucidate the impact of differences in family members' perceived roles and expectations in family interactions and guide the family through renegotiating behavioral expectations collaboratively may be helpful in SAA families.[56] Attachment-based family therapy (ABFT) may be another useful intervention in collectivistic cultures like SAA.[43] ABFT aims to repair ruptures in the attachment relationship, renew trust and promote autonomy through an attributional shift in how each family member views the problem and the solution. Treatment of trauma through bibliotherapy and psychotherapy can empower children with adaptive strategies. Spiritual healing practices such as meditation and yoga may be culturally acceptable tools to increase well-being.

Practical tips for working with South Asian American youth with intersectional identities

- Continually self-assess for bias and stereotypes about accents, language, body size, model minority status, and/or sexual exoticization in SAA youth[57]
- Display visual cues portraying SAA sexual and gender minority youth to indicate safe spaces
- Understand the basic history of discrimination against SAA and SGM in the United States
- Assure SAA sexual and gender minority youth of confidentiality
- Recognize that disclosure of sexual orientation and gender identity may be particularly difficult for SAA youth; also understand the struggle of parents to accept their child's sexual/gender identity
- Inquire how intersectional identities have affected youth and their interaction with clinical providers and staff
- Provide psychoeducation materials and services, including medical interpreters, in SA languages for parents if necessary

School interventions
Discrimination in schools often takes the form of bullying based on race, gender, sexual orientation, and/or religion. Educators, peers, parents, and communities contribute to the creation of safe school environments that prevent and address bias-based bullying. A model curriculum to address bullying in SAA youth consists of (1) learning about the history of SA migration to the United States; (2) the historical roots of xenophobia and manifestations of exclusion, examples of bullying in and outside of schools; (3) education about the harm caused by racism along with tools for countering xenophobia; (4) building respect, celebrating and engaging with differences and pluralism; (5) building empathy and teaching strategies to be effective allies; and (6) upstander skills.[58] Ethnic student organizations may enable sharing and working through racialized experiences, reconciling the views of outgroups with SAA youth's self-identity in a supportive environment. Of note, SAA transitional age youth may be more willing to recognize and accept treatment of mental illness when parents are no longer gatekeepers.[59] Implementing the principles of culturally relevant pedagogy and introducing ethnic studies curricula would heighten awareness and acceptance within educational institutions.

Community interventions that harness the protective factors of the close-knit social fabric of SA community can be a vehicle for psychoeducation, building awareness about mental health, treatment and addressing stigma.[60] Community-based participatory research may also provide data on the prevalence of mental health issues in SAA youth and inform culturally-responsive interventions.

In summary, SAA youth are a diverse, rapidly growing community, marginalized as "perpetual foreigner-model minorities," which masks their unique and unaddressed mental health needs. Historical trauma linked to colonialism, immigration and acculturation stressors, intergenerational conflict, structural racism, and discrimination related to intersectional identities confer SAA-specific risk factors for stress, anxiety, depression, suicidality, and trauma-related disorders at developmentally sensitive periods. Partnering with SAA communities and families to reduce stigma and engage in mental health treatment would cultivate inherent resiliency, bolster protective factors, promote well-being, and advance health equity for this new generation of American youth.

CLINICS CARE POINTS

General risk and protective factors for mental health conditions
- South Asian communities are diverse, with a large variance in sociodemographic status, immigration/migration history, premigration stressors, exposure to structural violence, and social determinants of health that impacts the development of mental health concerns in South Asian American (SAA) youth
- SAAs are subject to acculturative stressors, including intergenerational conflicts, role reversal and parentification of children, racism/discrimination
- "Model Minority" stereotypes compound stressors of parental expectations, extended family/community social norms, and influence relationships with non-SAA peers to see them as outliers
- "Perpetual Foreigner" stereotypes perpetuated by structural racism contribute to discrimination and related stress and anxiety, increasingly related to perceived religious affiliation
- Intersectional identities including gender and sexual identity and expression coupled with a racial, ethnic, and religious identity increase risk for bullying or discrimination, depression, anxiety, or trauma-related symptoms
- Microaggressions in combination with family, acculturation stressors, and overt discrimination converge during crucial developmental periods and contribute to psychological distress experienced by SAA children; these factors influence the detection and diagnosis of mental health conditions and help-seeking

Diagnostic considerations in assessment
- SAA with depression and anxiety may present with somatic symptoms, which contribute to underdiagnosis and undertreatment
- Primary Care Providers may be the initial point of contact for treatment because of somatic clinical presentation, referral bias, limited perceived need, structural barriers, and mental health-related stigma
- SAA youth identifying as female may present with elevated risks for suicidality
- Historical trauma related to colonialism and immigration-related stressors intersect with post-migration structural violence to confer elevated risks for intergenerational trauma and related sequelae

Considerations for engagement in treatment
- A nuanced approach to mental health treatment that begins with building a therapeutic alliance, psychoeducation, and harnessing family strengths would help clinicians regardless of background effectively engage SAA youth and families in treatment
- Effective patient–physician interaction entails eliciting and listening to experiences with humility and curiosity, intentionality on the part of the physician to explore patients' explanatory models and treatment goals while being aware of the explicit and/or implicit hierarchy in the physician–patient dynamic
- Psychoeducation is a powerful intervention that improves treatment engagement and addresses stigma, particularly when indigenous terminology is reflected back to families rather than stigmatizing language

- Mental health-related stigma, particularly affiliative stigma, contributes to the concealment of mental illness, prompting delays or prevention of help-seeking, resulting in negative mental health outcomes
- Culturally responsive approaches for working with SAA youth include assuring confidentiality, involving families, addressing stigma, eliciting explanatory models, using indigenous terminology, and incorporating spirituality

DISCLOSURE

The authors have nothing to disclose.

REFERENCES

1. Budiman A, Ruiz NG. Key facts about Asian Americans, a diverse and growing population. Pew Research Center; 2021. Available at: https://www.pewresearch.org/fact-tank/2021/04/29/key-facts-about-asian-americans/.
2. South Asian Americans Leading together. (2017). Demographic information. Available at: http://saalt.org/south-asians-in-the-us/demographic-information/. Accessed April 15, 2022.
3. Jang Y, Yoon H, Park NS, et al. Mental health service use and perceived unmet needs for mental health care in Asian Americans. Community Ment Health J 2019;55(2):241–8.
4. Rastogi P, Khushalani S, Dhawan S, et al. Understanding clinician perception of common presentations in South Asians seeking mental health treatment and determining barriers and facilitators to treatment. Asian J Psychiatr 2014;7(1):15–21.
5. Husain M, Waheed W, Husain N. Self-harm in British South Asian women: psychosocial correlates and strategies for prevention. Ann Gen Psychiatry 2006;5:7.
6. Choi Y, Tan KP, Yasui M, et al. Advancing understanding of acculturation for adolescents of asian immigrants: Person-Oriented Analysis of acculturation Strategy among Korean American youth. J Youth Adolesc 2016;45(7):1380–95.
7. Sirin SR, Ryce P, Gupta T, et al. The role of acculturative stress on mental health symptoms for immigrant adolescents: a longitudinal investigation. Dev Psychol 2013;49(4):736–48.
8. Chandra RM, Arora L, Mehta UM, et al. Asian Indians in America: the influence of values and culture on mental health. Asian J Psychiatr 2016;22:202–9.
9. Jensen KB. It's hard to balance it": cultural identity Production among youth of the South asian diaspora in metropolitan New York and Oslo. Middle States Geographer 2011;44:82–94.
10. Inman AG, Howard EE, Beaumont RL, et al. Cultural transmission: influence of contextual factors in asian indian immigrant parents' experiences. J Couns Psychol 2007;54(1):93–100.
11. Karasz A, Gany F, Escobar J, et al. Mental health and stress among South Asians. J Immigr Minor Health 2019;21(Suppl 1):7–14.
12. Chowdhury T, Okazaki S. Intersectional complexities of South Asian Muslim Americans: implications for identity and mental health. InMental and behavioral health of immigrants in the United States, vol. 1. Academic Press; 2020. p. 179–200.
13. Rai A, Choi YJ. Domestic violence Victimization among South Asian immigrant men and women in the United States. J Interpersonal Violence 2021. https://doi.org/10.1177/08862605211015262.

14. Ragavan MI, Fikre T, Millner U, et al. The impact of domestic violence exposure on South Asian children in the United States: Perspectives of domestic violence agency staff. Child Abuse Negl 2018;76:250–60.

15. Pizmony-Levy O, Kosciw JG. School climate and the experience of LGBT students: a comparison of the United States and Israel. J LGBT Youth 2016; 13(1–2):46–66.

16. Meyer IH. Prejudice, social stress, and mental health in lesbian, gay, and bisexual populations: conceptual issues and research evidence. Psychol Bull 2003; 129(5):674–97.

17. Ali SH, Mohaimin S, Dhar R, et al. Sexual violence among LGB+ South Asian Americans: findings from a community survey. Plos one 2022;17(2):e0264061.

18. Bi S, Gunter KE, López FY, et al. Improving shared decision making for asian American Pacific Islander sexual and gender minorities. Med Care 2019; 57(12):937–44.

19. South Asian Americans Leading together. (2019) A demographic snapshot of South Asians in the United States. Available at: http://saalt.org/wp-content/uploads/2019/04/SAALT-Demographic-Snapshot-2019.pdf. Accessed April 15, 2022.

20. Misra S, Wyatt LC, Wong JA, et al. Determinants of depression risk among three asian American subgroups in New York city. Ethn Dis 2020;30(4):553–62.

21. Perry B. Gendered Islamophobia: hate crime against Muslim women. Social Identities 2014;20(1):74–89.

22. Nadimpalli SB, Kanaya AM, McDade TW, et al. Self-reported discrimination and mental health among Asian Indians: cultural beliefs and coping style as moderators. Asian Am J Psychol 2016;7(3):185–94.

23. Tummala-Narra P, Alegria M, Chen CN. Perceived discrimination, acculturative stress, and depression among South Asians: mixed findings. Asian Am J Psychol 2012;3(1):3.

24. Rehman TE. Social stigma, cultural constraints, or poor policies: Examining the Pakistani Muslim female population in the United States and unequal access to professional mental health services. Research in Education. 2007;31:95–130.

25. Kim HJ, Park E, Storr CL, et al. Depression among asian-American adults in the community: systematic review and meta-Analysis. PLoS One 2015;10(6): e0127760.

26. Lai, D., & Surood, S. (2008). Socio-cultural variations in depressive symptoms of ageing South Asian Canadians.

27. Takeuchi DT, Zane N, Hong S, et al. Immigration-related factors and mental disorders among Asian Americans. Am J Public Health 2007;97(1):84–90.

28. Zhang W, Hong S, Takeuchi DT, et al. Limited English proficiency and psychological distress among Latinos and Asian Americans. Soc Sci Med 2012;75(6): 1006–14.

29. Huang KY, Calzada E, Cheng S, et al. Cultural Adaptation, parenting and child mental health among English Speaking asian American immigrant families. Child Psychiatry Hum Dev 2017;48(4):572–83.

30. Yang D, Oral E, Kim J, et al. Depression and perceived social support in asian American medical students [published online ahead of print, 2021 Apr 19]. J Racial Ethn Health Disparities 2021. https://doi.org/10.1007/s40615-021-01043-2.

31.. Sharma N, Shaligram D. Chapter 6.: suicide among South Asian youth in America. In: Pumariega AJ, Sharma N, editors. Suicide among diverse youth. Springer, New York; 2018. p. 83–97.

32. Bhugra D. Suicidal behavior in South Asians in the UK. Crisis 2002;23(3):108–13.
33. Patel SP, Gaw AC. Suicide among immigrants from the Indian subcontinent: a review. Psychiatr Serv 1996;47:517–21.
34. Supple AJ, Graves K, Daniel S, et al. Ethnic, gender, and age differences in adolescent nonfatal suicidal behaviors. Death Stud 2014;37:830–47.
35. Lane R, Cheref S, Miranda R. Ethnic differences in suicidal ideation and its correlates among South Asian American emerging adults. Asian Am J Psychol 2016;7(2):120–8.
36. Srinivasa SR, Pasupuleti S, Dronamraju R, et al. Suicide among South Asians in the United States: Perspectives, causes, and Implications for prevention and treatment. J Ment Health Soc Behav 2021;3(2):150.
37. Shanmuganandapala B. Mental Health and Well-Being Among Tamil Youth of Sri Lankan Origin Living in Toronto: A Mixed Methods Approach.
38. Guruge S, Butt H. A scoping review of mental health issues and concerns among immigrant and refugee youth in Canada: Looking back, moving forward. Can J Public Health 2015;106(2):e72–8.
39. Cai J, Hayden B. Intergenerational trauma and mental health in Asian American immigrant families. B.A. thesis. Dept of Cognitive, Linguistic, & Psychological Sciences. Brown University; 2017.
40. Yehuda R, Halligan SL, Grossman R. Childhood trauma and risk for PTSD: relationship to intergenerational effects of trauma, parental PTSD, and cortisol excretion. Dev Psychopathol 2001;13(3):733–53.
41. Scorza P, Duarte CS, Hipwell AE, et al. Program Collaborators for Environmental influences on Child Health Outcomes. Research Review: intergenerational transmission of disadvantage: epigenetics and parents' childhoods as the first exposure. J Child Psychol Psychiatry 2019;60(2):119–32.
42. Tummala-Narra P, Deshpande A. Mental health conditions among South Asians in the United States. InBiopsychosocial approaches to understanding health in South Asian Americans. Cham: Springer; 2018. p. 171–92.
43. Sharma N, Shaligram D, Yoon GH. Engaging South Asian youth and families: a clinical review. Int J Soc Psychiatry 2020;66(6):584–92.
44. Chadda RK, Deb KS. Indian family systems, collectivistic society and psychotherapy. Indian J Psychiatry 2013;55(Suppl 2):S299.
45. Cooper J, Husain N, Webb R, et al. Self-harm in the UK: differences between South Asians and Whites in rates, characteristics, provision of service and repetition. Soc Psychiatry Psychiatr Epidemiol 2006;41:782–8.
46. Bhikha A, Farooq S, Chaudhry N, et al. Explanatory models of psychosis amongst British South Asians. Asian J Psychiatry 2015;16:48–54.
47. Tiwari SK, Wang J. Ethnic differences in mental health service use among White, Chinese, South Asian and South East Asian populations living in Canada. Social Psychiatry Psychiatr Epidemiol 2008;43(11):866–71.
48. Shaligram D, Chou S, Chandra RM, et al. Addressing discrimination against asian American and Pacific Islander youths: the mental health Provider's role. J Am Acad Child Adolesc Psychiatry 2021;26. S0890-8567(21)02030-X.
49. Misra S, Jackson VW, Chong J, et al. Systematic review of cultural aspects of stigma and mental illness among racial and ethnic minority groups in the United States: Implications for interventions. Am J Community Psychol 2021;68(3–4):486–512. https://doi.org/10.1002/ajcp.12516.
50. Goyal D, Park VT, McNiesh S. Postpartum depression among Asian Indian mothers. Am J Maternal/Child Nurs 2015;40(4):256–61.

51. Chaudhry T, Chen SH. Mental illness stigmas in South Asian Americans: a cross-cultural investigation. Asian Am J Psychol 2019;10(2):154–65.

52. Thapar-Olmos N, Myers HF. Stigmatizing attributions towards depression among South Asian and Caucasian college students. Int J Cult Ment Health 2018;11(2): 134–45.

53. Spiegel J. An ecological model of ethnic families. Ethn Fam Ther 1982;31–51.

54. Kalia V, Aggarwal P, Raval VV. Buffering against parent-child conflict: exploring the role of biculturalism in the relationship between South Asian College students and their parents. InRe/Formation and Identity. Cham: Springer; 2022. p. 111–33.

55. Pandurangi AK, Shenoy S, Keshavan MS. Psychotherapy in the Bhagavad Gita, the Hindu scriptural text. Am J Psychiatry 2014;171(8):827–8.

56.. Shariff A. Ethnic identity and parenting stress in South Asian families: Implications for culturally sensitive counselling. Can J Counselling Psychotherapy 2009;43(1):41.

57. Tan JY, Xu LJ, Lopez FY, et al. Shared decision making among clinicians and Asian American and Pacific Islander sexual and gender minorities: an intersectional approach to address a critical care gap. LGBT health 2016;3(5):327–34.

58. Bajaj M, Ghaffar-Kucher A, Desai K. In the face of xenophobia: Lessons to address bullying of South Asian American youth. Takoma Park, MD: South Asian Americans Leading together (SAALT). 2013. Available at: https://saalt.org/wp-content/uploads/2013/06/InTheFaceOfXenophobia-Final-11.4.2013.pdf. Accessed October 12, 2021.

59. Jampala E, Radhakrishnan S. Finding community, creating community: South Asian Americans' mental health seeking and experiences of racial stress. (Sociology honors thesis). Wellesley (MA): Wellesley College; 2021. Available at: https://repository.wellesley.edu/islandora/object/ir%3A1588/datastream/PDF/download. Accessed March 12, 2022.

60. Roberts LR, Mann SK, Montgomery SB. Mental health and Sociocultural determinants in an asian Indian community. Fam Community Health 2016;39(1):31–9.

VIDEO REFERENCES

EthnoMed UW. Saving Face: Recognizing and Managing the Stigma of Mental Illness in Asian Americans. YouTube. 2019. Available at: https://www.youtube.com/watch?v=v8bvt642c5s. Accessed April 15, 2022.

Netflix Is A Joke. Hasan Learns What It's Like To Grow Up Desi In 2019. YouTube. Oct 14, 2019. Available at: https://www.youtube.com/watch?v=CFfNIsnScdc. Accessed April 15, 2022.

UW Video. A Parent's Understanding: Stigma in the South Asian Community. YouTube. Oct 10, 2018. Available at: https://www.youtube.com/watch?v=nn__1LAee50&t=350s. Accessed April 15, 2022.

Desis in Pardes. Desi Parents and Infant Development - Part 1 of 3. YouTube. Sep 26, 2021. Available at: https://www.youtube.com/watch?v=5ixm095IcRk. Accessed April 15, 2022.

Desis in Pardes. Desi Parents and Infant Development - Part 2 of 3. YouTube. Sep 26, 2021. Available at: https://www.youtube.com/watch?v=fcDsv560gZg. Accessed April 15, 2022.

Desis in Pardes. Desi Parents and Infant Development - Part 3 of 3. YouTube. Oct 9, 2021. Available at: https://www.youtube.com/watch?v=Q6vVUCgxp2c. Accessed April 15, 2022.

UNITED STATES POSTAL SERVICE ® Statement of Ownership, Management, and Circulation (All Periodicals Publications Except Requester Publications)

1. Publication Title	2. Publication Number	3. Filing Date
CHILD AND ADOLESCENT PSYCHIATRIC CLINICS	011 – 368	9/18/2022

4. Issue Frequency	5. Number of Issues Published Annually	6. Annual Subscription Price
JAN, APR, JUL, OCT	4	$358.00

7. Complete Mailing Address of Known Office of Publication (Not printer) (Street, city, county, state, and ZIP+4®)

ELSEVIER INC.
230 Park Avenue, Suite 800
New York, NY 10169

Contact Person
Malathi Samayan
Telephone (Include area code)
9 -44-42994507

8. Complete Mailing Address of Headquarters or General Business Office of Publisher (Not printer)

ELSEVIER INC.
230 Park Avenue, Suite 800
New York, NY 10169

9. Full Names and Complete Mailing Addresses of Publisher, Editor, and Managing Editor (Do not leave blank)

Publisher (Name and complete mailing address)

DOLORES MELONI, ELSEVIER INC.
1600 JOHN F KENNEDY BLVD. SUITE 1800
PHILADELPHIA, PA 19103-2899

Editor (Name and complete mailing address)

MEGAN ASHDOWN, ELSEVIER INC.
1600 JOHN F KENNEDY BLVD. SUITE 1800
PHILAELPHIA, PA 19103-2899

Managing Editor (Name and complete mailing address)

PATRICK MANLEY, ELSEVIER INC.
1600 JOHN F KENNEDY BLVD. SUITE 1800
PHILADELPHIA, PA 19103-2899

10. Owner (Do not leave blank. If the publication is owned by a corporation, give the name and address of the corporation immediately followed by the names and addresses of all stockholders owning or holding 1 percent or more of the total amount of stock. If not owned by a corporation, give the names and addresses of the individual owners. If owned by a partnership or other unincorporated firm, give its name and address as well as those of each individual owner. If the publication is published by a nonprofit organization, give its name and address.)

Full Name	Complete Mailing Address
WHOLLY OWNED SUBSIDIARY OF REED/ELSEVIER, US HOLDINGS	1600 JOHN F KENNEDY BLVD. SUITE 1800 PHILADELPHIA, PA 19103-2899

11. Known Bondholders, Mortgagees, and Other Security Holders Owning or Holding 1 Percent or More of Total Amount of Bonds, Mortgages, or Other Securities. If none, check box ▶ ☐ None

Full Name	Complete Mailing Address
N/A	

12. Tax Status (For completion by nonprofit organizations authorized to mail at nonprofit rates) (Check one)
The purpose, function, and nonprofit status of this organization and the exempt status for federal income tax purposes:
☒ Has Not Changed During Preceding 12 Months
☐ Has Changed During Preceding 12 Months (Publisher must submit explanation of change with this statement)

PS Form 3526, July 2014 [Page 1 of 4 (see instructions page 4)] PSN: 7530-01-000-9931   PRIVACY NOTICE: See our privacy policy on www.usps.com.

13. Publication Title	14. Issue Date for Circulation Data Below
CHILD AND ADOLESCENT PSYCHIATRIC CLINICS	JULY 2022

15. Extent and Nature of Circulation			Average No. Copies Each Issue During Preceding 12 Months	No. Copies of Single Issue Published Nearest to Filing Date
a. Total Number of Copies (Net press run)			148	144
b. Paid Circulation (By Mail and Outside the Mail)	(1)	Mailed Outside-County Paid Subscriptions Stated on PS Form 3541 (Include paid distribution above nominal rate, advertiser's proof copies, and exchange copies)	69	84
	(2)	Mailed In-County Paid Subscriptions Stated on PS Form 3541 (Include paid distribution above nominal rate, advertiser's proof copies, and exchange copies)	0	0
	(3)	Paid Distribution Outside the Mails Including Sales Through Dealers and Carriers, Street Vendors, Counter Sales, and Other Paid Distribution Outside USPS®	25	26
	(4)	Paid Distribution by Other Classes of Mail Through the USPS (e.g., First-Class Mail®)	0	0
c. Total Paid Distribution (Sum of 15b (1), (2), (3), and (4))		▶	114	110
d. Free or Nominal Rate Distribution (By Mail and Outside the Mail)	(1)	Free or Nominal Rate Outside-County Copies included on PS Form 3541	17	16
	(2)	Free or Nominal Rate In-County Copies Included on PS Form 3541	0	0
	(3)	Free or Nominal Rate Copies Mailed at Other Classes Through the USPS (e.g., First-Class Mail)	0	0
	(4)	Free or Nominal Rate Distribution Outside the Mail (Carriers or other means)	0	0
e. Total Free or Nominal Rate Distribution (Sum of 15d (1), (2), (3) and (4))		▶	17	16
f. Total Distribution (Sum of 15c and 15e)		▶	131	126
g. Copies not Distributed (See Instructions to Publishers #4 (page #3))		▶	17	18
h. Total (Sum of 15f and g)		▶	148	144
i. Percent Paid (15c divided by 15f times 100)		▶	87.02%	87.3%

* If you are claiming electronic copies, go to line 16 on page 3. If you are not claiming electronic copies, skip to line 17 on page 3.

16. Electronic Copy Circulation		Average No. Copies Each Issue During Preceding 12 Months	No. Copies of Single Issue Published Nearest to Filing Date
a. Paid Electronic Copies	▶		
b. Total Paid Print Copies (Line 15c) + Paid Electronic Copies (Line 16a)	▶		
c. Total Print Distribution (Line 15f) + Paid Electronic Copies (Line 16a)	▶		
d. Percent Paid (Both Print & Electronic Copies) (16b divided by 16c × 100)	▶		

☐ I certify that 50% of all my distributed copies (electronic and print) are paid above a nominal price.

17. Publication of Statement of Ownership

☒ If the publication is a general publication, publication of this statement is required. Will be printed ☐ Publication not required.
in the OCTOBER 2022 issue of this publication.

18. Signature and Title of Editor, Publisher, Business Manager, or Owner

Malathi Samayan

Malathi Samayan – Distribution Controller

Date 9/18/2022

I certify that all information furnished on this form is true and complete. I understand that anyone who furnishes false or misleading information on this form or who omits material or information requested on the form may be subject to criminal sanctions (including fines and imprisonment) and/or civil sanctions (including civil penalties).

PS Form 3526, July 2014 (Page 3 of 4)   PRIVACY NOTICE: See our privacy policy on www.usps.com.

Printed and bound by CPI Group (UK) Ltd, Croydon, CR0 4YY

03/10/2024

01040474-0006